AGE POWER

LESLIE KENTON

For Pat Kavanagh
whose beauty is ageless

AGE POWER

The revolutionary path to natural
high-tech rejuvenation

LESLIE KENTON

Vermilion
LONDON

12

Published in 2002 by Vermilion, an imprint of Ebury Publishing

Ebury Publishing is a Random House Group company

The Random House Group Limited Reg. No. 954009

Addresses for companies within the Random House Group can be found at
www.randomhouse.co.uk

A CIP catalogue record for this book is available from the British Library.

Typeset by Palimpsest Book Production Limited,
Grangemouth, Stirlingshire

ISBN 9780091857462

Copies are available at special rates for bulk orders. Contact the sales
development team on 020 7840 8487 or visit www.booksforpromotions.co.uk
for more information

To buy books by your favourite authors and register for offers, visit
www.randomhouse.co.uk

Penguin Random House is committed to a sustainable future for
our business, our readers and our planet. This book is made from
Forest Stewardship Council® certified paper.

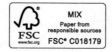

Printed and bound in Great Britain by Clays Ltd, St Ives plc

Author's Note

The content of this book is intended for informational purposes only. I am only a reporter. None of the suggestions or information are meant to be prescriptive. Any attempt to treat a medical condition should always be under the direction of a competent physician – preferably one knowledgeable about nutrition and natural methods of healing. Neither the publishers nor the author can accept responsibility for injuries or illness arising out of a failure by a reader to take medical advice. However, I have long sought to learn more about whatever can help us to live at a high level of energy, intelligence and creativity, for it is my belief that the more each one of us is able to re-establish harmony within ourselves and with our environment, the better equipped we shall be to wrestle with the challenges now facing our planet.

TABLE OF CONTENTS

AGE POWER

PART ONE:
AGE EXPLODES

TO AGE OR NOT TO AGE

The privilege of a lifetime is being who you are.

Joseph Campbell

During the eighteen-month period of writing *Age Power* I was asked to make a television documentary on ageing for the Southern Hemisphere. Called *To Age or Not To Age* it asked the question, 'Can we slow ageing by making simple lifestyle changes?' We also wanted to know, 'Might it even be possible to *reverse* age-related degeneration which has already occurred?' Finally we wanted to know, 'Can these things be verified in medically measurable ways?' What we discovered was mind blowing.

Our medical advisor, Dr Tony Edwards – a physician well trained in functional medicine – and I began the project with a search for a group of people who considered themselves generally healthy, were not on long-term drug therapy and who wanted to explore what might be possible in terms of age reversal. We invited forty such people to a day's seminar on the ageing process. At the end of the day, after interviewing each of them, we chose eight men and women aged between thirty and sixty to participate in the programme. Our choice was based on the intention to work with as diverse a selection of backgrounds, interests and ages as possible in so small a group. All we asked of them at this stage was that they were interested enough in improving their health to want to take part.

CHECK IT OUT

Deeply immersed in the work of Irwin H Rosenberg MD and William J Evans PhD, we were keen to establish the current state of each participant's biomarkers. We sent them to Wakefield Hospital in Wellington, New Zealand to have their biomarkers measured – from fasting insulin and blood sugar levels through cholesterol, triglycerides and blood pressure. We chose Wakefield Hospital because not only could it do all the standard blood testing, it also has a first rate physiology laboratory where exercise physiologists were also able to establish each participant's VO2 Max, body fat percentage and lean body mass to fat ratio. To our surprise every participant – including our 50-year-old top triathlete, Vic – showed abnormalities associated with Syndrome X.

We then introduced our group to Age Power's Insulin Balance Diet, supplementing it with a good multiple vitamin and flaxseed oil. We also suggested that our older participants would benefit from a supplement of good quality fish oil, and we asked that everyone take 230g of chelated magnesium a day, just before bed. We asked them to walk for 30 minutes a day and to use Michael Colgan's weight training videos four times a week (see Resources, page 482). Then we set them loose.

PROOF OF THE PUDDING

We expected some of our eight participants to drop out. Indeed, we planned for that to happen. We were making a one hour documentary which meant we would only have time to follow four people. Experience had taught us that in all of these kinds of experiments only half of the participants carry on with any programme right to the end.

Five weeks later our participants returned to Wellington Hospital to have their biomarkers checked. All eight of them. No-one had quit. This created a real challenge for us as suddenly we had eight stories to weave into an hour's show. Well, we would just have to see what happened when we re-measured their biomarkers. Perhaps some of the stories would be very short.

NEW MAPS FOR AGEING

The documentary set out to explore what the Age Power's post-modern Paleolithic diet, coupled with weight resistance and walking could do to help people grow younger. It looked at Syndrome X and the role of insulin resistance in age degeneration. It asked the question, 'Is this something over which we ourselves have control, both in terms of prevention and the reversal of degenerative changes after they have already occurred?' It explored natural methods for living long and *dying young, late in life*. In effect, the producer, director, myself and all of our participants worked together to see if we could create new maps of the ageing process and explode the negative beliefs that most of us hold. Beliefs which prevent each of us from experiencing a better and better life with the passing of each year.

PERSONAL REVOLUTION

The results were simply astounding. Before beginning the Age Power programme, most of the group had four or more biomarkers out of kilter. Some had as many as seven. But by the end of the four-week period, every biomarker had either already normalised or was well on its way there. This was true for every participant. This amazed us. We had no idea that change would happen so quickly. And the transformations were so great that we had to tell every story – all eight of them.

All of this was exciting enough – for these people's bodies had actually been rejuvenated in medically measurable ways. But what really excited me was the transformation we witnessed in the people themselves. Vitality increased. Every one of them lost fat and built muscle. Most important, in each of them, a sense of enthusiasm, boldness and fun had developed about their lives. Dreams and ambitions that had been lying dormant now surfaced as real possibilities. It was magnificent to watch. None of us dreamed the Age Power programme would have such life transforming power.

THE AFTERMATH

When the programme aired, the network was so swamped with hits on their website that the system went on a go-slow and many people could not get through at all. At the same time, my own website – www.lesliekenton.com – received 35,000 hits in 48 hours.

The whole thing made me aware of just how many people are passionate about taking action for themselves to transform their lives. It has always been my belief that the power to transform our health lies in our own hands and that the more responsibility we take for it, the more joy we are able to bring into our lives and to the lives of those around us.

We all know about age-related changes. You wake up one day and notice that you no longer have the energy you once had. Your skin and nails have lost their strength and glimmer. Your digestion no longer seems to work as well as it did. These things are so common an experience as we grow older we barely comment on them, nor on rises in blood pressure or diagnoses of high cholesterol and triglycerides. We simply accept them as inevitable. We have been taught to think that dysfunction and degenerative disease are a natural consequence of time passing. They most certainly are not.

BASE-LINE STUDY

Our documentary was a simple experiment – what is known in medicine as a *base-line study*. But it pointed the way towards an approach to ageing that works. It demonstrates that you can reverse functional deterioration and restore the homeostasis characteristic of young healthy bodies. It showed that the loss of vitality, impairment of function and the degenerative conditions our participants had each experienced were far from a normal consequence of chronological ageing. Even more important, we showed that they could be reversed by making simple changes in how you live and work and eat.

Age Power is what happened next. Fired by the extraordinary results we had achieved with putting eight people on what was simply a diet and exercise plan, I began to investigate further. This book is the result of these investigations. It gives you all the information you need to use Age Power's Insulin Balance Eating and to follow the sort of exercise regime the participants of the documentary were asked to follow. It tells you why as well as how, and leads you on past the basics into other exciting realms of scientific research and discovery. But much more than that, *Age Power* shows you how you can take control of your life, your health and your dreams. The goal of *Age Power* is to make you more truly who you have always thought you were, who you really are, and whoever you want to become.

Leslie Kenton
London 2002

AGE COMES OF AGE

I am ready to meet my Maker. Whether my Maker is prepared for the ordeal of meeting me is another matter.
Winston Churchill

Growing older means growing wiser. It can also mean growing healthier, more creative and more fulfilled as you move towards greater authenticity, personal power and freedom. *Age Power* looks at life as a process – the process by which you become more fully who you really are. It makes use of life-changing information, new ways of thinking, natural methods and powerful cutting-edge technologies, to slow degeneration and heighten vitality. Available to us now, how we use them is up to us.

Turning your experience of growing older into one of expanding joy, energy and fulfilment draws on the work of visionary scientists, leading-edge clinicians and pioneers in human development. Some of the techniques and discoveries you'll find within stretch back half a century. Others are so recent the media has yet to make them public. Here is just a taste of some of the exciting material you will find within.

MEASURE YOUR AGE

Age Power honours many exciting discoveries, including the work of farsighted American scientists William Evans PhD and Irwin Rosenberg MD – that when it comes to how old you are, it is your *biological* age that is important, not your *chronological* age. And unlike your chronological age which cannot be altered, how old you are biologically is fundamentally under your own control. Evans and Rosenberg created the now universally accepted measurements of biological age by which you and your doctor can measure your own Age Power regenerative process, month by month, as you follow the programme. It also looks at a collection of abnormalities as yet little known which lie at the core of degeneration in the body: Syndrome X.

SYNDROME X

Endocrinologist Gerald Reaven at Stanford University identified Syndrome X – the most destructive collection of age-
related abnormalities known to man, encompassing
high-blood pressure and distorted cholesterol and triglycerides. As yet little known, Syndrome X – or insulin resistance – makes us prone to obesity, heart disease, stroke,
diabetes and a myriad other degenerative conditions associated with growing older. Between 25 percent and 65
percent of people over 35 in the Western world show signs
of Syndrome X. Doctors who favour natural methods of
healing have worked with Reaven's findings and taken them
further, developing ways and means through simple changes
in how we eat and live, to reverse these abnormalities so we
live longer and healthier than ever before. These are changes
we can make ourselves. They form the core of Age Power.

PARADIGM SHIFTS

Researchers and clinicians from Mitsuo Koda in Japan to Richard
Weindruch in the United States are experimenting with nutrient-rich-
calorie-poor eating. Their work points the way to a whole new relationship between food and ageing. Meanwhile, an age power revolution in
science and in consciousness is happening in university and molecular
biology laboratories, in psychologists' consulting rooms and in rarefied
chambers where philosophers and physicists bring to birth new paradigms
in medicine and health. It threatens to change forever the way we think
about ageing. Age Power explodes most commonly held notions about
ageing. In the process it lays to rest more than a few sacred cows, not by
some trick of thought, but as a result of the most remarkable, verifiable,
scientific understanding about what causes degeneration in the body and
what we ourselves can do to prevent and reverse it. Leading edge work
in integrative biochemistry is beginning to revolutionise delivery systems
for natural anti-ageing elements. Products are being created so powerful
that they can counter major degenerative processes in the body. There
are even quantum leaps being made in cosmetic treatments that within
ten years will make the skin-care products we are using now obsolete.

ELECTRONIC BLISS

Musician Bill Harris has invented state of the art binaural technologies for meditation and brain enhancement. Using sound as a means of integrating brain functions, this dazzling electronic method provides what is one of the most powerful mind development and personal growth tools ever created. Meanwhile, simple mental exercises such as those developed by Lester Levenson, creator of the Sedona Method, can easily, and gracefully help us shed negative habits and thought patterns – even life-long emotional trauma.

HALT DEGENERATION

Recent research has identified four processes fundamental to the way in which your body ages – Oxidation, Glycation, Inflammation and Methylation. Look after these four processes and you slow down the ageing process. You will find natural means of doing this within. Ageing experts now insist that if we can also protect the energy factories within our cells – mitochondria – and keep them working efficiently, we protect ourselves to a significant degree from ageing and create life-long vitality. Following the discoveries of Nobel Laureate Albert Szent-Gyorgyi, Greek cell biologist Nicholaos Skouras investigated the power of coenzyme A and developed a remarkable natural supplement – Coenzyme A™ to help us do this. It is not just on a biochemical level alone that Age Power transformation is possible. All sorts of powerful new methods for transforming mind and emotion are also useful in de-ageing the body.

These are but a few of the visionary people who are changing the face of ageing so rapidly it can make your head spin. Until now, most life-changing benefits from their work has remained unavailable to ordinary people like you and me who want to make growing older a continually unfolding adventure. Thanks to the trailblazing work of these people and many others at the leading edge of natural ageing, it is possible at last to look upon growing older not as an experience of 'waiting in dread for the parts to fall off', but as a process of growth. By choosing to live each day and year of our lives as a passage towards wholeness, our enthusiasm for life, instead of diminishing, increases. So can our stamina and our capacity for joy as vitality and a sense of fulfilment expands.

QUANTUM ANTI-AGER

Eccentric American scientist Patrick Flanagan recently harnessed the power of the negatively-charged hydrogen atom to create what is one of the most powerful anti-oxidants known to man. It can help rid your body of dehydration characteristic of an ageing body while increasing the availability of nutrients and oxygen to cells, alkalinising the system and fuelling ongoing vitality.

SECRETS OF THE GENES

In no small part, the Age Power revolution owes its impetus to twentieth century discoveries that vie for importance with Darwin's own: the Human Genome Project. The Human Genome Project has been focused on analysing the almost six billion pieces of DNA which make up our human inheritance. Although very little of the human genome has so far been analysed, the volume of information about health and disease patterns already emerging is breathtaking. Even twenty years ago the idea that disease patterns could be identified in genes seemed like science fiction. It is happening as we speak.

CRY FOR HELP

Our ever-changing world cries out for the experience, wisdom and guidance of healthy, mature men and women in their prime – people whose lives have not been compromised by the discouragement and resignation too many still believe to be the inevitable consequences of growing older. Much fear and misinformation still abounds. It needs to be cleared. Fear alone undermines immunity and diminishes emotional, physical and spiritual health. Most fears about ageing are worse than old wives' tales. Forfeit your belief that growing old means degeneration and loss of vitality – a downhill ride all the way. It can mean growing stronger, more richly sexual, more radiant and rewarded in every area of your life.

GENE EXPRESSION

To the uninformed, the notion that health, biological age and death is written in your genes still sounds depressing. They look upon this discovery as something akin to asking that a dour clairvoyant predict the future, which you remain powerless to change. Such people know less than half the truth. For even more exciting than the discovery that specific genes make us either susceptible or resistant to specific illness, is a lesser known but far more powerful revelation to emerge from the Human Genome Project: Yes, the genes we inherit define our 'risk' of early ageing, degeneration and disease. But whether or not this 'risk' becomes 'fact' and negative events happen to us depends *far less on our genetic inheritance* than on *how we live our lives.* It is not the genes themselves that give rise to disease and degeneration. It is the way they are *expressed.*

What this means is that there are many possible versions of you tucked within your genes and chromosomes. Which versions become expressed – which *potentials* become 'facts' – depends almost entirely on the way you *live.* Age Power's simple, practical changes in the way you eat, use your body, handle stress and orient yourself spiritually and creatively, can help prevent degenerative conditions: Alzheimer's disease, many forms of cancer, heart disease, diabetes, arthritis, obesity – even overt signs of skin ageing. There is still better news: once signs of degeneration have already appeared, more often than not it is possible to *reverse* them – literally rejuvenating your body and mind in *medically measurable ways.*

There are many forms of 'you' encoded into your genes. The 'you' who is reading this book right now is the result of the experience of your life thus far bathing over your genes to produce the expression of who you are. Under a different set of experiences in life a different 'you' would be reading this book today. Your genes would be the same, but the way their message was expressed would be different.

Jeffrey Bland PhD

DO IT YOURSELF NATURALLY

To benefit most from the information you find within, forget magic bullet drugs which promise to restore virility when impotence occurs, or to lower high blood pressure in the face of hypertension. Choose instead natural means for lasting health enhancement from within. Age Power's Programme provides you with the wherewithal to enhance your own *biological terrain*. Detoxify your body and strengthen it physiologically and biochemically so that the life energy within rejuvenates your tissues, calling forth the highest levels of vitality from a cellular level, metamorphosising the way you function, feel and look into a new dynamic version of you.

Growing research and clinical experience show that what works best in almost every circumstance are *natural methods*. Make changes in your diet, and increase your body's production of coenzyme A to restore the flow of youthful hormones and improve mental and physical functions. Take part in the *right* kind of exercise. Make use of deep relaxation or meditation techniques every day. Explore what smart nutrients, or binaural sound technology has to offer your nervous system. They can help alter moods, improve sleep patterns and make you more resistant to stress. You can even call on consciousness-expanding techniques to transform your experience of reality or use consciousness-expanding exercises to replace a world view too limiting for you and to open up a new sense of what's possible.

Cosmetic companies stuff products with free radical scavengers to protect skin from age-related damage. Everywhere you turn one company after another is selling a new form of anti-oxidant. Things have moved on in the 20 years since my book *Ageless Ageing* appeared – especially in relation to the development of powerful natural methods you can employ to counter degeneration.

In the process of researching Age Power I came upon two stunning scientific discoveries. The first was that insulin resistance has reached epidemic proportions and is severely undermining human health, making us age rapidly as well as making us fat. The second was the work of the new scientific discipline palaeopathology, which is beginning to find out the kind of diet we, as human beings, are genetically programmed to thrive on.

I became so excited about these discoveries that I decided to test them out in a documentary I was filming. The success was so phenomenal, giving people the ability to shed fat from their bodies, that I felt the need to gather information specifically related to rebalancing the body's metabolic functions. This led me to write a book called *The X Factor Diet*, which was specifically geared to permanent fat loss. Here in *Age Power* you will find the crux of the discoveries I made in much greater detail, specifically

TAKE TWO

This is the second time in my life I have chosen to bury my head in books on biochemistry and in papers gleaned from scientific libraries, to spend endless hours listening to experts on ageing, consciousness research and personal growth. By interacting with doctors and biochemists, spiritual teachers and psychiatrists as well as researchers into non-ordinary states of consciousness, I sought to find out what is true and what is possible, and how we can make practical use of both, right now. My first foray into natural ageing took place more than twenty years ago. Then I wrote *Ageless Ageing* – the first best-selling book in Britain to explore the natural ageing process and the free radical theory of disease. At that time the world was so unfamiliar with 'free radicals' that to many they sounded like political dissonants. Now free radicals are common parlance and the importance of using anti-oxidants to protect from the damage they can cause is taken for granted.

oriented towards preventing degeneration and reversing biological ageing in medically measurable ways.

NOW IS THE TIME

Although virtually all of the research and clinical experience on which *Ageless Ageing* was based still holds, a veritable explosion of life-changing tools and techniques has happened in the last two decades. So life-changing is this collection of discoveries and so powerful are their practical applications that we can – if we so choose – make an exponential leap forward using them.

I believe that our making use of the material you will find in this book is a matter of urgency. Far too much human suffering ensues when we live in a way which does not support the finest expression of our genetic inheritance and does not foster the full development of our mental, spiritual and creative capabilities. When, out of self-neglect or being ill-informed, we undermine our potentials, we end up with all manner of physical, mental and emotional disabilities that we wrongfully assume to be a 'normal' part of ageing with which we have to 'cope'. Our society, our culture, our planet cannot afford to neglect the 'ripening' of human beings who have decades of experience, vision and wisdom to offer. These resources are profoundly needed in a world which continues to change out of all recognition.

AGE POWER PRINCIPLES

Age Power is based on 8 principles which I believe to be irrefutable:

❑ The human body is a multi-dimensional organism, not a machine: We are body, mind and spirit – so interrelated that they cannot be separated.

❑ Each of us is an utterly unique being. Health at its most profound level is a full expression of that uniqueness in everything we are or do.

❑ By improving our ability to adapt to stressors and maintain physiological balance and function, we can effectively prevent accelerated ageing as well as most degenerative diseases associated with it.

❑ Where negative changes in the body have already taken place, most can be reversed. This is measured by hard core parameters doctors use such as cholesterol levels, fasting blood sugar, insulin levels, triglycerides, blood pressure and all the rest.

❑ Natural methods work best for regeneration and rejuvenation.

❑ Age Power asks that we live and think in ways that encourage the best possible *expression* of our genes.

❑ Regeneration is a process by which the body and psyche rid themselves of whatever does not support the highest levels of gene expression, strengthen physical vitality and empower greater expression of your authentic nature.

❑ By living out our unique biological, spiritual and creative potentials we not only fulfil ourselves, we also bring the greatest gifts we have to offer our family, our community and the world as a whole.

Age Power is just what its name implies. It offers the possibility of living each passing decade at a high level of health and vitality. It enables us to 'die young late in life'. It offers practical tools which a man or woman of any age can use to live a life where excitement, joy, creativity and satisfaction, instead of diminishing with time, can actually increase as we grow older.

Your health at 80 is a profit or loss on the investment you make in health today.
Michael Colgan PhD

DE-AGE THE LOT

To live our values we need to *make use* of our genetic inheritance, physically and spiritually. We cannot afford to be hampered by less-than-optimal gene expression. We have the potential to experience well-being and fulfilment at a level most have never known before – both physically and spiritually – even if the world we live in seems to be disintegrating around us. As we do, we become more able to help others do the same.

These two realms – the spiritual and the physical – are really one. Age Power addresses regeneration and rejuvenation from both angles. Unless blood sugar levels in your body are balanced by good insulin sensitivity at a cellular level – virtually impossible for people over 30 who have been living on the high-carbohydrate-low-fat diet of convenience foods – your capacity for clarity of mind and creative work are vastly diminished. So is your overall vitality and your ability to resist degeneration. If you do not make use of some of the effective techniques for consciousness expansion and spiritual growth – from leading-edge binaural technologies to ancient methods for breath control or meditation, you miss out on the physical benefits as well as the emotional and spiritual ones such techniques offer.

PASSIONS OF THE SOUL

It has long been my belief that each of us comes on to this earth as a unique divine spark. Just as our genetic inheritance – whether our eyes are blue or brown, our bodies tall or short – is utterly individual, so is our nature and our spiritual orientation. Each of us has individual passions – unique values – things we have come here to do or be. The more we live them out in work, in play and in our relationships to each other, the richer, more satisfying and authentic our life becomes. After all, you can only collect so many PhDs, houses in the country and delicious lovers. Wonderful as these things may be, they come nowhere near to bringing the sense of satisfaction which we can get from living our core values and following our soul's passion.

THE POWER OF AGE

We live in exciting times – times when the breach between science and spirituality ushered in 400 years ago by the Copernican Revolution is rapidly narrowing. Age Power makes use of the gifts from this closing of the gap. Even if you have neglected yourself over the years – most of us have, by the way – it is never too late to change. Making simple alterations in the way you live can regenerate your health and rejuvenate our body and mind.

Take an Age Power approach to growing older and the suffering and loss that can enter your life becomes a wake-up call. It can lead you to discover deeper meaning and purpose in your life, and teach you more about how to help yourself and others. Like the Phoenix, it can help you learn to transmute suffering in a fire that consumes what no longer supports your life and growth – the full expression of your unique divine nature. Each encounter with life's flames can lead us upward towards another rebirth of health, creativity and joy.

Such is the power of age. Within I hope you will find the tools and techniques, information and inspiration to help you live out your own unique life more fully with each year that passes. The more you do, the more health and fulfilment you welcome into your life and the more you bring the very highest level of wisdom and friendship you have to offer to the lives of others.

AUTHENTICITY BRINGS FREEDOM

I view the whole of life, including health itself, as a process of unfolding, by which more of our unique divine spark is expressed in what we do and who we are. Age becomes a blossoming of authenticity and freedom from within. Its blessings are contagious. The more authentic and rich your life becomes, the freer the rest of us are to ripen into our own authenticity and to experience our own sense of freedom.

THE RACE IS ON

Collectively we are involved in a race against time. It has no precedent in human history. The stakes are high – ultimately the future of our planet. Scientific discoveries about the relationships between mind and body, about life changes which can alter our genetic expression, are all here to be understood and used. Experiential methods of self-exploration, healing and personal transformation emerging from humanistic and transpersonal psychologies offer enormous potential for taking control of our lives and creating the future we want. Making good use of what is already tried and tested can transform the whole way you experience life so that ageing becomes a process of growth and joy, instead of one of degeneration and disillusion. If a sufficient number of us undergo a process of deep phys-ical and spiritual transformation, we may in time reach a critical mass that enables us, working together, to envisage another, finer and more just, way of living together on the planet. Two things are certain: Now is the time. We are the people. May your own life be blessed with Age Power.

To orient your life around a structure of some other human being's understanding is to worship a false god. It is to lock yourself into a frame-work of someone else's prej-udice, however well intentioned. It is to prefer the past-oriented knowledge of another to your own present-moment perception. It is to doubt both yourself and the Creator who would, if you permit it, awaken within you.

Ken Carey

LIES, DAMN LIES
AND STATISTICS

It is now proved beyond doubt that ageing is one
of the leading causes of statistics.
Unknown

We have inherited an albatross. It hangs about our necks
in the form of a widely accepted, negative and highly
destructive view of ageing. To enjoy the rewards of growing
older we need to explode the false myths we carry about
ageing and uncover the surprising truths buried beneath
them.

In the nineteen seventies and eighties when interest in gerontology – the
study of ageing – began to be supported by government funding, age
researchers fell into a mire of confusion, primarily because they lacked
any conceptual foundation for understanding the nature of ageing in its
many faces – biological, psychological and spiritual. They became obsessed
with disability, disease and chronological age instead of seeing the experience of ageing itself as a whole, in all of its positive as well as its negative aspects.

NEGATIVE OBSESSIONS

The media almost always focuses on the weakness and pathos of the
elderly, just as scientific literature on gerontology is still obsessed with
the issues of nursing home admissions, frailty and the economic costs of
looking after our impaired elders. It is all part of the negative obsession
that we as a society seem to have developed with ageing, and very little
has been available that offers a positive understanding of how human
beings can function effectively in later life.

> The competitive edge in the coming decades will be held by those individuals and companies who can tap into new, life-driven sources of inspiration, creativity and vitality.
>
> *Carol Osborn*

How long you live rests largely in your
own hands. So does how *well* you live, how
much vitality you have and how good you
will look in 20 years time. Age Power is
not an accident of fate. Neither is it heavily
dependant on the kind of medical care you
get, nor on your genetic inheritance,
although certainly both have a part to play.

It depends upon how you choose, right here, right now, to live your life from here on out. And this is regardless of how much self-neglect you have poured on yourself in the past.

AGE CURSES

Almost everybody has heard of death curses. Psychological literature is laced with accounts of how Aboriginal witch doctors have brought about the death of the young and healthy by cursing them. No sooner do these people learn of the fate which has been cast for them than they begin inexplicably to sicken and eventually to die. It appears that through complex biological processes, their simple belief in the curse brings about destruction of their organism.

In civilized society we tend to look upon such phenomena as anthropological curiosities – products of primitive superstition which simply don't touch us in our more enlightened age. What we are not aware of however is that many of us in the civilized world are also under our own brand of 'death curses'. They may be subtler than those issued by witch doctors but they can be every bit as potent in bringing about the physical and mental decline which we have come to associate with ageing. Common (and usually unconscious) notions such as 'retirement', 'middle-age', 'It's all down hill after forty', and 'At your age you must start taking things more easily', are widely held. They can exert a powerful effect on the process of ageing by creating destructive self-fulfilling expectations about age decline. Instead of facing the future full of confidence and excitement about what lies ahead, optimism is replaced by anxiety as we are warned to 'Be careful', or 'Don't take chances on a new career at your age'.

WAGES OF FEAR

The list of commonly proffered 'sensible' advice is a long one. Such well-meaning suggestions often lead people to make changes in their lifestyle which encourage physical decline – for instance, decreasing the amount of exercise they get, altering their eating habits away from fibre-rich natural foods towards 'softer' foods, and even decreasing the amount of social and intellectual stimulation they have been used to. Worse, this kind of advice can undermine self-image and destroy self-confidence, which in turn interferes with the proper functioning of the immune system which plays such a central role in protecting your body from ageing. An essential ingredient

> Do you believe you're in poor or excellent health? What you believe and expect about your health may be more important than objective assessments made by your doctor.
>
> *Robert Ornstein, PhD and David Sobel MD*

in Age Power is a strong awareness of just how powerfully your emotions, state of mind and your unconscious assumptions can influence both your susceptibility to illness and the rate at which you age.

Most of us hold a lot of false notions about ageing and life expectancy. These ghosts need to be laid before we can make Age Power a workable part of our lives, for they are truly legends of the fall, and like many false legends, they carry the warning that if you believe in them, the belief itself goes a long way to making them true. So deeply entrenched are these negative legends in the worldview of our culture, that each one needs to be examined quite carefully before we can begin to transform them. Let's look at them one by one.

TRUE OR FALSE?
TO GROW OLDER IS TO FALL APART

The notion that age degeneration – including the loss of good looks, and the onset of long-term illnesses such as arthritis, coronary heart disease and cancer – is a 'normal' experience of growing older is simply untrue. These conditions develop primarily as a result of eating foods which the body has not been genetically programmed to deal with, the build-up of toxicity in the body over long periods, lack of physical exercise and/or crash dieting which shrinks lean body mass (the major measurement of how old your body is *biologically* rather than *chronologically*). Where these conditions develop, your lifestyle needs to be altered. And to a very great extent, if they have developed, they can be much ameliorated by altering the way you live now.

Throughout history most medical traditions – from China and India to ancient Sumaria – have taught that **degeneration is not a normal part of ageing.** Provided we recognise the biological laws by which we are constituted and live with respect for them, we can live to a great age free of arthritis, heart attacks, cancer, lung diseases and the rest. These traditions have also taught us that **great age can be matched by great vitality** so that we should be able to – as an editorial in the *Journal of the American Medical Association* suggested a few years ago – 'die *young*, late in life'.

What is so exciting about the research

> You can unlock the tremendous potential for good health that is stored within your genes. That potential may not be optimally realised at the present time due to a mismatch between what your genes need and what they are given… our genetic inheritance does play an important role in defining our risks to most age related diseases, but healthy ageing is even more controlled by how we communicate with our genes through our diet and lifestyle.
>
> *Jeffrey Bland PhD*

into ageing undertaken in the last 20 years is that we now have an abundance of scientific information about how such things as a diet low in sugar and starchy grains and vegetables can keep hormones balanced to youthful levels, while phytonutrients – recently discovered powerhouses of natural chemicals in some foods that we eat – can enhance immunity, protect from free radical damage, and improve the functioning of whole systems in the body.

TRUE OR FALSE?
MEDICAL MIRACLES HAVE LENGTHENED LIFE

The idea that medicine has already significantly extended life is as unfounded as the notion that degenerative diseases are inevitable. Our average lifespan (or life expectancy) which means the average age at which 50 percent of the population die, has indeed lengthened considerably. It is approximately 25 years longer now than it was in 1900. However, this is largely the result of the waning of infectious diseases in the first half of the century, which had little to do with drugs or vaccines. For instance, 80 percent of the decline in tuberculosis took place before any good drug therapy was developed for it in the 1950's, while the 90 percent decrease in the death rate from whooping cough and the more than 70 percent decrease in the mortality of scarlet fever and diphtheria, took place before effective vaccines were developed. In fact, polio is the only disease in the twentieth century whose decline shows a correlation between the development of a drug or vaccine designed to treat it and the lessening of the infection rate.

In Neo-Paleolithic times, around 15,000 years ago, man's life expectancy was 18 years. However, recent studies in Paleopathology show that this short lifespan was due to a high mortality rate at birth and the sheer violence and danger of their lives – not to ill health. Much scientific evidence now indicates that the maximum human lifespan appears to be 120 years, and that this has not changed considerably in the past 100,000 years. Mass immunisation, the development of drugs, and high technology hospital procedures have had little impact on the *real* life expectancy of anyone who has already reached adulthood, for they have had little impact on *maximum* lifespan. Despite all our efforts in genetic engineering it appears unlikely that maximum lifespan will change in the near future.

Each human being is biologically unique. We all share the same basic structure. But our individual combinations of genes make us unlike anyone else who ever lived. We all have our own biological needs and our own responses to the world around us. What works for one person may not work for another.

Michael Murray MD

NEW VIEW OF AGE

To most people in the West old age brings ghastly images of decrepitude – not pictures of vigorous and sexually active old men and women intensively involved in work and looking forward to what comes next. The potential for creativity and enjoyment which is wasted in age-degeneration in the developed countries of the world is shocking. So is the cost to the state in providing medical treatment, hospitalisation, food and care for people for whom ageing has become a nightmare of physical pain and emotional isolation. Few of us even come close to fulfilling our psychobiological potentials. Instead we look forward to a steady and inexorable increase in morbidity and mortality from one disease to another. Applying the principles of Age Power, however, will give you a very different view. For the same principles which help keep your skin smooth, your muscles firm and your vitality and creativity high, can also reduce the incidence of chronic disease and postpone degenerative illnesses so that if they occur at all, they come only very late in life.

TRUE OR FALSE?
IT'S DOWNHILL ALL THE WAY

One of the most persistent false notions about ageing is that as people get older their brains falter, they are unable to learn new things and they lose their creativity and their usefulness to society. The pervading image of the very old is of dull-witted wrinklies drooling in old people's homes. Research shows that young people do have better hearing and sharper vision than older people. Their reaction time is also faster, and so is their short term memory and their physical strength. But research also shows that many of these deficiencies can be overcome in older people simply by training. Researchers working with groups of elderly people have demonstrated that short-term memory loss is significantly improved simply by making lists and practising games for memory enhancement. In another area, researchers took older people whose inductive reasoning and spacial orientation had diminished and put them through five training sessions designed to improve these abilities. The results were phenomenal. Not

> There is dramatic research that links changes in feelings to the functioning of the immune system.
>
> *Robert Ornstein, PhD, and David Sobel, MD*

only did they improve, the improvements they made in only five sessions were permanent. In the workplace the false belief persists that old people cannot be innovative like their younger colleagues. Studies show that this, too, is not the case. Very often the seniority and security that comes with having done a job for many years gives older people an innovative edge – in short they dare to make changes that their younger cohorts would not dream of suggesting.

TRUE OR FALSE?
IT'S TOO LATE TO CHANGE

This convenient notion that goes with an idea such as 'I've been smoking all my life and it's too late to change now' is totally ridiculous. It is never too late to transform your health and your life. If you've been drinking too much alcohol and eating too much sugary fat-laden food, if you have neglected exercise for years, if you have forgotten how to look after yourself physically, it is never too late to make simple changes that can really alter your life. The risk of heart disease begins to fall from the moment you stop smoking, no matter how long you have smoked. Five years down the road, as an ex-smoker you are not much more likely to have heart disease than someone who has never smoked. Studies show that 34–55 year olds who had stopped smoking 2 to 4 years previously, were no more at risk of stroke than those of the same age who had never smoked.

Body Alchemy

Years without exercise, we know quite clearly, can lead to a lessening in nerve function and kidney function as well as heart capacity. It interferes with your body's ability to use oxygen effectively, not to mention diminishing your vision and hearing and decreasing both physical strength and muscle mass. All of these things are generally considered an inevitable part of ageing. Nonsense. Beginning an exercise programme of strength training and simply deciding to walk for half an hour a day transforms your life, rejuvenating your body in medically measurable ways. So can changing the way you eat. What you are likely to find surprising as you read this book is that none of the standard advice about low fat diets and lots of complex carbohydrates holds true. We have been fed this information for almost 20 years, during which time all of the illnesses generally associated with ageing such as coronary heart disease, diabetes and obesity, have soared. Yet like most of the research done into *positive* ageing, the information you need to change your diet in a way that will genuinely rejuvenate your body has largely been ignored under a

> What we need is more people who specialise in the impossible.
>
> *Theodor Roethke*

mountain of media dis-information and commercial hype from food manu-facturers, in whose interests it is to sell you yet another 'healthy' low fat food.

TRUE OR FALSE?
MOST AGEING IS GENETICALLY PROGRAMMED

While it is true that genetic diseases such as Huntington's Disease can shorten life, recent studies show that how you live and how you eat have the most powerful influence on whether you actually develop a disorder to which you have inherited a genetic tendency. This is great news, for while genes certainly play a role in the promotion of disease and in deter-mining the rate at which our body ages, they are less than half of the story. An inspiring set of dozens of individual research projects carried out from the mid-eighties onwards – known as the Macarthur Study – shows that heredity is far less important than environment and lifestyle in determining how and how fast we age. Further, as we get older our genetic inheritance becomes far less important and our lifestyle factors become far more important.

This means that in medically measurable terms – the hard-core parame-ters doctors use to register health and degeneration such as cholesterol levels, fasting blood sugar, insulin levels, triglycerides, blood pressure and all the rest – ageing can now be reversed, rejuvenating your body and de-ageing your life.

What was once a pipe-dream, followed by rich eccentrics who had them-selves injected with monkey glands or drank snake blood in an effort to grow younger, has become a real possibility. It can be done right here, right now. For me, these three facts add up to the most exciting information to come out of twentieth century science related to establishing and maintaining high level health. For the first time in history Age Power is possible for each of us – a journey into wholeness, authenticity and fulfilment. What could be better than that?

. . . only a small portion of the genetic information in our cells is expressed. Our diet, lifestyle and environment modify the nature of this information and how it is expressed. We are the prod-ucts of what and how well our genetic messages are expressed. Healthy ageing is accomplished when our genes continue to express healthy messages throughout our lives.

Jeffrey Bland PhD

AGE POWER STARTS HERE

So much for the myths of ageing. The next time you find your-self grunting when you get out of a chair, or refusing to play run around after a young niece or nephew on the grounds that you are too old, think again. Forget the myths and remember just three important Age Power *facts:*

FACT ONE: it is *biological* not chronological age, that matters.

FACT TWO: by improving your ability to adapt to stressors and maintain physiological balance and function, you can effectively prevent accelerated ageing and the degenerative diseases asso-ciated with it.

FACT THREE: There is even better news. Even when negative changes in your body have already taken place, by making alter-ations to the way you live and eat, many – in most people even *all* – of these changes can be reversed.

The goal of the hero's journey is yourself, finding yourself.

Joseph Campbell

PART TWO:
THE POWER OF AGE

MEET THE BIOMARKERS

The secret to staying young is to live honestly,
eat slowly and lie about your age.

Lucille Ball

Your age depends on your biomarkers. Biomarkers are
scientific measures of how old you are *biologically*, not
chronologically. Forget the birthdays. This is the only age
that matters. Make simple lifestyle changes and you can
reverse not only how old you look and feel but how your
body functions – *in medically measurable ways.*

Biomarkers show how well you function physically and mentally, regardless of what the calendar says. Whatever your chronological age, your
biomarkers are always changing for the better or for the worse. For over
30 years scientists have worked to identify the most important biomarkers
of ageing, examining dozens of potential candidates such as the degree
of skin dryness, the greying of hair, levels of blood cholesterol and liver
enzymes, and the incidence, time, and onset of cataracts.

CLEAR CUT MEASURES

For a long time researchers were not able to agree on just which biomarkers
should be considered the *major* measurements of biological ageing. Then,
in the late nineties, two brilliant yet highly practical American scientists,
Irwin H. Rosenberg MD and William J. Evans PhD, got together at the
United States Department of Agriculture's Human Nutrition Research
Centre on Ageing at Tufts University, and made age research history by
defining biomarkers on which everyone in the scientific world could agree:
once and for all.

Rosenberg, the director of the research centre, is a physiologist as well
as a physician. His special interest is in clinical nutrition and metabolism. A
former chairman of the Food and Nutrition Board of the National Academy
of Sciences in the United States as well as former president of the American
Society of Clinical Nutrition, he has held professorships at Harvard and the
University of Chicago. Evans was chief of the Human Physiology Laboratory
at the centre. His research has focused
primarily on the *physiology* of ageing and
sports performance. A fellow of the
American College of Sports Medicine as well
as the American College of Nutrition, Evans

> How old would you be if
> you didn't know how old
> you was?
>
> *Satchel Paige*

is also exercise advisor to many top sports teams, and is highly respected, not only for his scientific work but for his ability to communicate the value of it to the general public.

HARD FACTS

Evans and Rosenberg identified the biomarkers of ageing as clear-cut, scientific measurements doctors can use to determine how old an animal or human is. The biomarkers of age are valuable. They make it possible for you, your doctor, or health professional to assess your functional age right now, and then to reassess it as you make changes in your lifestyle designed to reverse it. In effect the biomarkers objectively measure the effectiveness of any change in diet or exercise you make, or any treatment. Working with them is a great way to increase your motivation to transform your life for the better. Week by week, month by month, you have objective proof that your body is rejuvenating itself.

EARLY DAYS

When Evans and Rosenberg began their work, they were dogged by the huge variety of changes related to ageing – from wrinkles to risk of stroke. They knew that they needed a much tighter definition if they were going to use the term 'biomarkers' in a way that had real practical significance. Sifting through the vast number of changes associated with ageing led them to eliminate its more superficial cosmetic aspects like sagging skin, hair loss and age spots, as well as some of the internal physiological functions which are difficult to measure. They were keen to emphasise the *positive* aspects of the ageing equation, and to identify the most significant age concerns. Their team of researchers had wanted to include the body's immune function for instance. For there is no question that a decline in immune function is associated with degeneration in the body. However, when the

> Defining aging from the perspective of increasing risk of death didn't strike us as fruitful either. It's like viewing a glass as half empty instead of half full . . . Instead of looking at aging from the negative side (what causes death), we've been concentrating on the positive (what maintains health). That is, our focus is not on postponing death but on maintaining health for the longest possible period of time.
>
> *William Evans MD, and Irwin Rosenberg PhD*

original studies were carried out, they were unable to identify enough definitive data to be able to make immunity part of the biomarker list.

DEFINITIVE LIST

The biomarkers finally agreed upon have only two characteristics: They describe critical biological functions which influence vitality. And, as numerous clinical studies now show, even if any of these functions have been compromised they can be, to a large degree, restored — even in very old people. You will notice that the actions you take to reverse one biomarker will often be the same needed to reverse others. The Evans and Rosenberg team finally came up with what is now considered the 'gold standard' — a list of ten biomarkers now widely accepted to indicate *biological* not chronological – age. These biomarkers have three important characteristics:

THEY ARE OBJECTIVE.
THEY ARE EASILY MEASURABLE.
THEY ARE ALTERED BY THE WAY WE LIVE.

TOP TEN BIOMARKERS

Think about your body in terms of these ten biomarkers and you are well on your way to Age Power.

- ❑ **Lean Body Mass**
- ❑ **Muscle Strength**
- ❑ **Basal Metabolic Rate (BMR)**
- ❑ **Body Fat Percentage**
- ❑ **Aerobic Capacity**
- ❑ **Insulin Sensitivity/Blood Sugar Tolerance**
- ❑ **Cholesterol HDL/LDL Ratios**
- ❑ **Blood Pressure**
- ❑ **Bone Density**
- ❑ **Body Heat**

BEWARE SARCOPENIA

The most important physiological degeneration involved in many of the biomarkers is that of *sarcopenia*. This is something you really need to know about. Most of us carry around far too much body fat and far too little muscle. Evans and Rosenberg coined the word *sarcopenia*. It is the shrinking of muscle mass and the distortion of muscle to fat levels. It's a great word. Remember it. Sarcopenia describes the overall weakening of your body as a result of gradual – usually decades long – changes in its composition and loss of muscle mass. The negative consequences this brings are loss of strength, and lowered basal metabolic rate – BMR, an increase in body fat percentage as well as other degenerative functional changes. This biomarker – how much of your body is lean muscle as opposed to how much fat (something which has nothing to do with how much you weigh, by the way) – is the most important degenerative change to reverse if you want to rejuvenate your body, restore a high level of vitality and enhance your good looks.

This fact is often not a happy thought to those of us who would rather spend our time looking for quick fix solutions to age problems. For changing one's life for the better asks that each of us take real responsibility. However, if you are one of a growing number of men and women excited about the prospect of rejuvenation at the deepest level, this is the best news to come out of a century of age research. If you carry too much body fat and too little muscle you need to reverse this to banish sarcopenia. Through weight resistance exercise or strength training you can increase muscle mass and strength more effortlessly than you think. This in turn helps normalise your basal metabolic rate and will dramatically shift your fat percentage. Pick up a pair of dumbbells. They can change your life.

BANISH FEAR

Many people, especially women, are frightened of the idea of building muscle. They think it will make them bigger. Just the opposite is true. When you work with muscle in a concentrated way through resistance training, your muscles don't become larger, they become more dense. Your body takes on a much more aesthetic shape and contour. Your body becomes leaner. So in case you have any fears of ending up muscle bound through strength training, forget it. What you may find is that you actually *gain* rather than lose weight, however, for muscle on your body is dense and compact, while fat is fluffy and bulging. Yet your clothes will be looser than before and you will be a much better shape.

Let's explore each biomarker one by one. For it is important not only to understand how each is specifically related to ageing and degeneration, but also how they are interrelated. Age reversal is not only a total *body* process, it is a total *person* process. Make changes to alter one of the biomarkers of vitality, and you invariably improve others.

Biomarker One
LEAN BODY MASS
Action Plan: Get Lean

Build Muscle

Body composition matters. It is the single most important biomarker of all. Your body is made up of two different kinds of tissue. Body fat — scientifically known as *adipose tissue* — and lean body mass. In the lean body mass category, scientists put everything that is *not* fat. This includes your bones, all of your tissues built of proteins such as your organs, your central nervous system as well as, the most important of all, your muscles. Muscle breeds vitality. Fat undermines it.

LOSE FAT GAIN YOUTH

It is not *weight* that is the issue. It is *fat* that we need to lose. Not by going on another calorie controlled diet either. Slimming diets don't just shed fat, they burn protein — that is muscle tissue. After being on a low calorie diet, more than 90 percent of people regain the weight they have lost within a year. But they don't regain precious muscle tissue lost. Muscle is hard to put back on the body. Fat is easy — just eat a few more muffins each week. The weight regained after a crash diet is going to be fat not muscle. Yoyo dieting creates a situation in which the ratio between muscle and fat on your body continues to be upset. More fat gets laid down, more and more muscle is lost, and sarcopenia plus the accelerated ageing that accompanies it develops.

Adipose tissue, that is stored fat, is metabolically *inactive*. Its primary purpose is to store energy for times of famine so humans can survive through the lean times until food is available again. People who, like me, have inherited what is known as the *thrifty gene*, have a genetic tendency to store fat. Our ancestors were the ones that lasted through those long cold winters while everyone else was dying of starvation. The trouble is, the thrifty gene is not of great benefit to those of us now in developed countries who are not starving. Storing excess fat in our bodies makes us highly prone to a lot of degenerative conditions, especially obesity and diabetes, and to developing sarcopenia.

People with a high percentage of muscle have a much higher metabolism. Like kids, they are capable of burning many more calories, so they don't have to worry about getting fat, sometimes no matter how much they eat. Most women find themselves in the opposite situation, often because of crash dieting. Although they may be thin, they may be technically obese because their ratio of fat to lean body mass is much too high. They still have far too high a percentage of fat. This weakens them and makes them haggard. Such people are forced to lower drastically the calories they take in to prevent themselves from getting fatter. So serious is this situation that many women live on a diet of 1000 calories or less a day just to prevent weight gain. Such a diet cannot supply the nutrients you need for adequate protection from degeneration. So these people, whose bodies by now are undergoing accelerated ageing, grow less vital and more haggard as the years pass, finding it harder and harder to lose weight and easier and easier to gain it, no matter how little they eat.

HOLD ON TO IT

Loss of lean body mass and an increase in the level of fat in your body, not only from dieting but also from living a couch potato life, is the single most destructive biomarker in relation to ageing anyone has so far been able to identify. In later chapters we'll look in depth at how to bring about a couch-potato-to-powerhouse transformation in your own body.

Reclaim Muscle

Fat in the body – adipose tissue – is highly inactive. Except for a small amount of fat which every one of us needs to cushion our organs and to offer some stored energy, we don't need it. Most fat is nothing but *dead* weight for you to carry around. It offers no vitality. The more you carry, the less energy you have and the less effectively the systems of your body can work. By contrast, muscle is highly *alive* biologically. It is vital tissue. It is in your muscle cells that energy is converted from the foods you eat to be burnt as fuel. Within each muscle cell, your mitochondria – the body's energy factories – take in blood sugar and through a complex process of oxidation turn it into your body's energy currency, ATP. The more mitochondria you have the more efficiently they work the more vitality you experience and the more resistant your body is to ageing.

A high level of muscle means a good metabolism, so you can easily burn body fat and continue to improve your body composition. Muscle also improves your ability to use oxygen, on which the health of your cardiovascular system – in fact your whole body – depends. Muscle in your body helps protect from insulin resistance – Syndrome X – the recently discovered collection of abnormalities associated both with early ageing and the onset of degenerative diseases. Prevent Syndrome X and you prevent accelerated ageing. Reverse Syndrome X and you quite literally rejuvenate your body (see page 59). A good percentage of muscle helps protect you from cholesterol problems too, so you maintain high levels of the beneficial HDL cholesterol in your blood. Between young adulthood and middle age, most of us in the West lose 3 kg of lean body mass – muscle – each ten years of our life. Muscle loss gets even faster after the age of 45. This loss, however, is by no means inevitable. It is not a *normal* part of ageing as we have come to believe. It occurs as a result of disuse.

Muscle, to a far greater extent than most people realize, is responsible for the vitality of your whole physiological apparatus. It's why muscle mass and strength are our primary Biomarkers and why we believe that building muscle in the elderly is the key to their rejuvenation.

William Evans MD, and Irwin Rosenberg PhD

Together with long walks four or five times a week, you can't do better than resistance training for de-ageing your body. There is more good news too. Lost muscle can be regained, steadily and slowly, simply by taking up resistance training and practising it for half an hour a time, four times a week. This kind of exercise not only rebuilds good lean body mass and lowers the level of fat, it also encourages the production of growth hormone and other anabolic youth-related hormones. Growth

THE POWER OF RESISTANCE

For many years we have been told that aerobic exercise is the way to maintain fitness and prevent degeneration. There is a certain truth in this. Regular aerobic exercise – running, walking, rowing, anything which gets your heart and lungs going – is important in protecting the cardiovascular system and bringing more energy to your body. But the most important of all in preventing and reversing 'age-related' degeneration, is not aerobic. New, widespread research shows clearly that resistance training or strength training – working out with dumbbells and barbells using a different muscle group each time – is by far the most important kind of exercise for overall health and to prevent muscle loss.

hormone levels are high when you are young. They are largely responsible for the high level energy athletes can call on whenever they need it. In the United States at the moment one of the big fads is growth hormone injections. It is a therapy which has not in any way been proven and is well out of reach financially for most people. Also, growth hormone injections can lead to disturbances in insulin resistance and blood glucose levels, both of which have a significant impact on degeneration. Much better to buy yourself a couple of dumbbells and do a simple workout routine for half an hour four times a week then shove them under the bed when you're not using them.

Responding to a telegram received by his agent inquiring: How old Cary Grant? Old Cary fine. How are you?

Cary Grant

Biomarker Two
MUSCLE STRENGTH
Action Plan: Go For Power

***

Get Into Strength

The second biomarker you will want to change for lasting youth is muscle *strength*. Building lean body mass means building strength. Muscle strength itself has huge implications for all the other biomarkers of ageing. The gradual muscle loss most of us experience as we get older not only results in a steady increase in the levels of body fat, it also brings about a decline in your aerobic capacity and overall vitality. Loss of strength lowers your blood sugar tolerance and increases insulin resistance – interfering with your body's ability to produce energy (see Biomarker Six, page 43). It also causes your bones to lose their density, making you susceptible to osteoporosis and it slows down your metabolism. Experts in sports medicine used to believe that once muscle strength was lost there was little chance of regaining it. Thanks to the work of a few American pioneers such as Walter Frontera, an expert in rehabilitation medicine, we now know that this is not the case. Frontera's findings are life-changing. They confirm that any work that we do to build strength – provided we work hard enough at it – can regenerate muscle and rejuvenate the body.

NEVER TOO LATE

Frontera looked at the effect of weight training on the size and strength of the muscles of elderly people. In the process, he and his team exploded negative myths about what is and is not possible in terms of rejuvenation. Until this time most sports physiologists believed that once you are past the age of 50 or 60, any gain in muscle strength was a result of learning how to use your body more effectively. It had, they thought, nothing to do with your muscles actually growing denser and stronger. This is why for many years we have been told – in fact we continue to be told – that as you get older the ability of your muscles to get stronger and denser in response to weight training inevitably declines. It just ain't so.

Challenge Yourself

Frontera and his team showed this in their research. They examined other research projects previously carried out with older people, and discovered that the researchers had made a fatal assumption when designing their studies: That the elderly could not withstand anything more than very low intensity exercise – training which demands only 30 to 40 percent of a person's maximal lifting capacity. It is well established that for a young person to improve in strength it is necessary for them to lift between 60 to 100 percent of maximal capacity. Frontera asked the question, 'Why should older people be treated any differently?' Why should they not have to make the same concerted effort that the young do if they are to bring about any significant gains in strength?

One of his studies took twelve older subjects between the ages of 60 and 72 and got them to train at 80 percent of their *one repetition maximum.* A one repetition maximum is the term used to describe the heaviest weight a person can lift doing a particular exercise once. His subjects worked out three times a week for twelve weeks. Each week this one repetition maximum weight was increased.

Double Your Strength

The results of Frontera's experience transformed the scientific beliefs about what is possible for older men and women. During the period of his study, the quadriceps strength in men taking part more than doubled, while the strength of their hamstrings tripled. In effect, Frontera and his colleagues succeeded where everyone else had failed, simply by eliminating the self-limiting assumptions about ageing, namely that older people should be treated with kid gloves.

Even more exciting, when they began to measure by CT scans (computerised tomography) how this muscle strength had been built, they discovered that these men had achieved an amazing 12 percent collective increase in the muscles. Muscle biopsies were taken before training began, after six weeks, and then at the end of the study. Examination of these tissues through a microscope showed that even the size of muscle cells had progressively increased from beginning to end (another thing previous researchers believed impossible). What I find delightful about the study is the fact that the men who took part were

Sam Semansky, a 93-year-old study participant, spoke for many of his peers when he observed, 'I feel as though I were 50 again. Now, I can get up in the middle of the night and I can get around without using my walker or turning on the light. The program gave me strength I didn't have before. Every day I feel better, more optimistic. Pills won't do for you what exercise does.'

William Evans MD, and Irwin Rosenberg PhD

stunned by their improvements. By the end of it, many of them were able to lift more weight than 25-year-old graduate students involved in other experiments in the same laboratory.

Later, another doctor – Maria A. Fiatarone, a specialist in geriatric medicine – decided to conduct quite different experiments with the elderly. Working with institutionalised people who were very frail indeed, she wanted to find out if she could help people grow stronger, improve the quality of their lives and increase their capacity to function day to day. Her study was conducted at a 700-bed hospital for chronic care. There she worked with ten men and women between the ages of 87 and 96, doing just as Frontera had done, getting them to train at 80 percent of the 1RM – the one repetition maximum – this time for eight weeks. Fiatarone's goals were different than Frontera's. She was interested in exploring the relationship between muscle strength and how quickly older people could walk. She hypothesised that the weaker your legs are, the longer it is likely to take to walk 20 feet. She too used CT scans to examine any changes of thigh muscle size. She found that during the study these muscles had grown by more than 10 percent within an eight week period.

These two studies, and others that have taken place since, have established categorically that you do not have to lose muscle strength as you grow older. And further, if you have lost it, you can regain it no matter what your age, through simple weight training.

Biomarker Three

BASAL METABOLIC RATE
Action Plan: Walk To Freedom

What's Your Burn Rate

The rate at which your body expends caloric energy from your foods when at rest is known as your basal metabolic rate, or BMR. It is biomarker three. This biomarker tends to decrease with age. As it does, the chemical processes by which your body releases energy, builds new tissue and eliminates waste no longer work so efficiently. You do not break down calories from your food as well. Nor do you absorb nutrients and eliminate waste as a healthy young person does. Until recently no-one knew why. Now we do.

> A good time to think about old age is when you are young, because you can then do much to improve the chances that you will enjoy it when it comes.
>
> *B.F. Skinner PhD*

COUCH POTATOES TAKE NOTE

If you are living a sedentary life as most people do, as you get older your body's need for oxygen declines. So does the amount of food you need to maintain your body weight. Yet most of us continue to eat the amount of food we ate when we were younger. As a result we gain yet more fat tissue. Our lean-body-mass-to-fat ratio shifts more and more in favour of fat. This causes our basal metabolic rate to fall.

In most people BMR decreases by about two percent every 10 years, beginning at the age of 20. The fall in BMR is part of a vicious circle that leads to yet more fat gain and more muscle loss, all of which further accelerates ageing. And unless you break through this degenerative cycle by making changes in how you eat and taking up the right kind of exercise to improve strength and increase muscle mass, the BMR function you have is lost and will only get worse with every year that passes. As muscle strength grows, your BMR increases. It's as easy as that.

Biomarker Four
BODY FAT PERCENTAGE
Action Plan: Eat For Youth

Lose the Fat

The tendency we have to gain fat year by year, even if we don't gain weight (most of us seem to manage that too) leads to a change for the worse in our lean-body-mass-to-fat ratio. Evans and Rosenberg concluded that the average sedentary 65-year-old women is about 43 percent adipose tissue, compared to only 25 percent at 25. Women lay down more fat tissue than men because their bodies are far higher in oestrogens. If a woman has taken The Pill or is on hormone replacement therapy, she is likely to struggle even harder to keep her weight down. The average body fat in a man at aged 25 is 18 percent, moving up to about 38 percent by the time he is 65. As this happens, his lean-body-mass-to-fat ratio goes askew and fat takes over.

> The body is a sacred garment. It's your first and last garment; it is what you enter life in and what you depart life with, and it should be treated with honor.
>
> *Martha Graham*

DISTRIBUTION MATTERS

Not only does the *amount* of fat on your body greatly determine your tendency to accelerated ageing and degenerative conditions, how the fat is distributed matters. Many researchers now believe that fat *distribution* is equally as important as lean body mass to fat ratio in predicting the likelihood of degenerative disease. Cholesterol levels by the way – another biomarker of age – are closely related to fat distribution. Just about the worst place you can carry your fat is right around the middle. If you have a trim waist and big hips you are much more likely to have increased levels of HDL cholesterol – a protective form of cholesterol. Whereas if your fat is stored around the waist area, you are statistically much more prone to heart disease, diabetes, and strokes, even if you are not particularly overweight.

One fact of life that must be faced if you have gained a considerable amount of fat over the last decade or two, is that it *is* harder for you to shed fat once it has accumulated than for your younger cousins. This has to do with the lowering of the BMR. And this is made worse for women for they are the worst yo-yo dieters. As a result they suffer all of the nasty consequences including loss of lean muscle tissue, and lowering of the metabolic rate, all of which leaves women with flabby bodies, even when they don't look particularly overweight. But take heart, it is by no means impossible.

TAKE HEART

Recent work with Age Power's Insulin Balance (see page 211) shows quite clearly that you can shed fat permanently without ever going on a low calorie slimming diet. Combined with the right kind of exercise (the same exercise that will shift Biomarkers One and Two), the more excess fat you shed, the better your lean-body-mass-to-fat ratio becomes in favour of muscle. Your BMR also improves. Then the more calories you burn from the foods that you eat. You are not only able to eat more without becoming fat because your metabolic rate speeds up, the fat burning process becomes an ongoing experience, more and more efficient all the time.

Biomarker Five
AEROBIC CAPACITY
Action Plan: Bump Up Your O_2

Oxygen Yields Energy

How well your body processes oxygen within a specific measured time is known as your *aerobic capacity* – the fifth biomarker. The greater your aerobic capacity, the more energy you will have available to your body, both to support its optimal functioning, to slow age degeneration and to provide you with the vitality that you need to live life to the full. A high aerobic capacity means you can, with ease, take in large quantities of air to oxygenate your blood, delivering this oxygen with each heart beat throughout your body to all its cells and tissues. This process all works well provided you have a good vascular network, a powerful heart and healthy lungs. You probably did when you were 18. But masses of studies show that most people's aerobic capacity diminishes with age. In men, the maximum oxygen intake begins to decline from 20 years onward. In women, for reasons as yet unknown, the decline happens later – not until the early 30's. By the age of 65, most men and women have lost 30 to 40 percent of their aerobic capacity. In older people who exercise, this decline is much less. But if you lead a sedentary life, even the size of your heart can shrink so that the quantity of blood that it is able to pump through your body in a specific length of time diminishes. As it does, so does your overall functioning and vitality.

Aerobic capacity is considered a good index of your overall cardio-vascular fitness too. There is absolutely no necessity for aerobic capacity – sometimes called VO_2 max – to undergo rapid decline as the years pass, provided you get enough exercise. Your VO_2 max tells how well the cells of your body are receiving the oxygen they need to function optimally. The passing of the years plus an inactive lifestyle actually interferes with capillary growth, so that your body ends up with fewer than optimal capillaries to carry oxygenated blood to its tissues. This diminishes your *oxidative capacity* – how well your muscle cells can make use of oxygen by converting it to energy instead of storing it as fat.

If, like most of us, you have spent too many years not getting enough exercise, don't worry, it's never too late to change.

The only exercise you ever get is jumping to conclusions.

Danny Kaye, The Secret Life of Walter Mitty

Double Your Power

Both aerobic exercise and weight resistance exercise, such as strength training, increase aerobic capacity. Aerobic exercise gets the heart and lungs working and increases your muscles' oxidative capacity. (This is particularly true as you grow older). Then, as you build muscle mass and shrink fat in your body through strength training – particularly if you train around 80 percent of 1RM (one repetition maximum weight) you actually create more muscle cells to consume oxygen. The more muscle mass you have calling for oxygen, the greater your utilisation of oxygen becomes and the better your aerobic capacity. The opposite is also true. When your musculature shrinks you have a much lower aerobic capacity for no other reason than you have fewer muscles demanding oxygen. This is the main reason why, as we grow older, we tend to huff and puff climbing stairs. But your body has a magnificent ability to renew and rejuvenate itself so any loss of aerobic capacity can be regained.

As you have probably figured out by now, the first five biomarkers of ageing are tightly interwoven. The major answer to reversing all five of them is muscle. Working to enhance muscle will rejuvenate you better than magic potions, expensive hormone injections or weird treatments. It will even change the way you think and feel about your life. So much for the external biomarkers; on to the internal.

TAKE COURAGE

A number of studies show that when a person whose aerobic capacity has declined begins to exercise regularly, they can reverse this decline. Within weeks, their VO2 max can return to that of someone 10 to 30 years younger biologically.

Don't say my last, you damned fool! Say my latest.

Sir Henry Parket, when he was congratulated at the age of eighty on the birth of a new baby.

FEAR NO MORE

Don't be afraid life will end; be afraid it will never begin.

Grace Hansen

Changes in the first five biomarkers identified by Evans and Rosenberg are easy to monitor – whether the changes are for better or worse – in the shape and tone of your body, in your energy levels and your overall sense of your strength and fitness. The second five biomarkers are more hidden. Because they are so hidden, it is often these biomarkers of ageing that we worry most about as we get older. Fear no more.

Getting a grip on them means measuring changes to the *inside* of your body in insulin sensitivity, cholesterol levels – the ratio between HDL, the so called 'good' cholesterol and LDL, the so called 'bad' – as well as changes in blood pressure, bone density and the body's ability to regulate temperature. Despite the belief that detrimental changes in the second five biomarkers are a normal part of the ageing process, this is untrue. These 'age-related' changes can also be reversed in most people through changes in lifestyle and diet.

BEWARE SYNDROME X

The first five biomarkers of ageing are so closely interlinked that altering one will significantly affect the others. The same is true of the second five. There is one biomarker in this group which it is critical to change to improve all the others: Biomarker Six – insulin levels/blood sugar tolerance. The reason detrimental changes in these 'internal' biomarkers can be reversed is because, far from their being part of a 'normal' ageing process, abnormalities in these biomarkers tend to occur together forming a sinister sounding condition known as Syndrome X. Not some recently discovered disease, Syndrome X is a term coined by a gifted endocrinologist at Stanford University, Gerald M. Reaven. For many years Reaven studied a phenomenon called *insulin resistance* which accompanies negative changes in biomarkers. Insulin resistance is a loss of insulin sensitivity, so the cells of the body, which depend on insulin to make energy, can no longer respond to the hormone as they do in a youthful, healthy body.

A fine scientist with the ability to bring together information from different disciplines, Reaven realised that insulin resistance and distortions in the body's blood sugar tolerance belong to a constellation of related symptoms, including a rise in blood sugar, elevated cholesterol and triglyceride levels, and a number of other known risk factors for coronary heart disease.

INSULIN RESISTANCE

Reaven coined the phrase Syndrome X to describe this cluster of abnormalities seen in an increasing number of people. It is also known as *insulin resistance syndrome*. This single abnormality links your body's mounting insensitivity to insulin at a cellular level with disorders such as diabetes, heart disease, arteriosclerosis, obesity and the inability to shed fat from your body no matter how hard you try, chronic fatigue, depression and anxiety.

Fifteen years ago scientists estimated that Syndrome X affected one in four people. Now many clinicians and scientists believe it may be more like two thirds of the adult population living on a diet of Western convenience foods. We will look at Syndrome X in a lot more detail in the next chapter, since an understanding of what it is, how it works, how it can be prevented and how it can be reversed, is crucial to altering not only the sixth biomarker, insulin sensitivity, but also the seventh and eighth – cholesterol levels and blood pressure. And good news: the measures you take to counteract these three biomarkers will also go a long way to address problems associated with the ninth biomarker – bone density – and the tenth – body temperature regulation. Let's examine the biomarkers themselves and see why they are important.

Symptoms are a way for your body to say 'Listen to me talk for a change'.

Carl A Hammerschlag

Biomarker Six
INSULIN SENSITIVITY/BLOOD SUGAR TOLERANCE
Action Plan: Eat for Age Power

Cut the Sugar

How well your body controls blood sugar is known as *glucose tolerance*. It has long been considered a biomarker of ageing since as we get older our bodies gradually lose the ability to take up and make proper use of the glucose carried in our blood stream which we derive from the foods we eat. As a result our fasting blood sugar levels tend to rise as we get older. With them, so does our chances of developing what is known as Adult Onset Diabetes or Type II Diabetes. By the time we reach the age of 70, 30 percent of all women and 20 percent of men have an abnormal glucose tolerance curve. As we grow older we tend to take less exercise than when we were young and become more and more sedentary. Combine this with a diet high in carbohydrates and sugars and most of us accumulate body fat. As this happens, the cells in our body tend to lose their sensitivity to insulin, so that the pancreas has to produce more and more to have any effect.

One of the great discoveries of the last century was the important role insulin plays in our health, yet most people – including most doctors – still primarily associate insulin with diabetes. Few understand the essential role that this hormone plays, not only in overall health but in protecting the body from accelerated ageing and degenerative disease. Here's how it works:

MASTER CONTROLLER

Glucose is burnt in your cells to produce energy. It is derived from the foods you eat and makes its way into the blood stream where it is ready to be taken up by your cells and used. It can only get into your cells, however, in the presence of the hormone insulin. Your pancreas releases insulin into the blood stream so that it is able to bind with receptor sites on your cells – in much the same way that a key fits into a lock. The door that insulin unlocks is the one through which glucose passes into cells. Without insulin the glucose from your food can try as hard as it likes to get into your cells but it won't find a way in. But when chronic high levels of insulin are present in the blood, the cell receptors stop responding to it and glucose can't get through to be turned into ATP – your body's energy currency. This is called *insulin resistance*.

Jaded Cells

Back in the sixties, researchers found ways of measuring insulin levels. In doing this they discovered that the illness known as Type II diabetes – adult onset diabetes – was not simply an abnormality of soaring blood sugar levels. You might expect that high levels of blood sugar would mean low levels of insulin – that the blood sugar was not able to travel out of the blood stream into the cells because there was not enough insulin to take it there. Instead they found that these diabetics have *high* levels of insulin compared to non-diabetics. From this discovery came an awareness of the phenomenon that Reaven studied so closely, known as insulin resistance. When insulin resistance occurs, your cells become jaded. In effect they stop fully responding to insulin so that it no longer unlocks the cell properly. Your pancreas just keeps secreting more and more insulin in an attempt to get the energy from the glucose in your blood stream into your cells. What this means in practical terms is that this energy is not available to your body, so you will tend to store the calories taken in through your food as fat rather than burning them for vitality.

As an awareness of the phenomenon of insulin resistance spread, researchers and clinicians began to understand that many of us who are not diabetic still experience insulin resistance, and scientists began to question what causes it. The discoveries they have made along the way are nothing short of revolutionary. They give us the power both to slow down the rate at which our bodies age and even to reverse degenerative changes in the biomarkers of blood pressure, insulin sensitivity and cholesterol HDL ratio, simply by changing the way you eat and live.

SYNDROME X

INSULIN RESISTANCE + GLUCOSE INTOLERANCE
(Elevated or erratic blood sugar together with high fasting insulin levels)

HIGH BLOOD PRESSURE
Hypertension. Look out if blood pressure is consistently higher than 140/90.

ABNORMAL BLOOD FATS
Elevated triglycerides and high LDL – high density cholesterol. Look out when triglycerides go above 160mg/dl and cholesterol gets above 160mg/dl.

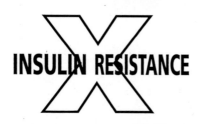

THE PAUNCH
Poor lean-body-mass-to-fat ratio in favour of fat – regardless of how much you weigh. Look out for excess fat around chest and stomach – the beer belly.

ENERGY SWINGS
Peaks and troughs of energy during the day – especially at 11am and 4pm – and mood swings that go with it. Look out for the urge to drink another cup of coffee or eat a sticky bun just to keep going.

Insulin resistance lies at the core of Syndrome X and predisposes you to all the other abnormalities that it encompasses such as obesity, elevated and distorted blood fats and high blood pressure. These abnormalities in turn predispose you to degenerative diseases and early ageing. They can be reversed through changes in how you eat and live, reversing age biomarkers and rejuvenating your body in medically measurable ways.

How It Works

How much insulin is released in your body is determined by *what you eat*. When you eat carbohydrate foods such as a baked potato, a piece of toast, a plate of pasta, a bowl of cereal, your digestion converts it into glucose very quickly. Now glucose is a simple sugar which causes your blood sugar levels to rise rapidly. As a response to this rise in blood sugar, the *islets of langerhans* within your pancreas secrete insulin. This is why insulin is often known as the *sugar processing hormone*. As soon as your body releases insulin in response to a rise in glucose, it turns some of this glucose into glycogen so you can store it as potential energy for future use in your muscle tissue and in your liver. Once there, glycogen, rather like a bank balance, can be turned back into glucose quickly and easily whenever you need energy. Meanwhile, whatever glucose has not been converted into glycogen continues to circulate in your blood stream for use as immediate energy.

At least this is how it all works when it works well. The problem is, as we get older it ceases to work well, and for some people it doesn't work at all. If there is a great excess of glucose in circulation, particularly if this happens day after day for many years, then when you eat a meal high in carbohydrates such as pizza and ice-cream, the insulin levels your body produces in response become abnormal. So your pancreas needs to secrete more insulin just to get the glucose into your cells and, as insulin increases further, it gradually fails to do so. It is this failure that results in mounting blood pressure levels, distortions in cholesterol and blood fats and, in many people, the development of obesity, arteriosclerosis and diabetes.

Silent Threat

The course of these unfortunate metabolic events is not only the primary reason that people in the Western world are getting fatter and fatter, but also why most of us are ageing too rapidly. In the last 30 years an ever more widespread number of people have experienced an alarming break-down in most of the metabolic processes which insulin controls. As a consequence we are experiencing a vast number of age related disorders and diseases. Our bodies develop far too much fat while our muscles shrink, producing what Evans and Rosenberg call sarcopenia. More than half the population of English speaking countries are now overweight. In the United States alone, millions of people have chronic high blood pressure – the seventh Biomarker of Ageing. Growing millions have elevated cholesterol levels too – the eighth biomarker of ageing. Syndrome X is responsible for spreading waistlines and growing obesity. It is also now considered

> It is never too late to be what you might have been.
>
> *George Eliot*

as a primary cause – what is known as a risk factor – for heart disease and many other conditions, and what is worse, insulin resistance like the other abnormalities associated with Syndrome X, such as hypertension and cholesterol and blood fat abnormalities, is a silent threat. Most people have no idea that they even have it.

Deadly Duo

The most direct causes of insulin resistance are two of the other biomarkers associated with ageing – increased body fat and inactivity. Generally they go hand in hand. The other important cause is a diet far too high in sugar, refined grains and all of the convenience foods made from them. Put these two causative factors together and you create a prescription for disaster. However, if you are physically active throughout your life, and provided some of your activity is designed specifically to build lean muscle mass, then most of the carbohydrates you eat are likely to be used, especially if they are complex carbohydrates such as those from non-starchy vegetables and low glycaemic fruits – not masses of sugar, pasta or breakfast cereals. You are unlikely to develop insulin resistance and you will probably be able to burn the glucose in your blood right away for energy.

If you have not been active however, and you eat a Western diet high in carbohydrates (and by the way this is what governments throughout the world are still encouraging us to do) then your body will tend to turn this glucose into fat through a process known as *lipogenises*. But fear not. Even if you have not being doing the 'right' things to prevent insulin resistance – even if you already have it – there is a great deal you can do immediately to rectify the situation simply by making changes in the way you eat and the exercise you take. Age Power's Insulin Balance is the way to go.

Biomarker Seven

CHOLESTEROL HDL/LDL RATIOS
Action Plan: Strength and Balance

Lower Cholesterol

It wasn't long ago that the first thing you would be asked at any American cocktail party was what your astrological sign was, and the second thing was what your cholesterol level was. These two subjects were just as mysterious and arbitrary as each other. Happily, in my experience, this attitude is changing. But still there is an enormous amount of confusion surrounding cholesterol, what is it, is it dangerous, must we cut all foods that contain cholesterol such as eggs and shellfish from our diet or not. To understand this biomarker and how to let it work for you rather than against you, let's go back to first principles and look at what cholesterol actually is, how it works in the body and what causes abnormalities.

SECRETS OF CHOLESTEROL

Cholesterol is a waxy sterol. It is manufactured by all animal cells and is a perfectly normal substance to be found in your body. Not only is it normal, cholesterol plays a number of vital roles without which your body cannot remain healthy. For instance, it's essential to the manufacture of new cell membranes. It also is the source or precursor of many of the body's most important sterol hormones from pregnenalone and DHEA to testosterone, oestrogens and progesterone. In the body, cholesterol flows through the blood stream together with proteins in packages known as *lipoproteins*. There are four main types of lipoproteins found in your blood: *chylomicrons, very low-density lipoproteins (VLDLs), low-density lipoproteins (LDLs)* and *high-density lipoproteins (HDLs)*. At one time it was believed that a high level of any of these cholesterol-containing lipoproteins was a risk factor in the development of heart disease. Although there is much more to be learned about the four forms of cholesterol, researchers know that each of the four major classes of lipoproteins function quite differently. The VLDL and LDL cholesterol for instance, contribute to heart disease by creating an obstructive waxy build up of plaque in the arteries of the heart, while HDL cholesterol has protective properties, amongst them the ability to cleanse the arteries of plaque and help prevent heart disease. So where once your doctor looked at what your total cholesterol count was to determine your risk of heart disease, now he looks at the primary ratio between HDL which he wants to see raised, and LDL cholesterol in your blood which he wants to see lowered.

HDL/LDL's

The way this is figured is to take the total cholesterol divided by the HDL cholesterol and this gives your cholesterol/HDL ratio, the most important biomarker of ageing in relation to cholesterol which is as yet understood by science. Age researchers have discovered that the passing of the years has little effect on HDL cholesterol levels, which tend to remain constant. Many studies indicate however, that the total blood cholesterol level, particularly in men, increases in the Western world as they get older, at least until they are around 50, at which point it begins to decline. However, since the total cholesterol levels tend to increase with age while the HDL levels remain constant, it is the harmful LDL or bad cholesterol and VLDL cholesterol which is not fully understood, but which also appears to exert some negative effect on ageing and heart disease, which are increasing. Most doctors insist that a healthy total cholesterol/HDL ratio for middle aged and older men and women should hover around 4.5 or lower. In fact the lower the better because it means that the negative LDLs are not increasing your risk for heart disease or stroke. The LDL – the 'bad cholesterol' – should never get higher than 60-70 percent of total cholesterol, they say, while the helpful HDLs should make up 20-30 percent and the VLDLs which no-one quite understands yet should be somewhere between 10-15 percent.

What Causes High Cholesterol?
Probably not what you've been told. For a couple of generations we have been warned against eating egg yolks and shellfish, both of which have good quantities of cholesterol in them, in the belief that they would raise the cholesterol levels in the body. In fact, high cholesterol foods have little effect on the body's cholesterol levels, for cholesterol is a natural substance that is manufactured by your liver. Levels of cholesterol in the blood are far more affected by a diet high in both fat and sugars than by eating foods which themselves have a high quantity of cholesterol in them. Your cholesterol levels also have little to do with genetic inheritance. For while we can inherit a tendency to high blood cholesterol, it is how we eat and exercise – or don't exercise – as well as how fat we are which determines whether or not that genetic tendency ever turns into a choles-terol problem. The important question is, genetic tendency or not, how do we both prevent and reverse cholesterol problems.

The factors responsible for raising HDL cholesterol and lowering the harmful LDL cholesterol can be changed by the same diet that helps elim-inate blood sugar problems and insulin resistance, and the same exercise – especially strength training or resistance training which increases lean body mass and decreases body fat. Giving up smoking and not taking hormone pills helps. As you get older it also becomes increasingly important to be careful of the medications that you take and to know that certain conditions can also increase your LDL cholesterol levels, such as thyroid disease, kidney disease, obstructive liver disease and adult onset diabetes. It is particularly important to avoid the long-term use of diuretics and anabolic steroids (body builders beware!)

Biomarker Eight
BLOOD PRESSURE
Action Plan: Beat It

Shun The Junk

The name of the game is *hypertension* which means nothing more than blood pressure that's far too high. We've all been warned against it but few people know what high blood pressure is all about. You probably won't even know if you've got it because there usually aren't any symptoms. Despite this, like Syndrome X itself, it can be extremely dangerous. It is also very widespread. It is estimated that one in four people in English speaking countries now suffer from hypertension which makes you prone to a number of serious conditions including heart attacks and strokes. A tendency to hypertension can be hereditary. However, like all hereditary tendencies, whether or not they become a reality depends almost entirely on how you live and eat. Too much sugar, junk fat and alcohol, too little exercise and smoking all make you prone to high blood pressure if you have inherited a genetic tendency towards it. When it comes to ageing, one of the most important things to remember about blood pressure is that epidemiological studies show that cultures living on simple diets largely free of convenience foods, whose members are physically active, do *not* experience the rise in blood pressure that we in the Western world consider a normal part of ageing.

UPS AND DOWNS

When your doctor measures your blood pressure he is concerned with two different components. Your *systolic pressure* and your *diastolic pressure*. The systolic pressure is the pressure that the blood imposes on the walls of your arteries each time your heart beats. The diastolic pressure describes the pressure exerted between contractions of the heart – in effect when your heart is momentarily at rest. It is the systolic pressure which is always registered first. For instance, normal blood pressure is considered to be less than 140 systolic and less than 85 diastolic. Such measurements are not necessarily indicative of high level health since many athletes have both systolic and diastolic blood pressure much lower than this level and they are far fitter and often healthier than the rest of us. Nonetheless it is generally a good rule of thumb.

Stiff And Thick

When your diastolic pressure is high, this means that your arteries never get a rest in between heart beats so they are continually stressed and this stress over a period of time can cause the walls, particularly of your smaller arteries, to stiffen and thicken. The other thing to know about blood pressure is that it is constantly changing so that in order to really establish what anyone's blood pressure is a doctor needs to take a few readings, not just one, and they should be readings where the person being examined has been sitting quietly for a few minutes before the tourniquet is put on his arm. A lot of people believe that high blood pressure is controlled by eliminating salt from your diet. Yet studies show that the blood pressure levels of only about 10 percent of people respond at all to the level of salt in their diet. Once again regular exercise, both aerobic and resistance training, dramatically decreases your likelihood of ever suffering from high blood pressure, while tackling Syndrome X through diet and exercise gives you the very best chance in the world of reversing it.

The bottom line is very clear: with rare exceptions, only about 30 percent of physical ageing can be blamed on genes.

Robert L. Kahn and John W. Rowe

Biomarker Nine
BONE DENSITY
Action Plan: Lift Weights

Use Resistance

As we age we lose minerals from our bones. This leaves our bones weak, brittle and less dense and makes us highly prone to breakages. So much is this true that broken bones are actually the leading cause of accidental death in frail elderly people, especially fractures to the hip. One in three women and one in six men end up with hip fractures. Fifteen percent of them die as a result while another 50 percent often live in pain and need protracted care to get them back on their feet. Osteoporosis is the name of the game. It means the progressive loss of minerals, bone mass and bone density and despite the media coverage that might make you think otherwise, it affects men as well as women. It results in fractures of the shoulder, hip, ribs, vertebrae, forearms and wrists. Statistically, bone loss in women begins several years before menopause and then gets worse afterwards, creating an ever increasing risk of debilitating breakages. In Britain, where the incidence of osteoporosis has increased more than six times in the past 30 years, one in three women now develop it and one in eight men. In the United States, the statistics are even worse. The illness costs the country more than 11 billion dollars a year. Twenty-five percent of women who have hip fractures die within two years, not always directly from the fracture but from ending up in nursing homes where inactivity, alienation and loss of control of their lives defeat them. In the industrialised world, more women die of fractures related to loss of bone density than from cancers of the womb, cervix and breast put together.

THE CALCIUM MYTH

A high calcium intake is often toted as essential in preventing bone thinning. We are constantly being told to drink more milk and take more tablets of calcium. Yet in the United States the intake of calcium by supplementation or through milk drinking is the highest in the world and they have the highest rate of osteoporosis. In Oriental countries such as China where milk is not drunk and the intake of calcium is one of the lowest in the world, osteoporosis is virtually unknown.

The Chinese get their calcium the way that cows do, by eating green plants. Calcium metabolism is a complex process and the absorption of calcium from water or mineral salts in general tends to be highly inefficient. Only somewhere between 20–30 percent of the calcium you take in through supplementation or processed food will actually be absorbed. Most of that will get filtered through your kidneys and then excreted in urine or sweat or eliminated through faeces.

> ## BEWARE DRUGS
>
> Users of prescription drugs have more osteoporosis than people who do not take medication, and perhaps it no longer comes as a surprise that couch potatoes are far more prone to the condition than men and women who get regular exercise. Bone loss is by no means inevitable as we get older, despite the fact that research carried out in the Western world shows that on average we experience about one percent loss of bone mass a year. Like hypertension and insulin resistance, bone loss or osteoporosis is another silent killer.

Bones Alive

Bones may seem to you like tough inanimate objects. They are far from it. They are actually living support tissue – constantly changing and growing. Your bones are made up of a combination of a flexible non-cellular collagen matrix which has been imbedded with hard and inflexible mineralised crystals. In fact, bone is a kind of mineralised cartilage. Without the flexibility of collagen your bones would be so brittle they would easily shatter. Without the crystallised hardness of minerals they would resemble the soft cartilage of a shark. Unless you spent your entire life underwater, your skeleton would be unable to support the weight of your body. The combination of both the tensile strength from minerals and the compression strength from collagen creates just about the finest structural resistance to breakage found anywhere in the living world.

Being seventy is not a sin.
Golda Meir

DOWN TO THE BONE

Your bones are constantly being renewed at an amazing rate. This is what makes it possible for breaks to mend or for a child's body to grow taller. There are two kinds of bone, *cortical* and *trabecular*. The heavy bones of your body such as the long bones of your legs and arms are cortical bones. They are designed to give great directional strength. They are densely cast in spirals around tiny tubular channels through which cells can travel. Cortical bones renew themselves completely about every two years. The other kind of bone – trabecular – is found in the vertebrae of your spine and at the end of the long bones of your legs and arms, in places where you need compression strength. Trabecular bone is more web-like in its structure and its turnover is even faster than cortical bone. Trabecular bone renews itself every two to three years.

Both can be thought of as similar to the fibres that make a scarf or a shawl – fibres that are knitted together with little spaces in-between. When bone loss or osteoporosis occurs, not only have the fibres become finer, you actually have fewer of them. In effect you have lost a number of bone strands and the strands that are left have become thinner. Under the microscope, sometimes even with the naked eye, you can see there are spaces in such bones which make them look spongy and porous. That's where the word osteoporosis comes from.

Turn It Over

The bones in a healthy body are constantly breaking down – being *resorbed* – and building anew. This ability to break down and reform depends on a process called remodelling which relies on two very special kinds of cells in the substrate out of which all bone develops. The first are called *osteoclasts*. If you have ever played the video game Pacman its easy to understand how they work. It's the job of the osteoclasts to travel through the spirals and web-like structure of your bone tissue like a Pacman, seeking out old mineralised bone and then to gobble it up or dissolve it away – resorb it – in order to make way

> Losing weight is the wrong goal. You should forget about your weight and instead concentrate on shedding fat and gaining muscle.
>
> *William Evans and Irwin Rosenberg*

for new bone. Minerals contained in the gobbled bone are released into general circulation and only empty spaces – called lacunae – are left behind. After the osteoclasts have done their Pacman work, along come other kinds of bone cells – the *osteoblasts*. These cells are drawn to the same sites and make their way to these lacunae. There they get busy creating new bone.

While you are young and your pituitary is pumping out growth hormone the action of the osetoblasts dominates and more bone is created than destroyed. Then at puberty the activity of the osteoclasts and osteoblasts becomes more balanced. Later on, however, the balance can shift in favour of the bone eating osteoclasts, while osteoblast activity declines. It is now that bone loss occurs. You get shrinkage in bone mass since more bone is being resorbed than is being built and more spaces are appearing than are being filled. If this goes on for a long time, too many minerals can be lost and bone gets less hard and less dense until at last it becomes honeycombed and highly susceptible to breakage.

OESTROGEN FIX

One of the half truths that has come out of twentieth century medicine is the notion that women need to take oestrogen after menopause to prevent bone loss. Actually, oestrogen has little or no affect on the making of new bone. The other female reproductive hormone progesterone, on the other hand, is the hormone that helps enhance the work of the osteoblasts whose job it is to create new bone. In recent years there have been a number of clinical studies that support the use of natural progesterone creams to slow the rate of osteoporosis in women.

Sugar Crunches Bone

Diet and exercise are by far the most important protectors against loss of bone density as we get older. Eating sugar in large quantities including even fructose, the sugar in fruit, increases the likelihood of your developing osteoporosis. At the US Department of Agriculture Research Service in North Dakota in the United States, Forrest H. Neilsen and David B. Milne put a group of men onto a diet that included five cans of decaffeinated fizzy drink (just to make sure that they eliminated any possible caffeine related influences) sweetened with high fructose corn syrup each day. They discovered that the high fructose drinks lowered the men's level of calcium and phosphorus which are both needed for healthy bones. Researchers also discovered that the effects of fructose on bone loss were made much worse when they also put the men on a magnesium deficient diet.

BANISH FIZZY DRINKS

It is important to know that the average Western diet of refined foods is low in magnesium because few people eat magnesium rich foods, such as leafy green vegetables, whole grains and nuts. Soft drinks rich in fructose or sweetened with artificial sweeteners are also high in phosphorus and bone density depends upon a delicate balance of calcium, magnesium and phosphorus. This too, contributes to the loss of bone density. Stay away from canned fizzy drinks and soft drinks, even if they are sugar free.

On The Move – On The Mend

A way of eating that reverses Syndrome X and restores insulin sensitivity and more normal blood sugar functioning also helps rebalance the hormones that protect your body from loss of bone density. But this is something that is still little recognised by doctors and even less so by the general public who are still looking for quick fix solutions to prevent and to reverse osteoporosis. Major shifts in the way you eat so that you are getting a high level of low density and low glycaemic carbohydrates – the kind that do not turn quickly into glucose in your blood and end up producing insulin resistance – as well as (and this may be the most important element of all) weight bearing exercise – are the best things you can do both to prevent bone loss and to reverse it.

Just two weeks of bed rest can result in as much calcium lost from bones as what is considered to be 'normal' in a whole years worth of ageing. The rate of mineral loss increases 50 times during long bed rest as a result of illness or injury. Even the stress which gravity places upon us as we walk around from day to day helps. For stressing the bones with weight causes them to get stronger rather than weaker, and many studies now show that weight

> You can adopt a pattern of activity and eating that maximises your ability to age more slowly.
>
> Irwin Rosenberg MD,
> William Evans MD

bearing exercise, including running, walking and cycling, carried out over periods of from six months to two years, effectively reduces the rate of bone loss. Some researchers believe that this is because exercise itself helps encourage the body's absorption and use of calcium from food. Meanwhile, a number of studies done within the last 10 years not only show that strength training or weight training can prevent osteoporosis, a few even indicate that it can help reverse osteoporosis or bone loss where it has occurred.

Biomarker Ten

BODY HEAT

Action Plan: Sweat It Out

Temperature Regulation

The final biomarker which Evans and Rosenberg and their team identified is the loss of ability to regulate temperature. As you get older your ability to tolerate extremes in temperatures decreases. This means that in the summer you become more uncomfortable and are less likely than a young person to be able to sweat to cool off. You also feel colder in the winter because less of your blood circulates to the limbs and fingers and toes. Low fitness and poor aerobic capacity are largely responsible for these effects. In part this is the result of a lowered metabolic rate that comes from eating a diet far too high in sugar and refined carbohydrates to upset insulin balance and also a lifestyle that does not include enough physical activity.

The lack of temperature regulation in the body is to a great extent controlled by the diameter of your vascular system in your skin, which is largely controlled by prostaglandins. When your insulin levels get high as a result of blood sugar disturbances from wrong eating and your cells develop insulin resistance, this results in the production of prostaglandins which constrict the diameter of the vascular system, resulting in impaired circulation and decreased temperature regulation. This in turn decreases the amount of oxygen that reaches your cells, lowers vitality and makes you more susceptible to degeneration on many different levels.

> ## DRINK UP
>
> One of the most important negative changes that happens as your body loses its ability to regulate its internal temperature properly is dehydration. Reduced kidney function and an inability to sweat contribute to older peoples' thermo-regulatory problems and create dehydration. By the time most people are 70 years old, their kidneys filter waste out of water only half as fast as they did when they were 30, which means that the body stores toxicity and becomes more highly prone to degenerative conditions and more accelerated ageing. This is one of the reasons why as you grow older it becomes essential for you to continue to drink much more water than you think you need. For the sensation of thirst in older people is very much diminished. As a result, they often neglect to replenish their body's water supplies in good quantity. This in turn dehydrates the body and further disrupts temperature regulation mechanisms.

Few of us, as yet, come close to fulfilling our psycho-biological potentials. Instead, we look forward to a steady and inexorable increase in morbidity and mortality from one disease or another. The exciting thing about the principles of Age Power on which this book is based, is that if you begin now to apply simple, scientifically or clinically validated changes to your life, you will not only be able to extend your life, but to improve its quality beyond all recognition. The facts are in, provided you care to dig them up: all the major causes of death and disability appear to be secondary to the progressive degeneration of ageing. The same principles which help keep your skin smooth, your muscles firm and your vitality high, also reduce the incidence of chronic disease and postpone degenerative illness indefinitely – so that if they occur at all, they come only very late in life.

> These are the times. We are the people.
>
> *Jean Houston*

SYNDROME X
– DEVIL AGER

You are about to be engulfed in one of the largest disease epidemics
ever to strike ... a disorder caused by your body's inability
to make the most of the food you eat.
Jack Challem, Burton Berkson MD, and Melissa Diane Smith

Say the word 'insulin' and what do you think of...diabetes?
We all do. But when it comes to Age Power, insulin is the
most important hormone in your body. One of the greatest
scientific discoveries to be made in the last 50 years is this:
The way insulin behaves in your body determines, more
than anything, how quickly or slowly you age.

Few people are as yet aware that Syndrome X exists, although it affects
the majority of us over 25 to one degree or another. You will remember
it forms the core of Biomarker Six. Those affected usually think that the
symptoms they experience, including aches and pains and the sense that
something is 'just not right' in your body and your life, come from other
causes – usually 'getting older'.

The collection of related abnormalities which Syndrome X – insulin
resistance syndrome – encompasses include high blood pressure and
triglycerides, high cholesterol and blood sugar disorders. In addition, it
carries with it an increased risk of just about every age-related disorder
you can name: from eye problems, heart disease, nervous-system disorders,
diabetes, cancer and Alzheimer's to chronic fatigue, exhaustion, anxiety,
irritability, depression and a poor sense of self worth. Insulin resistance
can even make you chronically bad tempered.

Syndrome X is a hidden
life-threatening perversion
of bodily metabolism that is
likely to hasten the end of
anyone who has it. It is
alarmingly common. What's
more, evidence is growing
that we can bring it on
ourselves, by the way we
eat.

Gail Vines in
New Scientist

KEY WORDS

Glucagon: important hormone released by the pancreas which works together with insulin to control blood sugar and create energy for the body. When blood sugar levels fall, glucagon encourages the release of glycogen – stored glucose – from the liver. It can also help turn protein into glucose when needed.

Glucose: simple blood sugar made to feed the mitochondria in your body's 60 trillion cells so they can produce ATP – the energy currency on which metabolism runs and on which vitality depends.

Glycaemic (high and low): the glycaemic index is a measure of how much a specific food will raise your blood glucose (blood sugar) levels and how fast. High glycaemic foods such as flour, sugar, corn chips and breakfast cereals make blood sugar soar and insulin levels rise encouraging Syndrome X. Low glycaemic foods such as broccoli, spinach, capsicums and melon cause only a gentle, slow-release, rise of blood sugar and help protect you from Syndrome X.

Hyperinsulinism: chronic abnormally high levels of insulin which results in Syndrome X and ages the body rapidly.

Insulin Resistance: chronic high levels of glucose in the blood stream trigger chronic releases of high levels of insulin to help remove it. Over time the body's cells become jaded and no longer respond to insulin's attempt to escort glucose into the cells to make ATP. Insulin resistance encourages blood sugar to remain high or to soar and plummet while your energy levels fluctuate greatly.

Insulin Sensitivity: the normal, healthy state of a youthful body at any age in which your cells retain their responsive-ness to insulin's call to energy so glucose can be shunted into the cells to create energy for your body.

Syndrome X: the collection of metabolic abnormalities that increase our risk of early ageing, diabetes, heart problems, obesity, mood disorders and many other degenerative cond-itions. Where you find Syndrome X you often also find glucose intolerance, a high-fat-to-muscle ratio in the body, abnormal blood fats and high blood pressure.

Syndrome X was first described by an endocrinologist, Gerald Reaven, at California's Stanford University in the late eighties. Reaven studied the phenomena associated with it for many years. Syndrome X will age you fast. Although Reaven was the first to identify and name Syndrome X, the work of clinicians – doctors and natural health practitioners working to release insulin resistance in their patients – since then has taken our understanding of both how it works and how to eliminate it way beyond Reaven's first assertions.

FAST TRACK TO DISASTER

The cause of Syndrome X is insulin resistance – a hormonal spanner in the works which screws up your body's ability to translate the food you eat into energy your body can use. Take one part insulin resistance, combine it with high levels of triglycerides and cholesterol, too much fat and too little lean body mass and presto, your risk of age-related and life-threatening diseases soars. In fact, Syndrome X affects virtually every disease process one way or another.

The cause of Syndrome X is not some virus or accident of nature. It is your body's inability to thrive on the kind of foods you have been eating plus a sedentary lifestyle that undermines vitality – especially on the high-carbohydrate, low-fat, inadequate-protein way of convenience food eating we have followed for twenty years. Sadly, government directives are still telling us we should eat this way. Yet all those bagels and muffins, breakfast cereals, pasta and sweets are literally killing us.

Impeccable scientific research indicates these directives are wrong. Eating this way screws up human metabolism. It is so contrary to what the human body, throughout the whole of human evolution has been programmed to thrive on, that it causes degeneration. A high-carbohydrate-low-fat diet of pop-it-in-the-microwave foods raises levels of the hormone insulin

'Now we recognise that our life-saving technology of the past four decades has outstripped our health-preserving technology and that the net effect has been to worsen the people's health, we must begin the search for preventable causes of the chronic illnesses which we have been extending . . . We will not move forward in enhancing health until we make the prevention of nonfatal chronic illness our top research priority.'

Ernest M Gruenberg

in your body, destabilising blood sugar, and rendering your cells unable to respond to the call of insulin, so they cannot take in the blood sugar they need to burn for energy. Such a diet affects, either directly or indirectly, virtually every degenerative disease process known to man.

WHAT CAUSES SYNDROME X

Nutritional deficiencies such as chromium, magnesium, selenium, taurine and/or essential fatty acids.

Lack of Exercise		HYPERINSULINAEMIA (Chronic levels of high insulin)		Prolonged Stress

Poor Nutrition
- Too many high carbohydrate and convenience foods
- Too little omega-3
- Too few phytonutrients from low glycaemic fruits and vegetables
- Too little good quality protein
- Too little fibre

By understanding the kinds of foods humans evolved on – and then learning how human diets significantly changed with the agricultural, industrial and fast-food revolutions – you will gain a much clearer picture of why Syndrome X has emerged as a widespread modern disease.

Jack Challem, Burton Berkson MD, and Melissa Diane Smith

MASTER HORMONE

Insulin does not just regulate your body's use of glucose. It helps control appetite. It tells your kidneys whether or not to retain fluid. It acts as a growth hormone which helps keep your body lean and young, and it regulates the liver's synthesis of cholesterol. An amazingly talented hormone, it even orchestrates the flow of essential nutrients like amino acids and fatty acids, vitamins and minerals, into the 60 trillion microscopic cells of your body.

And all these jobs which insulin carries out work perfectly well. That is, provided there is no great excess of glucose in circulation. When there is – you've just eaten a meal high in carbohydrates, like pizza and ice-cream – then the high insulin levels your body produces in response to that meal stimulates *lipogenesis*. What this means is that, instead of burning the glucose as energy in your muscle cells the way your body is meant to do, your body tends to store it within your fat cells producing more and more body fat. When, over time, you continue to eat a high carb diet, matters get worse and worse. You store more and more glucose and fat and have less energy in your day to day life. This creates a vicious circle as people get older – especially those who have insulin resistance. They lack the energy to exercise, which deepens Syndrome X. If they are not processing energy from their foods, they are only laying down more and more fat stores. For both obesity and physical inactivity aggravate insulin resistance even more. This course of unfortunate metabolic events is the primary reason that people are experiencing a vast number of age-related disorders and diseases, the most obvious of which is that we are getting fatter and fatter on the standard Western diet.

SYNDROME X SCREWS UP BLOOD PATTERNS

It causes:
- ☐ Low HDL – the 'good guy' cholesterol
- ☐ High LDL – the 'bad guy' cholesterol
- ☐ High total cholesterol levels
- ☐ Laying down of plaque deposits in veins and arteries as a result of oxidized LDL cholesterol damaged by free radicals
- ☐ High triglyceride levels
- ☐ Beer belly
- ☐ Energy swings

DEADLY EPIDEMIC

Gradually an awareness of the phenomenon of insulin resistance is spreading. When insulin resistance occurs, your cells become jaded and non-responsive to the presence of the hormone so your pancreas just keeps secreting more and more insulin in an attempt to get energy into your cells. In some cases, when the body's cells do not respond to even high levels of insulin, glucose builds up in the blood and the condition turns into a high blood glucose, Type II or Adult Onset Diabetes. When it was discovered that many non-diabetics also experience insulin resistance, scientists began to ask questions about what caused it. The answers they have come up with are nothing short of astounding: Insulin resistance develops over time as insulin levels get higher and higher when a body is fed on lots of high density carbohydrate foods which release glucose rapidly into the bloodstream. A potentially deadly phenomenon, Syndrome X is not only associated with a number of recognised risk factors for many degenerative diseases, it is also linked with loss of memory, mental decline, depression and anxiety.

Insulin resistance, whether or not it turns into Type II Diabetes, is also accompanied by an increased level of blood fats – elevated total cholesterol and triglycerides and decreased high-density lipoprotein (HDL) cholesterol – or what is known as 'good' cholesterol. This increases your risk of heart disease. It is now considered a prime cause – what is known as a 'risk factor' – for heart disease. It is also the bête noir behind cholesterol imbalances, elevated triglycerides, hypertension and some kinds of cancer. It is these discoveries that are bringing to greater public awareness the way in which insulin resistance undermines our health.

You don't have to have all of the symptoms associated with Syndrome X to suffer from chronic high insulin levels, or even to be overweight. Thin people also experience Syndrome X. Yet it can remain hidden for years, based on the belief that the symptoms which these people show, such as chronic fatigue, fluid retention, an intense craving for sweets and an inability to concentrate, are masquerading as symptoms of other conditions. So insidious is Syndrome X that it often goes unnoticed for 30 or 40 years until serious health issues begin to surface. In some people their pancreas is producing three to four times the normal amount of insulin, because it cannot keep up with demand while on a cellular level, sensitivity to the hormone has been lost so that more and more insulin is needed simply to maintain normal levels of blood sugar.

'. . . low-fat-high-carbohydrate diets should be avoided in the treatment of Syndrome X.'

Gerald Reaven MD

SUGAR AGES

SUGAR, NOT JUST ON ITS OWN BUT PRODUCED IN YOUR BODY BY EATING LOTS OF HIGH CARBS FOODS, CAUSES INSULIN LEVELS TO RISE.

- ❑ Eating high carbohydrate meals and snacks shunts massive doses of glucose into your blood stream.
- ❑ This triggers the pancreas to produce more insulin and keeps insulin levels far too high for long periods.
- ❑ This creates insulin resistance interfering with your body's ability to get glucose into the energy factories – mitochondria – of your cells where it can be turned into energy so you feel fatigued, gain weight easily and develop the abnormalities of Syndrome X.
- ❑ This also stimulates your liver to produce triglycerides in the bloodstream.
- ❑ Blood fats are converted into bad guy HDL cholesterol.
- ❑ This raises your risk of developing heart disease.
- ❑ And bombards your fat cells with extra calories to tuck away as glucose and triglycerides.
- ❑ This produces yet more insulin resistance and can even start destroying the insulin-secreting cells in your pancreas.
- ❑ If you don't change your diet and way of life you succumb to whatever age-related destructive diseases you are genetically susceptible to, be it diabetes, obesity, arthritis, rheumatism, mood disorders, not to mention sagging skin and other miseries commonly (and wrongly) assumed to be a 'normal' part of getting older.

CHANGE YOUR WAY OF EATING AND LIVING AND
GROW YOUNGER BY THE DAY

OTHER CAUSES OF SYNDROME X

Getting older, for one. Insulin resistance can be both a cause and an effect of ageing. Syndrome X is not exclusive to humans either. Animal research shows that elevated insulin together with increased glucose, cholesterol and triglyceride levels, obesity, and heart disease, also occur in a number of animals as they get older. Other contributors to Syndrome X are:

- ❏ nutritional deficiencies
- ❏ eating too much
- ❏ eating highly refined and processed foods
- ❏ drinking too much alcohol
- ❏ smoking
- ❏ not getting enough exercise

Unbeknown to them, even teenagers munching on a bag of chips are speeding up their own ageing process by consuming excessive high-glycaemic carbohydrate foods. It's important to remember that not only sugar and refined carbohydrates cause this. So can eating excessive quantities of the so-called 'good' carbohydrates, such as whole-grain breads and brown rice. For although the human body runs on glucose as its principal fuel, it was never designed to deal with a diet in which most of the calories we eat come from high density carbohydrates which rapidly pour sugar into the bloodstream when we eat them.

ENDLESS CRAVINGS

Insulin resistance is often responsible for the so-called compulsive eating and carbohydrate cravings which are now widespread and which cause suffering for so many people. Ongoing high levels of insulin can create a feeling that you are constantly hungry. For insulin also triggers the hypothalamus, the gland responsible for letting you know when you are hungry and thirsty. As a result you can find yourself eating a meal yet feeling hungry soon afterwards. You can experience a sense that no matter what you eat, nothing will satisfy you and your body ages at a rate of knots.

FAST TRACK TO AGEING

❑ When glucose is burned efficiently – i.e. there is no Syndrome X or insulin resistance – masses of energy in the form of ATP is created for vitality and efficient metabolism, you don't gain weight or lay down plaque in your arteries, and only a small number of free radicals are produced in the process. In short you protect your body from rapid ageing.

❑ When you eat masses of high carbohydrate foods – that is foods high on the glycaemic index (see pages 193–4) as opposed to fresh non-starchy vegetables like spinach and broccoli, herbs and non-sugary fruits such as melon or raspberries – you generate lots of free radicals which deplete your body's anti-oxidant pool and trigger degeneration.

❑ These excess free radicals damage your DNA, including the DNA of your mitochondria – the energy factories in the cells – deplete your body's anti-oxidant protecting enzymes like *glutathione peroxidase* and *catalase,* undermine your immune defences and derail your body's anti-ageing mechanisms. It's a fast track to ageing.

BEWARE THE RANDLE EFFECT

All of this is made worse for health by what has come to be known as the Randle Effect. The Randle Effect describes a situation when lots of fat and carbohydrates are eaten together as they are in the standard Western diet. When you eat these foods, the fats they contain tend to get burnt as fuel while the carbohydrates are converted to glucose. The glucose in turn is converted to body fat. This throws any overweight insulin resistant person into a terrible vicious circle where hunger and carbohydrate cravings lead to overeating, followed by an inevitable increase in blood sugar and insulin levels as well as body fat deposits and more cravings. The irony is that for a long time we have been blaming dietary fat for all this when this phenomenon is actually caused by a high carbohydrate intake in the presence of junk fats found in margarines, golden oils and processed fats in convenience foods.

Natural fats eaten on their own or together with protein but without an abundance of carbohydrates do not appear to cause the laying down of fat in the body. Nor do they cause Syndrome X. This is perhaps the most difficult thing for those of us who have been highly schooled in the high-carbs-low-fat approach to weight loss and age protection to grasp. Yet it is essential to grasp.

DO YOU HAVE INSULIN RESISTANCE?

Check out whether or not you have any of the signs and symptoms listed below:

Do you:

- ❑ Crave sweets?
- ❑ Eat a high carb low fat diet?
- ❑ Eat convenience foods?
- ❑ Need to urinate very frequently?
- ❑ Drink more than a cup of fruit juice a day?
- ❑ Avoid regular exercise?
- ❑ Have a low lean-body-mass-to-fat-ratio?
- ❑ Have an eating disorder?
- ❑ Go on and off slimming diets?
- ❑ Have a relative with Adult Onset diabetes?
- ❑ Have difficulty concentrating?
- ❑ Gain weight easily?
- ❑ Store fat around the middle of your body?
- ❑ Experience fuzzy mindedness?
- ❑ Have mood swings?
- ❑ Experience energy peaks and troughs throughout the day?
- ❑ Find yourself irritable or bad tempered frequently?
- ❑ Have trouble getting to sleep or staying asleep?
- ❑ Have blood pressure above 140/90?
- ❑ Have cholesterol levels higher than 240mg/dl?
- ❑ Have triglycerides above 160mg/dl?

If you answer yes to half or more of these questions you need to investigate what Age Power's Insulin Balance can do to change your body, your mind and your good looks for the better.

Having established that your biomarkers change as you age, and that there is a lot you can do to reverse these changes, we need to ask *why* they change. An understanding of the four major processes involved in age degeneration and how we can control them is as close as you can come to discovering the fountain of youth.

FOUR PILLARS
OF AGEING

*Every time I think that I am getting old, and gradually going
to the grave, something else happens.*

Lilian Carter

There are four major physiological processes which distort
your biomarkers and age your body. Take control of them
and you not only slow the rate at which you age, you can
reverse age related changes after they have happened.

The big four physiological processes associated with premature ageing are
oxidation, glycation, inflammation and methylation. When any of these four
processes get out of whack they bring about distortions at a cellular level,
resulting in physiological degeneration and those changes in the biomarkers
we all dread. These processes are intimately interrelated. When one of
these physiological processes – say oxidation – gets out of control it pushes
the other three off the rails, causing damage from altered gene expression, to distortions in the DNA, and cross-linking of body proteins. The
results? Wrinkling and sagging of your skin, obstruction of arteries, loss
of lean body mass, loss of hormone balance – in other words detrimental
alterations in all the biomarkers – as well as a build up of toxicity to
trigger neurological damage. To understand the devastation they can cause
we need to take a look at the miraculous structure that is the living cell.

SECRETS OF CELLS

A remarkable entity, the cell is the smallest structural unit in your body.
It moves, grows, reacts, protects itself and even reproduces. And despite
the most elaborate and learned research attempting to understand the
nature of that glorious aliveness, it remains a mystery.

Each cell in your body – and there are trillions of them – is a self-
contained centre of vitality. Your cells need a good supply of oxygen, nutrients, energy and enzymes. Each cell also needs protection from damage
and an efficient means of continually detoxifying itself. This marvellous
creation of nature – the tiny cell – is superbly *ordered* in its functions and
structure. On this order depends your body's youthfulness and longevity.
But because it is so complex each part of the cellular mechanism is also

highly subject to disorder. And when a cell becomes deranged, its entire function can be seriously impaired. Multiply one deranged cell by the thousand million million cells in your body and you experience what is known in modern medicine as degenerative disease and accumulated ageing.

At its outer edge each cell is surrounded by a protective membrane built mostly from lipids or fats. Through this membrane all nutrients and oxygen must pass to keep the cell alive and all wastes must be eliminated. Inside you find a gel-like ocean of cytoplasm which contains a variety of subcellular bodies – fat-protein complexes – called *organelles*, which take part in cell functions. The organelles include *microsomes* which make new proteins, *lysosomes* – which are like automatic waste collectors whose job it is to keep the cytoplasmic ocean unpolluted and, most important of all, *mitochondria* – minute energy factories where calories from the foods you eat can be burnt as fuel to yield vitality. Remember that word 'mito-chondria'. They are vitally important to an understanding of ageing and we look at them closely in the next chapter.

Each cell also has a nucleus in its centre. Here all the genetic details of its structure and functions are carefully locked away in molecules of DNA, so that when a cell gets ready to divide, another nucleic acid called RNA carries the DNA's coded instruction to get the correct amino acids for the synthesis of new proteins.

Disrupt the order of this system and chaos ensues: wastes leak into the cytoplasm causing the cell to poison itself, enzymes contained in the mitochondria can bring about serious biological disruption, and damage to both mitochondrial DNA and the total cell's DNA, within its nucleus. This leads to a mis-synthesis of protein. It can even mean the production of mutant or damaged daughter cells or to the development of cancer.

Theoretical data are suggesting that the major factor in Alzheimer's disease of the sporadic late onset type – that's 90 to 95 percent of Alzheimer cases – is a mutation in earlier life that affects mitochondrial function, either a mutation of mitochondrial DNA or of nuclear DNA that influences mitochondrial function.

Denham Harman MD, PhD

THE FOUR PILLARS OF AGEING

MORE OXIDATION
(free radical damage)

MORE GLYCATION
(cross-linking of proteins)

MORE INFLAMMATION
(compromised immunity)

REDUCED METHYLATION
(poor detoxification)

Abnormalities in these cause changes at a cellular level leading to:

- ❑ Poor gene expression
- ❑ Distortions in DNA
- ❑ Damage to cells
- ❑ Mitochondrial Dysfunction – poor energy production
- ❑ Damage to proteins – skin wrinkling, poor veins for example
- ❑ Loss of lean body mass
- ❑ Immune disturbances
- ❑ Hyperhomocysteinaemia – predisposing to heart conditions
- ❑ Loss of hormone balance
- ❑ Neurotoxicity

This results in

ACCELERATED AGEING
(negative changes in biomarkers)

It is important to understand the nature of each of these four processes, how they cause age-related changes in your body, and what you can do to reverse them if they have already happened. Lets look at oxidation first, since in many ways it is the most important of all. For oxidation and free radical damage form the core of destruction.

OXIDATION

FIRST PILLAR OF AGEING

❑ Free radicals alter physiological function in many ways, including cell, protein and DNA damage.
❑ Free radical damage increases as our biomarkers degenerate.
❑ The free radical theory of ageing says that continual damage from these molecular rapists results in rapid ageing and degenerative disease.

Let's look at oxygen first – a real double-edged sword for Age Power. For while your cells and your body as a whole can't function without adequate oxygen, it is also the worst threat imaginable to cellular order and overall health.

ENTER THE HERO

Two billion years ago – give or take a few million years – a profound change took place on earth which dramatically affected evolution: Plant life came into being. The first primitive plants, the algae, started to release oxygen into the atmosphere by breaking down water in the presence of sunlight through photosynthesis. In the beginning this 'new' element – oxygen – was lethal to virtually every living organism. The creatures who managed to survive did so only by continually adapting to oxygen's growing presence. Slowly these early simple animals evolved ways of doing this: they devised protective mechanisms against oxygen toxicity. The mitochondria in our cells were once such single celled organisms. Their solution to the oxygen challenge was to evolve into an oxygen-respiring purple bacteria lineage similar to rod shaped bacteria today. From there they metamorphosed into the energy transforming organelles in the cells of animals. They found ways of using oxygen to create energy – so successfully in fact that by now oxygen has become the potent impetus behind most metabolic processes that fuel complex forms of animal life on our planet. That is how we work.

STILL A VILLAIN

Yet oxygen's toxicity is still with us. Expose yourself to levels of oxygen beyond what you are used to – around one fifth of an atmosphere of pressure – and you will get sick. For instance, breathe in pure oxygen at one atmosphere for a few hours and you will develop inflammation in the trachea. Stay in such an atmosphere for days on end and soon you will die from a condition called *anoxia* which means, ironically, lack of oxygen. Even the oxygen we take in through the air we normally breathe is still highly toxic to many essential life processes on a cellular level. Oxygen has an obsession with combining with other substances. When it does so it often wreaks havoc with delicate cell structures, causing fundamental *disorder* at a molecular level to disrupt their integrity, and destroy the genetic information they need to reproduce accurately. Such cellular chaos is central to the whole process of human ageing.

STRESSED OUT ON O²

The trouble with oxidation as a means of energy production is that a number of highly reactive, potentially toxic and destructive species of molecules are generated when it occurs in the body. They are known as *free radicals* and they put us as human beings in the curious position of being dependent upon oxygen for our life energy and yet also susceptible to its toxic effects – what in biochemistry is known as *oxidising stress* or *oxy-stress*. It poses a continual challenge to the integrity of our cells and tissues and is a central cause of degeneration and illness.

SERIAL RAPISTS

Pathologist Alex Comfort once compared a free radical to a conference delegate away from his wife: 'A highly reactive chemical agent that will combine with anything that is around.' Other researchers liken free radicals to rapists who's union with other molecules, willing or unwilling, is nothing less than a clear attack. Free radicals can cut other molecules down the middle, chop pieces off them, destroy cellular information and generally wreak havoc with living systems. They can cause injury, inflammation and destruction to parts of the cells, cell walls and collagen fibres, the body's most important structural protein.

Because free radicals are species of atoms and molecules which are electro-chemically unbalanced, they are highly reactive. In stable molecules and atoms you find positively charged *protons* and negatively charged *electrons* in perfect balance so that the electrical charge an atom or molecule carries can be said to be nil. The molecule is neutral. Free radicals are different. Instead of having the usual orbitals occupied by pairs of electrons which spin in opposite directions, these renegades have an odd number. Therefore they carry a small electrical charge. Most retain a single unpaired electron in an outer orbital. This not only creates the electrical charge, it also gives the molecule astounding instability and makes it react with other atoms and molecules with which it comes into contact. It is a relatively simple matter to turn a stable molecule or compound into a free radical species simply by bringing it in contact with another free radical from which it gains or to which it loses an electron. The whole exchange takes place in microseconds. Once a free radical is present it tends to propagate by gener-ating other free radicals from chain reactions with the stable non-radical species which happen to be present. Sounds scary. But we *need* these beasties to maintain our lives.

OXY-STRESS AND FREE RADICALS CAUSE:

- ❑ Damage to your cells' DNA and to your mitochondrial DNA interfering with your ability to experience energy
- ❑ Poisoning – *excito toxicity* – to the brain and nervous system
- ❑ Dysfunction in the manufacture of energy within the mitochondria of your cells
- ❑ Damage to the cell membranes so that the cell cannot be properly nourished
- ❑ Damage to your body's proteins
- ❑ Compromise to your immune system

I have a detached retina.
Actually, it's not detached.
It's emotionally unavailable.
Nick Arnette

OXY-STRESS HAZARDS

Oxy-stress is the name for the potential negative pressure put on your body by free radicals created in the oxidation process on which life depends. It occurs when your body does not have the anti-oxidant wherewithal to protect itself from free radical damage. What causes oxy-stress? All sorts of things. Your body's own metabolic processes by which we eat, digest and assimilate food, triggers free radical production and can cause oxidation damage, particularly if the diet we eat is high in the kind of carbohydrates – muffins, pasta, bread and refined cereals, which produce poor control of insulin and disturbed blood sugar in the body. More about this in a moment. However, were the body's own metabolic processes the only trigger for free radical production, we would probably have little worry about age related degeneration caused by oxidation. Our protective mechanisms might be enough to protect our cells, proteins and lipids from damage. But a myriad external factors can initiate and accelerate free radical reactions.

RADIATION HURTS

Our environment is full of external triggers. These include radiation of all sorts, from the sun's ultra violet rays to emanations from nuclear power stations, and even electromagnetic fields set up by high tension electrical installations. They also include air pollutants such as ozone, nitrogen dioxide and sulphur dioxide as well as the xeno-oestrogens. Cigarette smoke is another major polluter, which produces free radicals and causes oxidation damage. So are solvents and drugs, heavy metals such as lead, cadmium and aluminium as well as many foods, particularly those which are lacking in freshness. Even the eating of too much food, and the toxic residues from illness or prolonged emotional stress, tends to increase free radical reactions and oxy-stress. Believe it or not, oxygen in the air we breathe can actually bring about free radical damage too. Not only because the majority of free radical reactions involve oxygen, but because oxygen in certain forms actually behaves like a free radical itself. Two forms of activated oxygen – *singlet oxygen* and *hydrogen peroxide* – although technically not free radicals themselves, nevertheless share with them a similar capacity to damage biological tissues and, therefore, age your body.

> Most researchers today agree that the underlying cause of ageing, especially the accelerated ageing that flows from the Western diet, is accumulated damage to our bodies from free radicals.
>
> *Robert Atkins MD*

FREE RADICAL TRIGGERS CAUSE OXIDATION DAMAGE

❑ Exposure to chemicals in food and air
❑ Exposure to household chemicals used for cleaning
❑ Not enough anti-oxidants in the body to counter free radical damage
❑ Any kind of inflammation
❑ Ionising radiation of any kind
❑ Long-term stress
❑ Not enough exercise or an excessive amount of exercise without extra anti-oxidant protection from supplements
❑ Surgery
❑ The build-up of toxicity in the body
❑ Syndrome X – poor control of insulin and blood sugar as a result of eating the wrong diet (see page 59)

INSULIN SCREW UPS

Oxy-stress and excess free radicals disrupt the hormone insulin's behaviour too. You will recall that insulin is the most important hormone in determining how rapidly or how slowly your body ages. Insulin communicates indirectly with your genes and faced with excess oxy-stress, can alter your gene expression. By doing this, it influences an enormous variety of other hormone and metabolic changes in the body. When healthy insulin behaviour is disrupted your body may deposit glucose as fat stores, fur up the arteries or create mounting toxicity, and further free radical damage. Excess glucose also produces destructive changes in skin, altering cells through the second pillar of ageing – glycation. More about this in a moment. If you value your body stay away from the low-fat-high-carb diet which elevates insulin levels in the blood, alters metabolism and creates the switched metabolic phenomenon that diverts the calories you eat from energy production to stored fat. Syndrome X is the single most important internal cause of ageing. The first thing you can do to control the rate at which your body is ageing is shift the way you are eating to Age Power's Insulin Balance diet and lifestyle, which improves insulin sensitivity, rebalances metabolism, gets rid of the

> Free-radical reactions can cause deleterious changes throughout the body. Anti-oxidants decrease this damage and hence contribute to health and longevity.
>
> *Denham Harman MD, PhD*

peaks and troughs of energy where you have to reach for a cup of coffee just to keep going, and sets you on the way to a dynamic Age Power way of being, year in year out.

FREE RADICAL REVOLUTION

What is amazing is just how extensive free radical activity is in the human body. One of the leading experts in free radical biochemistry, Dr Bruce Ames, at the University of California at Berkeley, estimates that every cell in our body experiences 10,000 free radical 'hits' every day. A well-nourished, healthy body is equipped to handle them.

We have amazing anti-oxidant defence mechanisms, and provided we are getting plenty of fresh foods, getting optimum amounts of exercise, and are not exposed to excessive amounts of chemical pollution, all should be fine. Unfortunately, most of us are subject to more free radical activity than our natural anti-oxidant mechanisms can detoxify. Then we find cataracts forming in our eyes, Alzheimer's disease being triggered, cholesterol building up in the arteries, and notice a thousand other negative changes associated with ageing.

PERFECT SYNERGY

Combine Age Power's Insulin Balance programme with extra anti-oxidants – not in the form of magic bullet tablets or great handfuls of vitamin pills – but rather in the form in which they come in nature. The advantages of getting anti-oxidants in natural form are many, particularly because the body has become genetically programmed to use the magnificent synergy of substances and compounds in plant foods. Natural, unprocessed, fresh foods are rich in anti-oxidants and in many other plant substances that in one way or another have anti-ageing properties. One of the interesting things about the anti-ageing substances in fresh foods is that they are also anti-cancer substances. The changes that take place in cancer are akin to the mutations to the cells, cell walls and genetic material which occur as the body ages. Eat foods rich in anti-cancer compounds and you automatically protect your body from free radicals.

> The typical American diet is a recipe for the one thing that will age you faster than anything: high blood sugar and the elevated insulin levels that invariably accompany it.
>
> *Robert Atkins MD*

There are certain foods such as particular herbs, mushrooms and other plant substances high on the list of powerful natural helpers. They include the algae such as chlorella, spirulina, the Australian Dunaliella Salina; the seaweeds – dulse, kelp, alaria and bladderwrack (see page 260); certain herbs that protect the body from stress, such as Fo-ti, astragalus, ginger and schizandra; cereal grasses; the immune supporting Oriental mushrooms such as reishi and maitake; as well as natural plant anti-oxidants such as those found in sage, rosemary and cloves. There are thousands of plant-based chemicals in natural foods, and some of them have even higher anti-oxidant activity than known anti-oxidant minerals and vitamins. Take grape seeds for example. Within the seed of red grapes you will find very high levels of *procyanidolic oligomers* (PCOs) which contain some of the most active free radical scavengers known.

PEROXIDATION PERIL

An important source of free radical harm occurs through a process called *lipid peroxidation*. Lipids – fats – are what makes up most of a cell's membrane. This is one of the reasons why we need to take in an adequate supply of unsaturated fatty acids. Unfortunately unsaturated fatty acids have a strong tendency to react with oxygen in the body to form *peroxides*. Peroxidation also occurs in the presence of oxygen in the atmosphere, turning butter or cooking oils rancid. Once formed in the body peroxides, like free radicals, tend to join with more lipids and propagate yet more peroxides and free radicals. They cause serious damage to organelles in the cells and to cell membranes.

Recent findings in the field of oxidation and free radical pathology – the study of free radicals 'gone wrong' – are nothing short of revolutionary. They make it possible for the first time in scientific terms to formulate a uniform theory of disease. Thanks to free radical biochemistry doctors well versed in the subject are able to make sense of what until now appeared to be contradictory clinical and epidemiological observations, and to create a scientific rationale both for

> Anti-oxidants in the diet come primarily from fresh vegetables and fruits and unrefined carbohydrates. A diet high in sugar and refined carbohydrates has little room for these foods.
>
> *Robert Atkins MD*

the treatment and the prevention of a number of the major causes of degeneration and death: arteriosclerosis, cancer, arthritis, heart disease, dementia and other age related problems. Free radical damage now appears to underlie the pathology of all these conditions despite the differences in their manifestation in the body.

The discovery that oxidation or oxy-stress – free radical damage and peroxidation – can bring about disease and degeneration in the body, and the development of ways and means of counteracting it, are providing scientists with coherent and workable methods. These include methods for preventing illness – from allergy to mental disorder – and for restoring much of the degenerative damage associated with ageing. So much for the first of the pillars of ageing. Now let's look at the other three.

GLYCATION
SECOND PILLAR OF AGEING

This is the process by which sugar is added to chains of proteins. The binding of glucose to any biomolecule causes it to change its nature and undermine its function. This in turn impedes cellular functions, causes inflammation and further free radical production.

It works like this:

Excess glucose damages proteins

AGES (advanced glycation end products) form in your body

Cause havoc with cells

Cells lose integrity, become disordered and are damaged

Your body ages faster

Degenerative diseases occur

EFFECTS OF GLYCATION INCLUDE:

❑ More oxidation stress
❑ More inflammation
❑ Kidney, eye and nerve degeneration
❑ Accumulation of advanced glycation end products in blood vessel walls
❑ Accumulation of *amyloids* leading to Alzheimer's disease

THE PERILS OF SUGAR

The degenerative actions of glucose on the body go far beyond the dangerous role it plays in insulin resistance and Syndrome X. Sugar, in fact all forms of standard sweeteners from high-fructose corn syrup to sucrose – the crystalline stuff you put in your coffee and all the rest – is one of the most dangerous substances you can put into your body. All common forms of sweetening – from malt extract to honey to table sugar – break down through digestion and turn into glucose. Glucose is meant to be transformed into other energy-containing compounds, the most important of which is as *adenosine triphosphate* (ATP) through a specific burning process which scientists call the Krebs Cycle, also known as the citric acid cycle and which takes place in the mitochondria. The energy from glucose burning is carried on subatomic particles – electrons – through the various energy producing steps that lead to the formation of ATP. ATP is the end product of oxidation metabolism on which our life depends.

MITOCHONDRIA – ENERGY FURNACE

What makes energy-yielding metabolism possible is the ability we have evolved to convert nutrients taken in through our foods into chemical energy – glucose and fats. We convert this blood sugar into energy to fuel our life processes by turning it into ATP in the mitochondria – the little energy factories – of our cells. This is a process known as *aerobic metabolism*. And it is a highly efficient means of energy production and release. Specifically, it involves the transfer of electrons from one molecule to another. In scientific terms this occurrence is what is known as an *oxidation-reduction* or *redox reaction*.

When your body's cells are overloaded with glucose, the containment of the energy-producing chemical processes of the Krebs Cycle becomes breached. Massive amounts of free radicals are formed. They leak out to play havoc with your cells and tissues. This is one of the major reasons why the Western diet, full of carbohydrates and convenience foods based on them, deplete your body's anti-oxidant reserves and age you. You lose protection from these free radicals which can damage the DNA both in your mitochondria and in the cells themselves, undermining immunity, depleting you of energy and hurling you towards degeneration. A diet replete in sweet foods and hidden sugars generates vast numbers of free radicals – very much the same way that being exposed to ionizing radiation, cigarette smoke, drugs and poisons do. It also increases your need for anti-oxidant nutrients – vitamins and minerals as well as phytonutrients – in an attempt to compensate for the damage. There is even more to the nasty sugar story than this.

AGES AGE YOU

Excess glucose causes your body's proteins – in skin, muscles, arteries and the brain for instance – to fuse with it and form *advanced glycation end products* abbreviated as AGES. AGES are formed as a result of free radicals. Once present, they encourage yet more free radical damage. They screw up the proteins of your cells by cross-linking them. This leads to countless problems from skin sagging and wrinkling to cataracts, damage to the lens of your eyes so you have to put the menu on the floor to read it and countless other destructive processes associated with rapid ageing.

BARBECUE YOURSELF

Glycation, which causes the formation of AGES, is the second major process involved in ageing. The damage AGES cause is just as detrimental to Age Power as are excessive free radicals. It triggers a cascade of destructive changes increasing free radicals formed in your body by a factor of as much as fifty. AGES are the chemical equivalent to the blackening of food on a barbecue or browning bread in the oven. And – here is the really bad news – AGES are *irreversible*. Despite ongoing attempts to create drugs that will dissolve away AGES, so far no one has succeeded. Once you've got AGES, science knows no way of getting rid of them. When AGES accumulate they leave brown patches here there and everywhere, just the way baking bread and searing meat does. A good example are the 'age spots' or 'liver spots' (in truth nothing to do with the liver) that mar skin as it grows older.

AGES denature proteins and cross-link them so badly that they cannot be broken down or eliminated. As the presences of AGES in your body expands, your blood sugar levels rise, as does the length of time it remains high. As blood sugar levels remain high long-term, this in turn causes the formation of yet more AGES to undermine insulin sensitivity, encouraging Syndrome X. As damage from AGES gets worse and collagen continues to be cross-linked, you can experience joint problems, loss of muscle strength, and consistently low levels of energy. AGES is also a major contributor to memory loss, mood disorders and Alzheimer's disease.

AGES AND RAGES

The receptor sites to which AGES attach in the body are called RAGES (Receptors for AGES). And there is yet more bad news here. For when AGES bind to RAGES this creates further oxidation damage from free radicals. Further, this binding process tends to be self-amplifying. The more AGES bind to RAGE binding sites, the more RAGES are created in the body – creating a kind of negative feedback loop so that tissue damage from glycation and all the age-related consequences of it spread like waves of degeneration in the body. This is a major factor in the spreading of *amyloid-beta* – the senile plaque found in Alzheimer's disease.

AN END TO AGES

How do you stop AGES from forming? The answer is simple but not palatable to the average person addicted to the high-carbs Western diet of convenience foods: Stop eating sugar and carbohydrate foods like breakfast cereals and pasta, sweets and white breads. All of which push your glucose levels too high. Get plenty of phytonutrients from low-glycaemic fruits and vegetables – sulforophane from broccoli, quercetin from green tea and courgettes, lycopene from tomatoes and garlic (see chapter 15). Control oxidation through diet and the use of anti-oxidant supplements such as alpha lipoic acid, pycnogenol, prosnthocyanidins from grape seeds, the vitamins A, C, and E, and the minerals zinc and selenium.. But pay attention to the way you cook your foods too.

Scientists have known for many years that cooking proteins with sugars in the absence of water forms advanced glycation products that can damage tissues in the body. Diabetics suffer a very high incidence of nerve, artery and kidney damage because high blood sugar levels in their bodies markedly accelerate the chemical reactions that form advanced glycation products.

Dr Gabe Mirkin

STEAM HEAT

Cooking protein foods together with sugars – as in chicken teriyaki for instance – is a bad idea. It creates advanced glycation products which, when we eat foods prepared this way, can damage our own tissues. Diabetics and people with many signs of Syndrome X are especially susceptible to this kind of damage. When you cook with water this helps prevent sugars from binding to proteins to form AGES. Steamed vegetables do not contain significant quantities of advanced glycation end products. Brown foods, including crusty baked breads and biscuits, basted or crusted meats and even roasted coffee encourage nerve damage and other destructive consequences (see page 82).

Now onto the third pillar of ageing – inflammation – which so many people still believe is an inevitable event once you pass 40. Far from it.

INFLAMMATION
THIRD PILLAR OF AGEING

Excessive immune activation which results in oedema, cell damage and free radical production: Any condition associated with increased activation of the immune system.

Inflammation is the body's natural reaction to infection and injury. All inflammatory reactions involve the release of free radicals in the body. Inflammatory reactions are typically seen in auto-immune disorders, chronic infections, allergies and exposure to toxicity. As your body ages the tendency to inflammation increases especially in the gut where food-borne chemicals, viruses, parasites and an overgrowth of pathological species which interfere with the body's ability to detoxify itself, cause defects in the gut barrier and further interfere with effective liver detoxification. The inflammatory cascade which is so damaging to the body acts like a feedback loop increasing yet more inflammation. It goes something like this:

Infection, stress, trauma, or exposure to toxins

Formation of cytotoxic compounds
(cell destroying chemicals)

Activation of inflammatory cascade

Pain, swelling, immobility

Accumulation of toxic response chemicals in area
(swelling, redness, breakdown of cellular functions)

Increased metabolic activity

Cellular catabolism
(breakdown of cellular structure)

Fatigue and further damage to cells and tissues

Interference with endocrine, nervous and immune functions

Leaky Gut Syndrome   Sore joints and muscles:
- arthralgia (joint pain)
- myalgia (painful muscles)
- fibromyalgia (pain in
   fibrous tissues)

Increased toxicity and
free radical damage

Release of alarm   Laying down of
chemicals from white   calcium in tissues
blood cells (leukotrienes)   (rheumatoid and
                                arthritic conditions)

Toxicity, hypersensitivity,   Yet more inflammation
mood disorders, allergy,
inflammation of blood
vessels (indicated by the
marker C-reactive protein [CRP])

Yet more inflammation

POISON FEEDS THE FIRE

Once inflammation is present in any form in your body, it tends to perpetuate itself. All inflammatory reactions involve the release of free radicals as well as the activation of yet more free radical damage. Inflammation is your body's natural response to infection or injury. White blood cells are released, irritated tissues swell and redden. If there are not enough antioxidants in your body to quell free radical damage to your cells and tissues, then chronic inflammatory conditions set in and your immune system goes into a state of prolonged overload. The chronic pain of arthritis, rheumatism, myalgia, fibromyalgia and arthralgia are typical inflammatory responses. So are chronic gastrointestinal disturbances – from poor digestion to diverticulitis, colitis and inflammatory bowel diseases – even excessive skin sensitivity.

Our tendency to inflammatory reactions and pain – swelling, redness, heat, digestive disturbances – increases as we get older when we are not living well. Millions of people regularly take medication in an attempt control it. In fact, pain and inflammation are some of the most common reasons people go to their doctors. Prescription and over-the-counter drugs – from antacids to the non-steroidal anti-inflammatory drugs (NSAID) including aspirin, ibuprofen, naproxen and others – are designed to suppress symptoms. They can have serious side-effects. For one thing they tend to cause damage to the gastrointestinal tract including bleeding and what is known as Leaky Gut Syndrome, which allows toxic substances including yeasts and fungi into the blood stream and puts an excessive toxic load on your liver.

DESTRUCTIVE CYTOKINES

As we grow older, our bodies have a tendency to release *inflammatory cytokines*. These are destructive cell-signalling chemicals that trigger degenerative conditions such as rheumatoid arthritis. In recent years biochemists have begun to identify natural substances that can reduce levels of inflammatory cytokines which contribute to autoimmune disorders characteristic of chronic inflammation. *Docosahexaenoic acid* (DHA) found in fish oils is the best documented supplement to suppress the production of cytokines. Studies both on healthy humans and those with rheumatoid disease indicate that fish oils are capable of suppressing cytokine production by as much as 90 percent.

CALMING INFLAMMATION

High levels of cytokines contribute to many degenerative diseases including autoimmune disorders, cancers, arterio-sclerosis, and rheumatic conditions. Inflammation of any kind causes an increase in free radical damage as it triggers oxidation. DHA – an omega 3 fatty acid found in fish oils – helps counter inflammatory processes. More powerful in their actions are the new non-steroidal anti-inflammatories NSAIDs. Researchers at Glasgow's Royal Infirmary have recently discovered that the common NSAID, ibuprofen, helps normalise anti-oxidant levels. But not without cost as NSAIDs damage the stomach lining.

BREACHING THE BARRIER

Poor diet – including the typical high glycaemic convenience foods most people eat – stress and exposure to toxic chemicals in the environment and in our foods, bring about the breakdown of an important system of defence called the *gastrointestinal mucosa*. If you do not get enough good quality protein in your diet or not enough vitamins and minerals which act as co-factors to the enzymes needed for digestion and other metabolic processes – zinc for instance, pantothenic acid (5B), vitamin A and C or the amino acid L-glutamine – the integrity of the gastrointestinal barrier begins to thin and break down and Leaky Gut Syndrome develops. Toxic compounds then leak into your bloodstream. They are carried to the liver for detoxification. Meanwhile you find yourself with all sorts of gastro-intestinal problems, while the result of mounting toxicity in the body shows itself in any number of ways.

PROTECT YOURSELF FROM BARRIER BREAKDOWN

All sorts of illnesses and problems occur as a result of the breakdown of the important barrier of defence known as the *gastrointestinal mucosa*. These disorders are often misunderstood and treated symptomatically with drugs – many of them dangerous – instead of detoxifying the body and restoring gut integrity. Here are only a few which become more common as we get older:

- ❑ Headaches
- ❑ Arthritic pain
- ❑ Rheumatic conditions
- ❑ Joint aches
- ❑ Chronic muscle pain
- ❑ Back pain
- ❑ Foggy brain
- ❑ Chronic fatigue
- ❑ Aberrations in immune functions with a tendency to chronic infections
- ❑ An overgrowth of yeasts and fungi (Candida Albicans) (page 114)
- ❑ Alterations in brain chemistry that result in memory loss, anxiety, depression
- ❑ An inability to handle stress
- ❑ Hormonal imbalances leading to PMS, menopausal problems in women and prostate troubles in men.

HEED THE WARNING

Chronic inflammation in any form is your body's way of warning you that you need to take action *now* to modify whatever the *causes* are. They may be poor diet. They may be exposure to toxins in your environment – anything from cleaning materials and laundry detergents to herbicides and pesticides in the foods you eat or heavy metals and chemicals in the water you drink. Trauma, too, can produce an inflammatory reaction. So does prolonged stress. You might need to have some bodywork regularly (see page 262). The trigger to inflammation can also be poor blood supply to your tissues or constipation and poor elimination of wastes because you are not getting enough simple exercise such as walking. You might even be allergic to some food or substance which needs to be identified and removed from your diet. Because few people, including most doctors, do not understand inflammation and its role in degeneration, they tend to turn towards symptomatic treatment by taking drugs that only suppress the problem while making the body yet more toxic and even more prone to inflammatory responses.

EASE INFLAMMATION

There are better ways: Follow Age Power's Insulin Balance Programme to restore digestion, increase the elimination of wastes, lower free radical production and eliminate chronic high levels of blood glucose. Then explore what natural help can do for you. Here are some of the best nutritional supporters to counter inflammation and autoimmune problems. Each of the following is a daily dose:

❑ Coenzyme A™: One capsule three times a day on an empty stomach

❑ Health Joint Image™: 3–9 capsules

❑ Natural fish oils EPA-DHA: 2–6 capsules

❑ Vitamin C (ascorbyl palmitate or ascorbic acid): 500–1500mg

❑ Lactobacillus acidophilus and Bifidus: 1–2 tsp a day with food

❑ Mixed carotenoids: 25,000 IU three times a day

❑ Vitamin E (dry vitamin E): 400–800 IU

❑ Pantothenic Acid (B5): 2000–4000mg (unnecessary if you are using Coenzyme A™ or Health Joint Image™)

❑ Selenium: 200–400mcg

❑ Vitamin A (palmitate): 25,000 to 40,000 IU

❑ PABA: 500–1500mg

❑ Licorice root extract: 1–2 capsules

❑ Mixed bioflavonoids (high on quercitin): 500–1000mg

❑ Milk thistle: 150–300mg

❑ Vitamin B6 (in the form of *paradoxyl 5 phosphate* which is the active metabolic form of the vitamin): 50mg–100mg three times a day

❑ Ginger tea

❑ Turmeric: 100mg of standardised extract three times a day

❑ Green tea

GOOD METHYLATION MEANS SLOW AGEING

Methylation is a good guy. It helps oxygenate your cells and makes sure your genes replicate themselves identically. Methylation reactions are crucial in the manufacture of many of your body's most important metabolites, including brain chemicals. Methylation is one of the most important ways your body clears itself of xenoestrogens – oestrogen mimics – taken in from the environment and from the residues of hormone-based drugs like the Pill that end up in the drinking water of many countries. When a methyl group attaches itself to these chemical hormones, it is methylation which makes it possible for your body to process and eliminate these troublemakers. The methyl group – a carbon atom plus three hydrogen atoms – is needed in order for methylation to take place. It can come from various biochemicals such as Coenzyme A, *N-Acetyl-L-Cysteine* and *Dimethylglycine* (vitamin B$_{15}$) each of which supply what is known as active *thiols* which induce methylation and potentiate it.

FOUNDATION SUPPORT

Coenzyme A is essential for methylation. Without an adequate supply of CoA – the most important enzyme in your body – you cannot detoxify toxic substances. Neither can your body synthesise sex hormones from cholesterol. CoA plays a major role in enabling your body to cope with stress. It also strengthens immunity. It helps protect the human cell from everyday exposure to ionising radiation from business machines, computers, television sets and mobile phones thanks to its active thiol which protects RNA and DNA and also helps to repair damage. All of the defence systems of your body need adequate coenzyme A to work. Coenzyme A initiates methylation in the body. Phase 2 detoxification cannot be initiated without coenzyme A. Yet the levels of CoA in twenty-first century bodies tends to be frighteningly low. CoA is the single most important natural supplement you can take for Age Power.

METHYLATION
FOURTH PILLAR OF AGEING

The process by which a methyl group (a carbon atom plus three hydrogen atoms) is added to proteins, hormones and DNA to empower biochemical reactions needed to prevent disease and premature ageing. Where methylation is impeded, this demeans gene expression, prevents efficient detoxification of excess hormones, toxic chemicals and heavy metals, and increases homocystine levels in the blood, increasing your risk of vascular and heart diseases.

HONEST MISTAKE

The nutrients which work together in methylation processes – folic acid, vitamin B_6, B_{12}, and choline – are in short supply in the population as a whole, in even shorter supply as we get older. Our Paleolithic ancestors got high levels of these nutrients as hunter-gatherers. The modern diet has far too little to promote the highest quality gene expression. To make matters worse, more than half a century ago – when the US government was busy trying to work out how much folic acid a supplement could contain – they made a mistake, for very little was understood at the time about folic acid deficiency. They knew that folic acid deficiency together with a lack of B_{12} created *megaloblastic* (pernicious) *anaemia* and that just a tiny quantity – from 400 to 800 mcg – overcame it. The problem was that too much folic acid, when taken on its own, could actually mask a B_{12} deficiency. So they set the folic acid limit in supplements far too low. Now we know that much more is needed to protect from birth defects, heart disease, intestinal disorders, depression, skin troubles and a host of other diseases.

SULPHUR HELPERS

Foods rich in sulphur such as eggs, garlic and onions support methylation. So does an important chemical in the body known as *S-adeniosylmethionine* – SAMe for short. SAMe is involved in more than 40 essential biochemical reactions necessary for preventing age-related degeneration. Your body makes SAMe by combining the essential sulphur-based amino acid *methionine* with ATP in the presence of coenzyme A. But for this to take place you need optimal supplies of nutrients which are key to the process: vitamin B_{12}, folic acid, vitamin B_6, and choline as well as the amino acid methionine. Through the methylation process SAMe clears toxicity. As we get older we typically have low levels of these essential nutrients and as a result end up suffering from conditions such as osteoarthritis, depression and numerous liver abnormalities as a result of poor methylation and low levels of CoA. If you decide to take supplements of SAMe, make sure you get plenty of folic acid, B_6 and B_{12} with it. When you are lacking in folic acid, B_6 and B_{12}, the SAMe in your body is converted into homocysteine (see pages 316–7) – a major trigger for cancer, cardiovascular disease and other degenerative processes.

SAMe – GOOD METHYLATOR

You might think that just by getting more of the amino acid methionine your body can create more SAMe. But this is not the case. High doses of methionine won't increase SAMe. Supplements of SAMe – which is one of the hottest new anti-ageing supplements – are now available over the counter in most countries. Together with CoA – which is even *more* important – they are being used to enhance methylation, improve detoxification and protect from high levels of homocysteine. SAMe is also a safe drug-free treatment for depression, arthritis, fibromyalgia, liver disorders and migraine. SAMe can also help enhance the clearance of various drug residues from the body. All of these positive effects are directly related to SAMe's ability to enhance methylation in the body:

❑ **Osteoarthritis**: 400mg three or four times a day (see caution on page 94)

❑ **Depression**: 400mg three or four times a day (see caution on page 94)

❑ **Migraine**: 200mg to 400mg two times a day (see caution on page 94)

❑ **Fibromyalgia**: 200mg to 400mg twice a day (see caution on page 94)

❑ **Liver disorders**: 200mg to 400mg two or three times a day (see caution on page 94)

Since SAMe works together with vitamin B$_6$, B$_{12}$, folic acid and choline in producing methylation reactions it is vital to ensure an adequate supply of these nutrients when taking a supplement of SAMe. When you are lacking in these nutrients SAMe can be converted into homocysteine which predisposes the body to cardiovascular disorders and cancer. The beneficial effects of SAMe are much heightened by using it in conjunction with Coenzyme A™ (3 capsules a day on an empty stomach).

Caution: It is important to begin slowly with SAMe when using it for osteoarthritis or depression since in a few people SAMe supplementation can cause temporary digestive upset. Start with 200mg doses for a day or two and then increase to 400mg doses over a period of a couple of weeks. No significant side effects have been reported from taking SAMe supplements orally. However, in the case of manic depression – bipolar disorder – take SAMe only under medical supervision as it can increase the manic phase.

B VITAMINS HELP

If you decide to supplement your diet with SAMe to empower good methylation make sure you take a good B complex as well as extra help from these nutrients:

- ❑   Vitamin B$_{12:}$ 180–240mcg
- ❑   Folic acid: 800mcg twice a day
- ❑   Choline: 300–600mg
- ❑   Vitamin B$_6$ (pyridoxal-5-phosphate)6: 50mg twice a day

WATCH YOUR PILLARS

When the first three pillars of ageing – oxidation, glycation and inflammation – run too fast, they bring about all sorts of age-related wasting and dysfunctions. When the fourth pillar, methylation, slows down similar decay sets in. And defects in the processes of each of the pillars only undermines the other three making you prone to all these things:

- ❑ Neurotoxicity (damage to the nerves from poisons in the body)
- ❑ Immune dysfunctions (see page 75)
- ❑ Sarcopenia (see page 29)
- ❑ Dysfunctions in energy production
- ❑ Damage to your cells
- ❑ Alterations in DNA
- ❑ High levels of homocysteine (see page 316)
- ❑ Hormonal and reproductive disturbances
- ❑ Altered gene expression (gene potential not fulfilled)
- ❑ Protein damage (see page 215)
- ❑ Toxicity build up

The net result of all this is to promote the development of degenerative disease and early ageing. Age Power's Insulin Balance helps prevent it from happening. What works superbly well with it are techniques for enhancing the body's master enzyme coenzyme A. Let's look at this next.

PRIMORDIAL POWER

I am the heat Hephaestus used to forge lightening
bolts and fashion jewellery for the gods.
Spirit of Creation from Journey to Freedom

Scientists tell us that metabolism recapitulates *biogenesis* –
the origins of life. In other words, what goes on in your
cells mirrors the creation of the universe. Within your own
mitochondria, your body's master enzyme – *coenzyme A* –
continually initiates the production of ATP. Enhance CoA
levels and de-age the body.

Enzymes matter. Without them there would be no life. An enzyme is a
compound which initiates or accelerates specific metabolic processes by
acting as a catalyst. You find them in all living things – from daffodils
to buffalos. So far science has identified thousands of enzymes which
help the human body function. One stands out above all the rest – coenzyme A.

ENERGETIC MASTER

Coenzyme A is your body's most active and most important catalyst. It's
needed to trigger hundreds of chemical reactions from the production of
energy and hormones to the detoxification of dangerous chemicals. When
CoA is in plentiful supply, your body is vital. When levels fall, your vitality
and resistance to ageing plunges. CoA also works its life generating magic

---

UNIVERSAL CATALYST

Every organ in your body has coenzyme A in its tissues.
Together with *polynucleotides* and *acetyl carrier proteins,* CoA
emerged from the primordial soup to provide matter with
the hydrogen and sulphur based chemical reactions it
needed to create life. When you have optimum levels of
CoA, this makes you highly resistant to fatigue and degeneration. The problem is that coenzyme A is constantly being
gobbled up by all the metabolic processes it looks after. This
is why it needs replenishing.

---

in your blood and in your brain. Most important of all, adequate CoA protects your mitochondria from the genetic damage that can cause your body to age rapidly.

Many age researchers now believe our mitochondria are not only the focal point of life but also of degeneration. For when our mitochondria get out of whack, degeneration gets the upper hand

SHEER GENIUS

Interesting things, mitochondria. These organelles, found inside each of our cells and whose job it is to provide us with life energy, were once denizens of a primordial world – purple photosynthetic bacteria. When oxygen appeared on the earth, instead of falling prey to its dangers, they learned to exploit its chemical and energetic reactivity. Like quantum physicists looking for a new source of power, these microscopic beasties invented ways of taking in a potentially lethal gas and transmuting it into a radical opportunity.

Slowly but inexorably purple photosynthetic bacteria evolved into masters of energy transformation. They learned to oxidise materials at hand by trapping the energy of light. Over endless eons, they honed their skills until at last they had learned to create life's energy storage compound, ATP. So successful was the energy currency they created that it could be used by every cell of virtually every living thing. And so efficient were their means of creating it through oxidation, that other early forms of life, like the yeasts and fungi – which rely on fermentation as an energy source – could never match them. Fermentation, practised by yeasts and fungi, produces only two molecules of ATP from each molecule of sugar. Mitochondria can take the same molecule of sugar and coax 36 molecules of energy from it – 15 times more than their oxygen-hating cousins.

Let's take a closer look at the energy creating process these little geniuses came up with.

ENERGY CYCLE

The *tricarboxylyc-acid-cycle* or TCA cycle, also known as the Krebs Cycle or citric acid cycle, consists of a number of chemical reactions within the mitochondria whereby nutrients from the foods we eat are oxidised to get energy. The complex chemical reactions involved in the TCA cycle were formulated in 1937 by Sir Hans Krebs, who won a Nobel prize for his work. So important is the TCA cycle that, in one form or another, it takes place in virtually every type of life-form. Each step on this cycle is catalysed by specific enzymes, arranged in such perfect sequence that energy creation happens with remarkable grace. Without adequate CoA it doesn't happen.

Before long the ancestors of our mitochondria gave up their bacterial independence and settled happily into larger organisms. By then they had so drastically changed that they would never again be able to live outside. There they have remained ever since – nurtured and safe within our living bodies.

BEWARE FREE RADICALS

Mitochondria have a remarkable distinction: They possess their own DNA. Even though they can no longer live alone, your mitochondria still reproduce very much the way bacteria do within our cells. It was not until the late sixties that scientists discovered mitochondrial DNA. They noticed that our mitochondria divide in completely different cycles than do the cells in which they reside.

In recent years mitochondria have come under close scrutiny by age researchers. First, they are the cauldrons in which ATP, our life energy, is made. Second, since the creation of ATP is an *oxidative* process, the DNA of our mitochondria is ten to twenty times more susceptible to free radical damage than the nuclear DNA of our cells.

The revelation that our mitochondria, these ancient monsters we thought were tame and benign, are in fact our silent executioners, has reinvigorated the field of mitochondrial research, putting it at the forefront of biological and medical research.

Guy Brown

THE MITOCHONDRIAL THEORY
OF AGEING

❑   Mitochondria create life energy to fuel healthy metabolism.
❑   Good functioning mitochondria are essential to preventing age degeneration.
❑   Mitochondrial DNA is highly susceptible to oxidation damage.
❑   Respiratory electron transport in mitochondria is accompanied by the generation of high levels of free radicals and associated with chronic degenerative diseases.
❑   Defective mitochondrial functions and damage to the mitochondrial DNA are major factors in speeding up the ageing process.
❑   A depletion in coenzyme A leads to mitochondrial dysfunction, producing an energy deficit in the body and fostering degenerative processes.

MUTATION MEANS TROUBLE

Now, this is serious business. For when mitochondrial DNA undergoes injury, daughter cells – the new mitochondria created – become mutated and progressively less able to produce energy. Without a continual supply of high level energy, our metabolic processes can't work properly. Our cellular messages get garbled. This alters the expression of our genes and causes changes in our biomarkers. Cellular physiology is undermined.

That our mitochondria's ancestors were oxygen-respiring purple bacteria has been shown beyond a doubt by DNA sequencing. Like a village ransacked by barbarians who ultimately became civilised, fermenting organisms were stalked by oxygen using predators that become mitochondrial labourers.

Lynn Marguils and Dorion Sagan

Rubbish accumulates – in our cells and eventually our tissues – so much that our immune system can become sensitive to the body itself, creating auto-immune disorders – from arthritis to food allergies and systemic lupus. Neurological functions and neuroendocrine functions are undermined. Hormones fall and serious metabolic imbalances can ensue, making it easy for degenerative processes to take hold.

It is little wonder that many scientists believe that at its core, ageing is the result of an accumulation of mitochondrial DNA mutations. As these DNA distortions accumulate they interfere with our bodies ability to produce ATP. Insufficient ATP in turn impairs system functions. That's where coenzyme A and its cohort coenzymes come in.

COENZYME POWER

Coenzymes are chemicals – biologically active forms of vitamins in fact. It is their job to potentise enzymic reactions. For a long time scientists believed that, like the enzymes they support, coenzymes could be recycled as substrates. Now we know that this is not true. Destroyed in performing the functions they are designed for, coenzymes such as the master CoA, CoQ10 and NADH – all necessary for the production of energy in the mitochondria – need to be continually replaced. Each has a specific role to play in the creation of energy via the TCA cycle.

ACTIVE METABOLITES

Unlike the enzymes they potentise, coenzymes are biologically active forms of vitamins. Often they are made from the B vitamins, thiamine, riboflavin, niacin, pantothenic acid and biotin, all of which help release energy from carbohydrates, fats and proteins and also help synthesise new proteins from amino acids. B_6 for instance aids in the metabolism of amino acids, while B_{12} helps cell multiplication. Coenzyme-A is made within your cells from the most active form of vitamin B_5 – pantothenic acid. This active form of B_5 is called *pantethine* and, among other things, it exerts an enormously beneficial effect on the utilisation of fats and carbohydrates in energy production as well as in the manufacture of adrenal and sex hormones and red blood cells. It also has significant cholesterol and triglyceride lowering activity. When incorporated into the CoA molecule these powers are increased significantly. While your body can synthesise some coenzymes such as Q10, which is a downstream metabolic product initiated by the presence of coenzyme A, those that it cannot make – such as the master CoA itself – need to be taken in through the foods you eat.

ENGINE FOR ENERGY

Think of your mitochondria as a car engine. Coenzyme A is the ignition switch. It triggers all other enzymic and hormonal biochemical reactions involved in energy making. CoQ10 acts as the carburettor. It keeps feeding oxygen for the process. Coenzyme1 – also known as NADH – acts like the sparkplugs. It keeps the electron transport moving.

In recent years CoQ10, also known as *ubiquinone*, has made biochemical news as a highly effective natural treatment for high blood pressure, periodontal disease and immune deficiencies. It enables the body to make better use of oxygen. NADH, a special form of the B vitamin niacinamide, has recently become available in supplement form too. It is being used to treat people with Parkinson's disease as well as chronic fatigue syndrome. NADH is also being used to enhance mental function.

PREVENTATIVE POWER

Since its discovery in 1947, coenzyme A's crucial importance in maintaining high level health and preventing degeneration has been intensively studied. Apart from its central role in initiating the TCA cycle, coenzyme A triggers the manufacture of a vast number of other substances that the body needs for high level health. These include *acetylcholine* – the calming neurotransmitter in the brain which dilates blood vessels, slows heart rate and improves digestion, learning and memory. Coenzyme A also initiates the production of steroid hormones in the adrenal glands: *aldosterone* and *hydrocortisone*, as well as many other hormones such as *pregnenalone*, DHEA, oestrogen, progesterone and testosterone. Hormones fall dramatically with age when the body becomes deficient in CoA. When it is supplied by nutritional supplement – which until recently was believed to be impossible – hormone levels often return to normal, literally rejuvenating the body.

PALEOLITHIC REFERENCES

Found readily in raw fruits and vegetables in minute quantities, pantothenic acid – B_5 – is needed for your body to make coenzyme A. CoA is easily destroyed by exposure to light, heat or radiation. The word pantothenic comes from the Greek word *pantos,* meaning *everywhere.* Vegetables and fruits are sources of B_5; meats, fish, eggs and all animal foods are rich in CoA. The most abundant source of CoA in nature are the raw glands and organs of animals. One of the reasons why the tradition in natural medicine of using animal glandulars in the natural treatment of human illness has been so successful is likely to be because these products are rich in

CoA and its substrates. Our Paleolithic ancestors got plenty. They were hunters and gatherers and, like the modern Inuit, on killing an animal, they immediately consumed the raw viscera. They also ate massive quantities of fresh raw vegetables, herbs, grubs and insects – all good sources of CoA which their bodies could then break down into its component parts through digestion, providing the cells with the wherewithal to synthesise new CoA for the body. Today, our CoA levels are low by comparison and our tendency to degeneration high.

CoA MASTER ENZYME

Here are a few of the ways that CoA protects your body from degenerative damage:

❑   CoA initiates the TCA cycle which produces 95 percent of the energy your body needs to stay alive and resist ageing.

❑   CoA increases your body's ability to deal with stress and inhibits degenerative processes associated with it.

❑   CoA initiates the manufacture of specific neurotransmitters and hormones which play a critical role in brain health and adrenal support.

❑   CoA acts as the 'universal acetate carrier'. This is the primary biological co-factor used in important *acyl* group transfers which initiate the metabolism of fatty acids as well as support detoxification.

❑   CoA supports critical functions of your immune system.

❑   CoA facilitates the repair of DNA, RNA and injury to both mitochondria and cells, helping to protect them from oxidation damage.

❑   CoA empowers the manufacture of connective tissue.

❑   CoA helps form and repair cartilage.

❑   CoA greatly enhances physical performance.

Studies show that people with rheumatoid arthritis, as well as gout and auto-immune disorders, have very low levels of CoA. In order for your body to manufacture it you need to be provided with good quantities of pantothenic acid either through foods or dietary supplements. Leading edge age researchers have long known that if we could find a way to raise the levels of CoA in the mitochondria, production of ATP would be enhanced, mitochondrial DNA would receive greater protection from damage, and the degenerative processes in the body could be slowed.

But, unlike CoQ10 and NADH – both of which now exist in supplemental form – no-one has ever been able to figure out how to create a nutritional supplement of CoA. For CoA can only be manufactured in the cells of your body. And no matter how much pantothenic acid you put into your body, because of an inhibiting enzyme within the cells, only a certain percentage of it will be turned into coenzyme A.

FAT BURNING

Coenzyme A is also your body's 'universal acetate carrier'. This enables CoA to initiate fatty acid metabolism by adding or removing an *acyl* group from their molecules. Efficient fatty acid metabolism is essential to protection from raised cholesterol and triglycerides. CoA must be in adequate supply for your body to be able to *burn* rather than *store* fat as well. Thanks in part to its role as universal acetate carrier, CoA also initiates the detoxification of many dangerous substances like acetaldehyde, protecting the body from age-related destruction caused by the build up of dangerous wastes. It also enhances immune functions and activates white blood cells whose responsibility it is to destroy and eliminate invaders. It spurs the formation of haemoglobin needed for new red blood cells. Finally, CoA both initiates and facilitates the manufacture of important components such as *chrondroitin sulphate* and *hyaluronic acid* necessary in the formation and repair of cartilage and collagen – essential for youthful skin.

The mitochondrial theory of ageing proposes that our mitochondria continually produce toxic free radicals that inexorably attack our mitochondria, mutating its DNA. The mitochondrial damage may cause an even greater production of free radicals, in an increasingly vicious circle. For mutant mitochondrial DNA is associated with a frightening range of progressive degenerative diseases, including Alzheimer's, Huntington's, and Parkinson's, diabetes, atherosclerosis and, of course, ageing itself.

Guy Brown

BREAKTHROUGH

In the mid-nineties, expert in coenzyme A metabolism Nicholaos Skouras and his colleagues made a significant breakthrough in the search to enhance levels of CoA within the human body. He created a unique delivery system which enables the body to make more CoA itself within the cells. And he did this in a way that is completely natural.

A Greek, who currently works in the United States, Skouras is an integrative biochemist. He looks upon the human body as a flow of energy, information and communication between its cells, tissues and organs. Impatient with the way nutrition and biochemistry is taught and lamenting the communication barrier between different scientific fields, he worked intensively for many years developing practical theories and incorporating them into clinical nutrition before discovering a way of supplying in supplemental form the wherewithal for CoA production. Since then he has created some of the best natural health care and skin products in the world – each of which, in its own way, makes use of the universal catalyst CoA.

INTEGRATIVE APPROACH

Looking at an anti-ageing programme from the point of view of integrative biochemistry asks that the biochemist work with nutritional substrates as highly biologically active substances – vitamins, minerals, amino acids, nucleosides, nucleotides and even special five-carbon sugars which act as communicators. These raw materials, found in foods or in the living body, are used to create a complexity of effects. These effects contribute to well-being by making it possible for the body's own metabolic systems to support health and good looks in the most natural and effective way possible.

Skouras believes that, supplied with optimal quantities of essential nuts and bolts in a highly active form which it can use at a cellular level, the human body manufactures its own hormones and enzymes from whatever metabolites it most needs. He insists it is better to support the body's own biochemical mechanisms for producing energy, hormones, anti-inflammatory and anti-ageing effects, than to supplant them by offering artificial hormones which eventually undermine the body's ability to create them. For hormones introduced from outside can, Skouras insists, undermine the body's ability to manufacture its own.

Preventative gerontology now aims not just to retard disease but to prevent functional decline. Health and functional status in later life are increasingly seen as under our control. Stages are set for major community based intervention studies designed to enhance the likelihood of older persons, not only to avoid disease and disability but to truly age successfully.

John Rowe MD

NUTRIENT MATRIX

Recognising that the synthesis of coenzyme A begins in the cells, Skouras set out to find a way of supplying direct to the cells exactly what they need to enhance production of the master catalyst. It was by no means a simple task. The problem was this: When a nutrient such as pantothenic acid, or even CoA itself, is taken in through foods – fresh raw organ meats for instance, or vegetables, herbs and seeds – it comes packaged synergistically in nature, in a matrix, with other related substances and compounds in a magnificent and ordered balance. The fresh food carries structural information of the highest quality and complexity. A food may contain enzymes, vitamins, minerals and phyto-chemicals of which the particular nutrient is only a part. Plant matrices have an affinity for the human body. For we have eaten plants throughout our own evolution and our body is programmed to welcome them. When nutritionists or doctors try to give a particular vitamin on its own – pantothenic acid for arthritis perhaps – the substrates that came packaged with it in nature are missing and the body cannot therefore make optimal use of the vitamin.

You might think that you could simply give large doses of pantothenic acid – or even of its most active form, *pantethine* – and this would enable your body to make its own CoA. Or perhaps you could create an artif-icial molecule of coenzyme A, a drug, and introduce it into the system thereby raising levels of the master CoA in the cells.

Great plan, but it just doesn't work that way. Both approaches have been tried many times without success. The first approach is undermined by an inhibitory process in the body's cells so that the amount of CoA they can make from pantethine in the presence of other substrates becomes strictly limited. The second approach fails because vitamin B_5 or CoA them-selves are simply broken down when they reach the body so that there is no way of ensuring they will ever reach the interior of the cell where CoA could be manufactured. The other problem is that, even if you could devise a way of accomplishing that task, there was no known way to get the CoA to cross the mitochondrial barrier which it needs to do to initiate more ATP energy production.

LIVING EXCHANGE

Cells maintain their individual integrity thanks to their semi-permeable membrane – their 'skin' if you like. This membrane stops the cell from dissolving into the fluid that surrounds it, however it also comes between the cell and what it needs to survive – the nutrients in the extracellular fluid. The *delivery system* by which the cell gets the nutrients it needs and gets rid of the wastes it produces is called *diffusion*. (Osmosis is probably the best known of the passive transport systems which use diffusion.)

When the fluid surrounding the cell has more of a particular nutrient in it than the fluid inside the cell, the molecules of that nutrient pass through the cell membrane until there is the same concentration of the nutrient inside the cell as outside. The *concentration gradient* – i.e. the difference

> We humans are a vast system of systems and sub-systems; to make conscious use of the complex wisdom of the body is to achieve a sublime orchestral exper-ience of the self and its many ecolologies.
>
> *Jean Houston*

between the concentration of a nutrient outside the cell to inside – determines how quickly this type of diffusion takes place. A high concentration gradient means that nutrients will pass quickly into the cell, or wastes pass out of it. For the cell's wastes are removed in just the same way, from a high concentration inside the cell to a low concentration outside it.

ACTIVE TRANSPORT FOR HEALTH

There is also a system of diffusion called *active transport* which behaves quite differently. Active transport takes place when a cell makes use of its own energy to draw a molecule across a membrane regardless of the concentration gradient. The work of active transport is performed by specific proteins which are part of the cell membrane and which use ATP to supply the energy they need to draw the molecules through the membrane. It is not easy to *create* an active transport mechanism to deliver specific nutrients to the cells when they have become depleted of them. The transport mechanism has to have a bioelectric attraction for the proteins in the cell walls and, when it comes to creating active nutraceuticals, it requires the building of a highly complex matrix of interacting chemicals to make it happen. This matrix becomes a kind of womb or cage in which active ingredients can be carried into specific cells where they can do the greatest good. Such systems are sometimes used in advanced drug delivery.

THE MATRIX

Biochemist Nicholaos Skouras has created a unique and entirely natural matrix which makes it possible for his formulations to deliver powerful nutraceuticals and substrates where they are needed most by the body. His work, much imitated by other scientists, has enabled him to create the only reliable method for enhancing CoA production in the cells and for ensuring the CoA produced naturally within the body finds its way within the mitochondria. There it encourages high levels of ATP production and the hundreds of other essential metabolic events – such as hormone production and detoxification processes. It is one of the most powerful anti-ageing tools available.

Skouras' matrix ingeniously mimics the way nature does things. Created through a complex series of chemical reactions and bonds, it performs not one but three impossible feats:

❑ It joins together nutrients and substrates, in exact amounts and balance, which your body needs to create its own CoA within the cells.

❑ It bypasses the inhibitory processes which limit the amount of CoA cells can produce.

❑ Once the cell has made CoA, it is transported across the mitochrondrial barrier where it can initiate production of high levels of ATP there.

CHEMICAL OBSESSION

Skouras lives and breathes his work. Interviewing him, one has the impression there is nothing he would rather do than spend the wee hours of the morning, with no telephone to ring and no administrative duties to perform, playing with his passion: inventing new ways to perform other apparently impossible feats – always naturally, and with respect for the human body's ability to heal itself. His *piece de resistance* is a product called simply Coenzyme A™. It is probably the world's best kept anti-ageing secret. Biochemists who grasp the complexity of its formulation praise it. Doctors who use it can often turn patients' lives around. But, because of the complexity and the ingeniousness of the way it has been formulated, very few people in the general public are as yet aware of how transformative it can be.

Except for those who have used the product of course. Reports from them of enhanced vitality, increased capacity to handle stress, more rapid healing from both acute and chronic conditions, and improved skin and hair, joints and muscles are legion. Men and women previously on hormone replacement therapy report their bodies are now producing their own hormones. Others speak of Coenzyme A™'s ability to enhance immune functions and repair physical injuries and claim using Coenzyme A™ has made them highly resistant to illness and to ageing. Skouras' looks on his inventions not as magic bullets but rather as useful adjuncts to a health-enhancing way of eating and living. They are part of a natural approach to countering ageing. And they address directly the biomarker issues.

DETOX AND REBUILD

Using Coenzyme A™ together with Age Power's Insulin Balance can be powerfully detoxifying thanks in no small part to its ability to enhance *acetyl transfer*, central to the body's Phase II detoxification processes. But, unlike a juice fast or most of the standard programmes designed to cleanse your system, it does not weaken it. Coenzyme A™ and Age Power's Insulin Balance actually *strengthen* metabolism while they are cleansing. I have experimented with it myself for several months and monitored the experience of many others who have used it. I find there is a surprising pattern of change which seems to occur. Although each human being is utterly unique, there appears to be a deep process of regeneration which occurs in a characteristic way for most people.

CoA FOR AGE POWER

Using Coenzyme A™ (together with Age Power's Insulin Balance) three times a day on an empty stomach for three to six months at a time enhances health in surprising ways. It usually happens sequentially, step by step, something like this:

❑ A subtle growing rise in energy occurs coupled with a noticeable improvement in your ability to deal with stress. Life may be as challenging as ever but you feel more on top of things.

❑ As your body clears itself of acetaldehydes and other toxic chemicals you feel mentally clearer.

❑ Strength increases.

❑ Libido rises and with it often creative energies of other kinds. (This can be especially helpful to perimenopausal, menopausal and post menopausal women, whose many years of reproductive hormonal cycling has depleted their body energy and suppressed hormone production.)

❑ The body gains metabolic momentum. Everything from digestion to physical movement seems to take place better and more easily.

❑ Mental acuity is heightened.

❑ A sense begins to grow that some kind of emotional or spiritual reawakening may be happening.

PRIMORDIAL TRANSFORMATION

It is almost as though the whole process of improving CoA levels on a biochemical level parallels the process of clearing and strengthening the psyche on a spiritual level described in the chapter DARKNESS INTO LIGHT on page 372 through meditation, Autogenics or good binaural technology. I have yet to experience anything quite like it. It gave me the opportunity to experience within my body and my being a little of what scientists mean when they insist that metabolism recapitulates biogenesis. You feel it happening progressively within your own life.

Central to the evolutionary processes which created cellular life, co-enzyme A is capable of bringing about profound regeneration in living systems. Race horse owners have long experimented with ways of increasing CoA in their animals in the hopes of helping them run longer and harder without lactate build up in muscles to undermine speed. For me the experience of what CoA enhancement brings to the body was like a personal lesson in just how all-encompassing the primordial elements which created life can be when let loose within the body.

TASTE OF ENERGY

A simple and easy-to-carry-out 10 day's experience of CoA's potential is the 10 Day Apple Detox and Rebuild (see next page). You can do it while working or while on holiday – really anywhere or any time.

Our own generation is simply the one to emerge at the time when human consciousness has become subtle enough and complex enough to awaken to what the universe has been telling us from the beginning.

Brian Swimme

10 DAY APPLE DETOX AND REBUILD

The processes involved in regeneration and rebuilding based on CoA take time to reap full rewards – a few months at least, more for some. But it is remarkable how quickly you can begin to feel the benefits in how you look and feel by combining Age Power's Insulin Balance Programme with Coenzyme A™ supplements. Take it three times a day on an empty stomach together with a good quality high potency B vitamin supplement and an apple (preferably organic). The apple is not only rich in pectin which helps remove heavy metals and other pollutants from your body, it is also a good source of *malic acid* which further empowers the energy-making and initiatory processes CoA carries out in living systems. It is essential you drink a 300ml (10 fl oz) glass of clean water with each dose of supplements. The only way to find out is to do it yourself.

HERE'S HOW:
- On rising (at least half an hour before breakfast):

1 Coenzyme A™ capsule
1 High potency B Complex
1 apple
300ml (10 fl oz) glass of spring water or filtered water

- Your Insulin Balance Breakfast (see page 228 for suggestions).

- ½ hour before lunch:

1 Coenzyme A™ capsule
1 High potency B Complex
1 apple
300ml (10 fl oz) oz glass of spring or filtered water

- Your Insulin Balance Lunch

- ½ hour before dinner:

1 Coenzyme A™ capsule
1 apple

300ml (10 fl oz) glass of spring or filtered water

- Your Insulin Balance Dinner

The 10 Day Apple Detox and Rebuild is an ideal way to start Insulin Balance. It helps your metabolism make major shifts away from the standard diet full of high-glycaemic carbs with greater ease and efficiency. It can also give you an inkling of what Coenzyme A™ might do to enhance your energy and life as a whole used longer term.

SCOURGE OF POWER

Bernard was right, the pathogen is nothing, the terrain is everything

Louis Pasteur on his deathbed

Syndrome X is not the only silent plague stalking twenty-first century health. There is another – equally virulent – and even more insidious. No investigation of ageing should ignore this scourge of power. It is caused by a visitor from the underworld and it hides beneath diseases with other names. It invades your body, distorts your brain functions, produces addiction and emotional miseries as well as mass biological degeneration. It undermines personal power until it can prevent you from taking control your life.

The earliest forms of life – yeasts and fungi – do not respire the way we do. Our bodies live by *aerobic* metabolism. We take in oxygen and give off carbon dioxide. They rely on *fermentation*, taking in sugars to produce alcohol as a waste.

ENTER THE UNDERWORLD

Yeasts and fungi get lumped together with plants only because they are not animals. The Japanese poet Jun Takami wrote, 'And fungi were fungi . . . they were like nobody on Earth.' We associate these primitive life forms with dank places, witches brews and smelly feet. Not without reason. Vampire-like organisms, they live off whatever is at hand. They eat sugar and high density carbs really turn them on. Yeasts and fungi have the ability to make loaves rise and to brew beer as they reproduce. At other times they attach themselves to animal skin, to hair, and to the inner secret folds of the human body. Among the earliest organisms to populate terra firma, yeasts and fungi boast powerfully protective cell walls made of *chitin* – a nitrogen-rich carbohydrate somewhat different from the cellulose found in the cell walls of plants or from our own.

SHAPE SHIFTERS

These denizens of the lower realms possess a magical ability to change from one form to another. Incredibly successful organisms, yeasts and fungi are master survivors. For more than 400 million years they have been devouring stuff that other forms of life eschew – breaking down corpses, munching faeces and invading the dark warmth of living bodies. Unable to produce food, they rely entirely on the generosity of other living things to nurture them. Meanwhile, these underworld wonders carry out essential tasks for the biosphere, turning wastes into reusable matter. They provide us with the alcohol for champagne, they ripen our Camembert, and give us fluffy rolls for the table.

MICROBEASTIES

In a healthy human body between 4–5kg (9–11 lbs) of micro-organisms – bacteria, yeasts and fungi – make their home. A few thousand, some believe as many as ten thousand, different species of micro flora inhabit your intestinal tract alone. There, these micro-organisms live together in a delicate and ever-shifting balance. Most are very different from the disease-causing bacteria which give micro-beasties a bad name. Some, like *Bifidobacteria* and *Lactobacillus* produce vitamins and other nutrients to help support our immune system. Others help us digest our food. Some forms of bacteria and yeasts, however, are parasitical and can be highly toxic to the human body – especially when their colonies overgrow and displace the good guy bugs and they begin to communicate signals to their host – the human host – which are actively detrimental to its health.

MOB RULE

The bad guys include *Clostridia, enterotoxigenic E. coli* and *Salmonella*. These beasties produce toxic chemicals, activating the body's alarm system and nudging it into chronic inflammation. Certain other micro organisms – like the water and food-borne amoebic organism *Guardia* for instance, as well as certain yeasts which metamorphose into fungi like *Candida albicans* – can utterly destroy health and life when they get out of hand. In the twenty-first Century world of junk foods, alcohol, drugs and ubiquitous poisons, they often do.

Recent research carried out at Washington University School of Medicine has shown that our intestinal bugs have a remarkable ability to send out signals which enable them to communicate their needs to our human body. When levels of the carbohydrates on which they feed get low, they shout for more. Obedient to their insidious calls, we respond unknowingly by reaching for yet another bar of chocolate or piece of pizza. The epithelial lining of the human gut is almost 5 cm (2 in) thick with bacteria. Even beasties with virulent potentials can live happily and benignly in the intestines of a normal healthy body. Then one day, things change – too much sugar, a course of antibiotics given for flu, an illness which suppresses immunity – and all hell can break loose.

OVERGROWTH

These are but a few of the symptoms connected with an overgrowth of Candida albicans on the human body:

- ❑ Weight gain
- ❑ Chronic fatigue as a result of impaired metabolism
- ❑ Brain and nervous system dysfunction
- ❑ Headaches
- ❑ Poor memory, fuzzy thinking, inebriation
- ❑ Heart problems – rapid pulse rate, palpitations, pounding heart
- ❑ Vaginitis and lack of bladder control – this can lead to frequent urination, itchy rashes and vaginal thrush
- ❑ Stomach troubles: diarrhoea, bloating and gas, gastritis, gastric ulcers, constipation
- ❑ Allergic reactions

A QUESTION OF BALANCE

Candida albicans is a form of yeast which occurs naturally in the human body, flourishing in the warm folds of the digestive tract, the vagina and the skin. There it absorbs certain quantities of heavy metals, and by doing so removes them from the human bloodstream where they could cause problems to our body. In a healthy body, the population of Candida is kept in check by the good guy bacteria that live in the same area. But when these normal, helpful, bacteria are disrupted, by the use of anti-biotics – which not only destroy the bad guy bacteria they are designed to destroy, but wash away the good – then Candida albicans can take on a very sinister form indeed. It can overgrow in the gastrointestinal tract, producing a complex medical syndrome known as *chronic Candidaisis* – also called the *yeast syndrome*. The most common place in the human body where yeast proliferates is the vagina of women, where it produces redness, burning on urination, a yeasty odour and itching, but it can also over-grow in the mouth where it is known as thrush, and inside babies nappies, causing nappy rash. In these places it can be irritating but really only causes minor problems.

DIVING DEEP

In people, however, who eat a high carbohydrate diet which provides the yeast and other bacteria and fungi in the body with an abundance of glucose, not only do they survive, they overpopulate and become an inva-sive and dangerous organism. When the immune system has been compro-mised, or when the normal lining of the gut becomes damaged, the yeast, instead of remaining within the intestinal tract where they belong, can metamorphose into its fungal form sending out *rhizomes* to penetrate the walls of the gut, opening it to the absorption of yeast cells, particles of cells, and the toxins these micro-organisms produce enter the interior of the body and pass into the bloodstream.

Although chronic Candidaisis was clinically defined back in the early eighties when Orion Truss published his excellent book *The Missing Diagnosis,* followed by William Crook's better known *The Yeast Connection,* neither the public nor the medical profession had any idea of the magni-tude of the problem.

A BLIND EYE

Almost 25 years ago, researchers in Japan discovered that there are many other – some as yet unidentified – organ-isms which proliferate with Candida albi-cans and are equally destructive to the body. These organisms produce toxins. When these toxins are injected into animals they cause immuno-suppression and can produce the symptoms of osteoarthritis and rheumatoid arthritis, as well as a myriad other illnesses. Candidaisis also produces food allergies, Leaky Gut Syndrome, and many other destructive processes in the body which are blamed on other diseases.

> Candida's presence, normally contained on the skin, mucous membranes, or in the bowel, can be compromised by immuno deficient states usually induced by diabetes, preg-nancy or certain drugs. The latter includes antibiotics, steroids, birth control pills and chemotherapy. Thrush, common in infants before the full development of their immune systems, is frequent in immuno-compromised individuals, regardless of their age or status.
>
> *Raymond Keith Brown MD*

FOOD ALLERGIES

Candidaisis can cripple an immune system so that it is no longer able to protect itself from invading chemicals and destructive organisms. It also produces a leaky gut making you highly prone to chemical poisoning and food sensitivities as toxins from micro-organisms and protein molecules enter the bloodstream. For your body sees them as foreign antigens – invaders – and this brings about a phenomenon known as *cross reactivity* producing yet more food allergies.

Conventional medicine has only begun to acknowledge the existence of overgrowth of Candida albicans and its opportunistic behaviour. Investigations in the last few years by physicians who are aware of the widespread nature of Candida overgrowth – by the latest, highly conservative counts, tens of millions of people in the United States are believed to have a Candida overgrowth – verify Truss's findings. Gradually Candidaisis is being accepted by an ultra conservative medical establishment, although few still understand either its nature or its cause.

ACETALDEHYDE POISONS

Yeasts feed on sugars and carbohydrates which easily turn into sugars. The chemical products they produce as wastes during the fermentation process by which they live contain high levels of ethanol – alcohol. This is why there are many cases on record of people who do not drink alcohol, yet continue to live in a state of drunkenness that alters consciousness. As the alcohol produced by the yeast begins to be broken down it creates *acetaldehyde*, a chemical which is six times more toxic to the brain than ethanol itself, which insidiously undermines brain functions and damages neurological structures.

Acetaldehyde is a dangerous chemical which enters the body in four main ways:

❑   Drinking alcohol
❑   Inhaling exhaust fumes
❑   Inhaling cigarette smoke, either actively or passively
❑   Having an overgrowth of Candida in our body

When we drink alcohol, it is broken down in the liver where an enzyme known as *alcohol dehydroginese* converts it into acetaldehyde. Then another enzyme, *aldehyde hydroginese*, is meant to break it down further into acetate, which is meant to fuel cellular energy. The problem is that in the body of alcoholics or people with a high level of toxicity – of which there are vast numbers these days living on the planet given our exposure to toxic chemicals in the environment and our diet of junk foods – the body's ability to convert acetaldehyde into acetate is undermined. High levels of this chemical remain in the body and can cause a kind of poisoning which not only does physical damage but can severely distort mental perceptions.

TOUGH JOB

Cleaning acetaldehyde from your system is no easy task. No matter what the cause, you need truly adequate supplies of coenzyme A, niacinamide and pyridoxal-b-5-phosphate (the active form of vitamin B_6):

- ❑ Coenzyme A™: 3 capsules a day
- ❑ niacinamide: 1000mg three times a day
- ❑ pyridoxal-b-5-phosphate: 50mg twice a day

INSIDIOUS DESTROYER

Acetaldehyde can combine with your red blood cells, enzymes, proteins and even the gut lining itself, travelling through the bloodstream where it has devastating actions on the brain. Cigarette smokers are continually at risk of acetaldehyde poisoning, which alters the structure of blood cells and interferes with the body's oxygen carrying capacity. It also screws up the body's ability to produce 'feel good' prostaglandins like prostaglandin E1. Another of its disturbing effects on the brain is that it alters normal brain function by combining with two key neurotransmitters, *dopamine* and *serotonin*.

Dopamine is the neurotransmitter essential for good motor coordination, motivation, insulin regulation, immune function, short-term memory, clear thinking, physical energy and balance in motion. Serotonin is one of the two neurotransmitters that look after learning and memory, calming the brain and the rest of the body. It plays a vital role in regulating appetite and sleep. When high levels of acetaldehyde are secreted into the system by yeasts and fungi who produce it as a waste product, it can turn emotional behaviour upside down, altering some people's perceptions so greatly that the whole of their lives become distorted. Yet very seldom is such an experience traced back to its cause. Instead, people tend to be filled full of anti-depressants, tranquillisers and other drugs which only serve to make the body more toxic.

MASTER ADDICTOR

Acetaldehyde reduces the level of coenzyme A in your body, impairing your cells' energy producing capacity. It also promotes addiction to toxic substances from cigarettes and alcohol to drugs because of its ability to combine in the brain with dopamine and serotonin. So powerful can be the addictive prompting that comes from high levels of acetaldehyde that many experts believe this phenomenon is responsible for other addictions as well those not apparently chemical in origin, such as eating disorders and compulsive behaviour – perhaps even religious fanaticism.

In 1977, I was a graduate student at the University of Texas Medical Centre (School of Public Health) in Huston, Texas. I had the opportunity to observe many cancer patients at the M D Anderson Tumour Institute . . . Many (perhaps most) had Candidaisis. The Candidaisis was not the cause of their cancer, rather it was part of their lowered resistance that had likely contributed to the cancer itself. Most sick people have yeast overgrowth . . . so as our population continues to develop more and more degenerative ailments, what do we do? As a culture ultimately, in addition to treating the effects of our lifestyle e.g. the yeast, at some point the way of life in this country led by so many folks has got to be changed in some very fundamental ways.

Paul A Goldberg

CANDIDAISIS TAKES HOLD

Candidaisis frequently takes hold after any kind of surgery, mostly because large doses of antibiotics are used in order to prevent post-operative infection. This is also true of antibiotic treatment given for various conditions in the body. What happens is the antibiotics don't just kill of the bad guy bacteria they are supposed to target, they also wipe out the good guys needed by our intestinal tract for the colony of flora to maintain a balance beneficial to our health. After any form of antibiotic treatment – and except in life threatening situations I believe there is little reason to use antibiotics – your intestine needs to be recolonised with the good guy microbes such as *Lactobaccillus acidophilus* and *Bifidis*. Candida albicans and the other yeast and fungi are opportunistic organisms. They invade at the first sign of immune weakening. Doctors, aware of the ubiquitous nature of Candidaisis, report the problem exists in numerous patients apparently suffering from other illnesses. Just how much the Candidaisis is a result of these organisms and how much the perpetrator, no-one yet is sure.

GUT INSTINCT

Few people realise we have a *second brain*. Called the *enteric nervous system*, it was only articulated less than five years ago by Michael D. Gershon MD, Chairman of Anatomy and Cell Biology at Colombia University College of Physicians and Surgeons. This primitive nervous system, located in our gastrointestinal tract, is incredibly complex. It boasts hundreds of millions of nerve cells – more than all the rest of the body put together – and is colonised by thousands of different species of micro flora. Depending on whether they are 'goodies' or 'baddies' they either help protect our bodies from illness and degeneration, or toss us headlong into it. Fatigue, depression, addictions, obesity, hormonal disturbances and mental disorders can all develop when the second brain gets out of whack. For it is responsible for maintaining the biological terrain that protects us from illness and degeneration.

Candida is best controlled through a combination of diet and medicines, either prescription, or non-prescription. One of the reasons Age Power's Insulin Balance works so quickly to enhance energy levels and improve the way most people feel, is that in addition to countering insulin resistance and blood sugar problems, it also encourages a decrease in any Candida overgrowth that may be present. It stops feeding these beasties the carbs and sugars on which they thrive. However, in moderate or serious overgrowth of Candida, more than this alone is needed. The standard anti-fungal prescription drugs used often address the symptoms rather than correcting the problem. For this can only be done by changing the biological terrain of your body so that it no longer lends itself to Candida's continued growth and reproduction.

THE STRESS FACTOR

Severe or chronic stress, the loss of a job for instance, or the exposure to various chemicals, emotional upset and allergies – even constipation or diarrhoea – are all factors that, because they influence your resistance to infection, can also encourage an overgrowth of Candida.

AMAZING ADAPTOR

What few are as yet aware of – even the growing number of physicians who do address the Candida issue – is that Candida albicans has six switching mechanisms and seven viable forms, thanks to the amazing ability of yeast and fungi to metamorphose. In effect, they change shape and function according to their surrounding environment. There is even a form of Candida which is cell wall deficient. In this form it is not recognised by the human immune system so that it floats around freely in the bloodstream. When it finds a suitable place to reproduce, it then changes into one of the other six forms, providing a constant focus of infection. One of the problems with only treating the intestinal tract for Candida – as most doctors still do – is that, because of this ability to migrate around the body unnoticed, you still get a constant return of the organisms even after a 'cure' is supposed to have taken place.

THE WHOLE NINE YARDS

Someone who is systemically affected with Candidaisis can have the organism spread throughout his or her tissues in any of these possible forms. For each different form tends to thrive in specific tissues and systems of the body.

MASTER SURVIVORS

Candida albicans and other primitive organisms of opportunity like it, have been gifted with so many switching organisms because they, like the rest of life, have a passionate need to survive. And a powerful species they are, even more powerful than cockroaches and sharks (who appeared on the scene much later in evolution). They are able to thrive almost anywhere. Yeasts and fungi, which have successfully populated the earth for hundreds of millions of years before the human body arrived, know how to hold on.

Gus J Prosch, an American physician and expert on Candida's behaviour, has written a fascinating paper called *System Candidaisis – The Fungus Amongus*. He says, 'Every human being from the day of birth lives in a sea of bacteria. Infectious germs known as microbes swim throughout our bodies at all times. These microbes can live in our throat, mouth, nose, gums, gastrointestinal tract, blood, bladder, vagina and numerous other body tissues. These micro-organisms which may be bacteria, viruses, fungi, or parasites, are as much a part of every human being as foods and chemicals. Figuratively speaking, they are constantly trying to "eat us alive". In some people they succeed and death follows. Even if we die of causes other than infection, they eventually eat our physical remains. Only healthy cells and tissues within our bodies can effectively defend against infectious microbes.' Since the Candidaisis syndrome produces so many symptoms that involve multiple organs and systems in the human body it is now being labelled *Polysystemic Chronic Candidaisis*.

LESSONS FROM AIDS

Like all primitive micro-organisms, Candida has a powerful will to survive. It will breach normal defence systems invading the skin and decreasing the level of protective white blood cells, to invade the deep tissues and the blood stream. Until the past ten years, most doctors did not believe that Candida could invade the body's tissues. Since AIDS, this has changed. Autopsies on AIDS victims – whose bodies become riddled with the organisms as their immune system is so compromised – show that it *can* invade. It ends up destroying the brain tissue, the lungs, the liver and just about everything else. As a result savvy physicians are working hard to take a second look at the Candida problem to try to learn more about how to treat this condition.

All arthritics, by virtue of their weakened immune system, suffer from Candidaisis, or 'organisms of opportunity similar to Candidaisis'.

James P Carter MD

The point that Prosch is making in relation to the dangers of micro-organism infestation is important. He is pointing out that in the world in which we live, infectious illness attacks our bodies not just because the germs are there, but rather because the biological terrain within us is nutritionally deficient and debilitated in ways that *allow* these microbes to set up residence. To put it simply, an opportunistic germ only produces disease when the circumstances in our bodies are favourable to its growth.

FINDING OUT

The classical test still used to identify Candida albicans overgrowth, a stool culture, seldom gives accurate results. Orian Truss reports that where Candidaisis is suspected because a patients' symptoms suggest it, a clinical trial of an anti-Candida programme is best carried out, since stool cultures often lead to misdiagnosis. Some doctors use a urine test known as the *indican test* to diagnose the condition since it is known that as Candida overgrowth clogs up the villi of the intestinal mucosa, it produces a gas known as *indol*. When Candida is present, this gas is absorbed into the blood stream and carried through the kidneys so it can be detected in a patient's urine. Some doctors believe this gives them a fairly good idea of whether or not Candida is a problem. Most who work with Candida, however, insist that the best way to identify it is through symptoms alone. These include nervousness, depression, fatigue, muscle aches, problems with the genital/urinary system as well as food sensitivities and sensitivities to chemicals in the environment and to perfumes. Fungal and yeast toxins play a major role in causing allergies, prostate, vaginal and bladder infections as well as headaches and nervous system problems. Arthritis and rheumatic conditions strongly point the finger towards Candida.

CANDIDA OVERGROWTH FACTORS

Here are some of the factors which are most common in people with chronic yeast syndrome. How many apply to you?

- ❏ Acne
- ❏ Blood sugar disorders
- ❏ Chronic digestive problems such as bloating or gas
- ❏ Constipation or diarrhoea
- ❏ Craving for alcohol
- ❏ Craving for high glycaemic carbs
- ❏ Cravings for sweets, breads or alcohol
- ❏ Decreased libido
- ❏ Depression
- ❏ Diabetes Mellitus
- ❏ Eating a lot of sugar
- ❏ Emotional mood swings, confusion and depression
- ❏ Endocrine disturbances
- ❏ Eczema
- ❏ Food reactions such as food allergies
- ❏ Frequent or long-term use of antibiotics for recurrent infections or the treatment of acne
- ❏ Frequent use of cortisone related drugs and ulcer drugs
- ❏ General malaise
- ❏ Insufficient digestive secretions
- ❏ Impaired immune function
- ❏ Irritable bowel syndrome
- ❏ Irritability
- ❏ Lack of digestive enzymes
- ❏ Long-term fatigue
- ❏ Long-term use of the Pill in women
- ❏ Multiple allergies
- ❏ PMS
- ❏ Rectal itch
- ❏ Recurrent skin fungus problems such as athlete's foot or nail problems or genital itching
- ❏ Recurrent vaginal yeast in women and recurrent problems in the prostate in men
- ❏ Sensitivity to cigarette smoke
- ❏ Sensitivity to dampness and smells
- ❏ Syndrome X

YEAST FREE OR NOT

The medical diagnosis of chronic Candidaisis is difficult to make because there is no single specific diagnostic test for it and because many doctors still know very little about it. Their medical training has taught them to diagnose and name specific diseases – 'arthritis', 'diabetes', 'manic depression'. Such naming is often only useful in identifying groups of symptoms and prescribing drugs for them. Many physicians are not trained to recognise the underlying clinical distortions to your body's biological terrain that has allowed these disease symptoms to develop. It is your body's biological terrain that must be changed to genuinely cure a disease. That is what an effective anti-Candida programme needs to do.

Here are also some common symptoms that give a strong indication of whether or not there is a Candida overgrowth in your body.

CHECK YOUR SYMPTOMS

Score yourself: 1 = seldom; 2 = sometimes; 3 = often. Ignore those which do not apply to you.

❑ Blurred vision	❑ Low libido
❑ Cough	❑ Light headedness
❑ Depression	❑ Menstrual irregularities
❑ Diarrhoea	❑ Mood swings
❑ Drowsiness	❑ Muscle or joint aches
❑ Dry mouth	❑ Muscle weakness
❑ Exhaustion	❑ PMS
❑ Flagging memory	❑ Poor concentration
❑ Genital itch	❑ Prostatitis
❑ Headaches	❑ Recurrent infection
❑ Heartburn	❑ Tingling or numbness
❑ Impotence	❑ Tummy ache
❑ Indigestion	❑ Vaginitis

PAST IMPERFECT

Now let's look at your present and your past. For each yes answer to the questions below, add ten points.

- ❏ Are you a sugar lover?
- ❏ Do you react badly to the smell of perfumes and chemical fumes?
- ❏ Do you take or have you taken the Pill?
- ❏ Have you taken or are you taking HRT?
- ❏ Have you taken broad spectrum antibiotics for more than 10 days in the past three years?
- ❏ Do you crave alcohol?
- ❏ Have you taken steroid drugs in the past year?
- ❏ Do you frequently feel helpless?
- ❏ Has your interest in sex decreased?
- ❏ Do you often feel weak?
- ❏ Do you get mouth ulcers?
- ❏ Do you get pain in your stomach?
- ❏ Do you have trouble thinking clearly?
- ❏ Do you often feel light-headed?
- ❏ Does your heart beat irregularly?
- ❏ Do you get cramps with your periods?
- ❏ Do you feel worse when the weather is damp or you are in a damp house?
- ❏ Does cigarette smoke make you feel unwell?
- ❏ Have you ever had athletes foot or fungal infections on hands or skin?
- ❏ Do your muscles ache often?
- ❏ Do you often feel depressed?
- ❏ Do you get regular headaches?
- ❏ Do you have more than two mercury amalgam fillings in your teeth?
- ❏ Do you have joint aches sometimes?
- ❏ Do you have a poor memory?

Now total the number of points from both quizzes. If your score is less than 60, Candida overgrowth is unlikely to be a problem for you.

If it is between 60 to 100, you probably have more Candida in your body than is healthy. Staying away from sugar, sweets and too much fruit may well be enough to clear it within a few weeks.

If your score is above 150, you may need to take serious action to clear Candida from your system.

RECLAIMING POWER

Clearing Candida requires a major life change. The good news is that change that comes about through a good anti-Candida programme can be so health-enhancing, that many people who experience it claim it quite literally changes their life. People who had not been able to think clearly, who suffered from aches and pains and from allergies to chemicals in the environment as well as food sensitivities, find they can lead a normal life. They can think more rationally and they no longer experience unpredictable emotional upsets. People who have long been overweight find, often for the first time in their life, they have shed excess fat. People whose candidaisis has been cleared often report that the sense that they have long had that they had no control over their lives and who were unable to make clear choices, is now gone. They now move into an experience of personal power that they seldom dreamed possible. Clear headed and emotionally balanced with energy to spare, they now look forward to a life in which they are at the helm.

TO EAT OR NOT TO EAT

There are certain foods you need absolutely to avoid when fighting Candida. They include any gluten containing grains such as wheat, oats, rye and barley. The fungus grows on and is fed by yeast moulds and yeasty foods which cross-react with it.

Eat plenty of garlic and onions (yeasts don't like them either) and only lean cuts of meat (preferably organic) and fresh fish as well as game. For salads and vegetables, don't use vinegar. Instead, go for lemon juice for your dressings. Eat only real butter. Steer clear of all of the margarines and butter substitutes.

HOW TO CLEAR IT

The successful treatment of an overgrowth of Candida needs a four pronged attack. All four aspects need to be strictly followed otherwise, experience shows, it just won't work. This is not always the easiest thing to do either. For people with an overgrowth of the yeast/fungus sometimes have difficulty sticking to the commitment they make to change their lifestyle. Their brains are sometimes so much at the mercy of the confusion, muddled thinking and lack of clarity that accompanies the high levels of ethanol and acetaldehyde produced by the Candida, that it can be difficult for them to take consistent action. The four steps to clearing Candida are:

❑ Starve out the fungus with a proper diet, at the same time using natural forms of treatment to wipe out the ineffective agent.

❑ Rebuild your immune system and restore the integrity of metabolism using specific vitamins, minerals and fatty acids which Candida overgrowth has created.

❑ Recolonise normal gut flora. To keep Candida from re-establishing its hold on the body, it's essential to use a *good quality* form of Lactobacillus acidophilus and other good guy bacteria – preferably in powder form – to build up the good bacteria in the intestine as well as in the mouth and throat. Capsules don't do this as well as the powder. These probiotic supplements need to be refrigerated at all times. They are living organisms.

❑ Stay away from the perpetrators of Candida overgrowth. This means avoiding all forms of antibiotics – except in life and death situations – hormones and steroids as well as any foods that you might be allergic too.

MAJOR THINGS TO AVOID

☐ Don't eat any standard form of sugar or any foods containing it including fructose, glucose, maltose and lactose.

☐ Don't eat corn, barley, oats, rye or wheat or anything made from it and steer clear of rice, potatoes, buckwheat, beans and corn until your body is completely clear of the infection. (Have a bowl of porridge made from steel cut organic oats once a day if you like.)

☐ Stay away from milk and all milk products except butter and plain unsweetened natural yoghurt.

☐ Eat nothing with yeast in it – this includes bread, pastries, cakes, rolls, hamburger buns, crackers and biscuits.

☐ Avoid all foods – except whole apple cider vinegar – which have been fermented, smoked, cured or contain yeast. This includes smoked fish, proprietary mayonnaise, most salad dressings, tomato ketchup, pickles and other condiments.

☐ Don't drink fruit juices or colas – even those without sugar.

☐ Be sure to choose top quality vitamins and mineral supplements that are yeast free and do not contain unnecessary additives.

☐ Avoid high glycaemic fruits – including dried fruits – and use low glycaemic fruits like berries only in limited amounts until the Candida is cleared. (See page 219.)

☐ Steer clear of melon, such as cantaloupe, rockmelon and watermelon as their skins accumulate mould during growth.

☐ Don't eat chocolate, honey, maple syrup and nuts – they tend to accumulate mould.

☐ Eat no mushrooms or fungal products of any kind.

☐ Black tea is notoriously loaded with yeast – steer clear of it.

☐ Do not drink alcohol of any kind, as it contains sugar and yeast.

GREAT VEGETABLES

These vegetables are great on any anti-Candida programme:

Artichokes	Endive
Asparagus	Fennel
Aubergine	Green beans (fresh)
Bamboo shoots	Green herbs (fresh)
Bok choy	Kelp and seaweeds
Broccoli	Mung bean sprouts
Broccoli sprouts	Parsley
Brussels sprouts	Peppers
Cabbage	Rocket
Cauliflower	Silverbeet
Celery	Snowpea sprouts
Chicory	Spinach
Dandelion	Watercress

Age Power's Insulin Balance forms the basis of anti-Candida eating because it supports the body at such a high level of well-being, keeps blood sugar and insulin low and is free of high glycaemic carbs. It is rich in the omega-3 fats DHA and EPA which yeasts and moulds hate. It is essential during the period of Candida clearance that you avoid the list of foods on page 130. Three months or more down the road, once the Candida has been cleared, you can experiment by introducing some of the good foods (not the ones that are excluded, in any case, from Age Power's Insulin Balance) and see how you get on with them. Everyone is unique. You have to play this by ear and feel your way.

GO FOR ENERGY

Most of the things you do on the Age Power programme – from Age Power's Insulin Balance to enhancing lean body mass – make your body into an unfriendly home for Candida. Like the beer-bellied TV sports enthusiast, these primordial beasties prefer crisps and colas. Green vegetables are anathema to them. So are the omega-3 fish oils DHA & EPA. If you suspect Candidaisis, it is useful to take note of the following advice since it does not contradict the general guidelines for good eating and has made an enormous difference in the lives of many people who, unbeknownst to them, are being made miserable by this condition:

Drop the drugs: Don't take antibiotics, steroids, birth control pills or standard drug-based HRT unless there is an absolute medical necessity.

Change your diet: Don't feed Candida on foods they love. This means avoid like the plague any refined carbohydrate foods like white flour, refined sugars such as corn syrup and glucose, fruit juices and honey. Steer clear of milk products, baked foods made with wheat flour, and all foods to which you suspect you might be allergic or sensitive.

Never eat foods which have a high yeast content: Avoid alcohol, cheese, peanuts, dried fruits, grapes and yeast breads.

Eat lots of low glycaemic fresh vegetables: and eat as much as you like of fish and game, lamb, turkey, chicken (all preferably organic), eggs, lemon, garlic and butter.

Limit fruits: to no more than two pieces a day chosen from apples, berries and pears, until symptoms have gone.

Check for food sensitivities: Food sensitivities are common with Candida. The things you crave are frequently what the yeast itself craves. Try to identify any possible sensitivities and weed them out. This can help a lot.

Drink Pau d'Arco: This tea from the South American tree has a long folk use in the treatment of infections probably thanks to its *lapachol* content. Both lapachol and other compounds from Pau d'Arco have demonstrated anti-Candida effects. Drink some several times a day.

Add a good probiotic supplement (see Resources, see page 482).

Get help: If these things do not make a significant difference then seek out a good nutritionist or nutritionally orientated doctor who is genuinely knowledgeable about the treatment of Candida.

Use digestive enzymes *amylase, protease, lipase* **and** *bromelin*: These are essential to break down the foods you eat into usable nutrients, especially where there is a Candida overgrowth which depletes hydrochloric acid and digestive enzymes in the stomach.

Take heart: Once the Candida is under control you will probably be able to eat almost everything you like so long as you continue to steer clear of unnecessary drugs and highly processed convenience foods. But be patient. It takes time for nature to rebalance your body from inside out.

SUPPLEMENTAL HELP

Specific natural products – from psyllium husk fibre, which helps clean the inside of the gut, to anti-oxidants such a *alpha lipoic acid* and even the old fashioned bismuth, which helps heal the intestine – are an important part of a good anti-Candidaisis programme. Here are some of the most important:

Zinc piccolinate or citrate	25mg or more a day
Alpha Lipoic acid	100mg or more twice a day
L-glutamine	1–6g a day on an empty stomach
Essential oil of oregano	2 drops under tongue twice a day

Olive leaf extract	100mg twice a day with food
Omega Fish oils	3 capsules or more twice a day
Digestive enzymes	2 capsules after every meal
Caprylic acid	600mg with each meal
Cellulase enzymes and Hemicellulase enzymes	100,000 IU of each an hour before breakfast and just before bed
Flaxseed oil	2 teaspoons a day

A good multiple vitamin and mineral formula is also important to help restore levels lost to the invading micro-organisms. When choosing a supplement it is best to go for a food-based multiple such as *Vita Synergy for Men* or *Vita Synergy for Women*. They are lower in nutrient doses than chemically made vitamins but far more bioavailable so you can get away with less. Whatever you do, don't use any supplement with *steric acid* in it. Read labels.

Don't forget, you will not be able to get rid of Candidaisis unless you continually clear acetaldehyde from your system using supplements of Coenzyme-A™, niacinamide and pyridoxal-b-5 (see page 117).

BE AWARE

The chemicals which are by-products of yeast and fungi metabolism have opioid characteristics. They create a situation of *substance abuse* within the body. They affect the hypothalamus in the brain so that your appetite becomes changed. Instead of longing for good quality food, you find yourself reaching for junk stuff and sugars. In the presence of someone smoking, you may find yourself wanting a cigarette thanks to the reaction of your body to the acetaldehyde in cigarette smoke. You may find yourself taking up the practice without understanding why. Nicotine also replaces nicotinic acid in the body. The body will eventually get to the point where it opts for nicotine over nicotinic acid – further increasing addiction and depleting your system of this essential B vitamin. So long as the yeast and fungi are being fed the yeasts and sugars they thrive on, things can remain relatively calm in a body. It is much the same way the alcoholic can be charming so long as he's sipping a drink. When yeasts become deprived of these goodies, however – as when you first switch over to Age Power's Insulin Balance eating – these beasties which have been exerting major levels of control over your behaviour and thoughts, can raise their ugly heads to make you feel worse temporarily. This is called a *die-off reaction*. It is akin to the detoxification that takes place in the alcoholic during the dry-out period. It will pass soon leaving you much better.

PAINFUL IRONY

One dreadful irony about the way our modern medicine developed from the time that Louis Pasteur created the germ theory of disease – and something that very few doctors are aware of – is this: For many years, Pasteur and another great French scientist Claude Bernard, debated over whether or not disease was caused by an invasion of a pathogen (as Pasteur claimed) or whether disease was caused primarily by a disruption in the body's biological terrain and metabolic processes which allowed microbes to grow. As far as nineteenth- and twentieth-century science is concerned, Pasteur won the argument. Yet on his deathbed, the great scientist repudiated everything that he had ever written and insisted that Bernard was right. The pathogen is nothing, terrain is everything.

An overgrowth of Candida albicans is a perfect example of how accurate Claude Bernard's view can be. The mistake that Louis Pasteur made created contemporary orthodox medicine, which primarily addresses the symptomatic treatment of a condition rather than seeking to restore good quality biological terrain so that no pathogen can take hold. Missing this point is a major reason why so many contemporary treatments for degenerative diseases fail miserably. Despite all of our high tech methods, we still have a lot to learn.

Let's take a look at the lifestyle demands our genetic inheritance place upon us when it comes to establishing the best biological terrain.

> Conventional treatment for Candida infections primarily involves antifungal agents such as clotrimazole, administered locally for thrush and oesophageal involvement, nystatin, for bowel therapy and other drugs for systemic infections. To avoid the side-effects of these agents . . . many practitioners use natural substances, herbals, homeopathy and acupuncture as possible alternatives.
>
> *Raymond Keith Brown MD*

PART THREE:
LIFE
SOURCE

ANCESTRAL GIFTS

By understanding the past, we have a starting point by which to understand
our basic dietary requirements. From that starting point, we can gain a
sense of direction for the present and the future. It is important to
remember that human beings co-evolved with their foods. In other words,
we all grew up together, in effect, on the same street on Earth, and we are
genetically dependant on the nutrients in simple, whole foods.

Jack Challem, Burton Berkson MD, Melissa Diane Smith

We need to look back in time to our Paleolithic ancestors
who lived 15,000 to 40,000 years ago, to find the answers
to the question, 'What kind of diet will promote the finest
genetic expression in our bodies, protect them from premature ageing and reverse degenerative changes when they
have already happened?'

Countless studies in paleopathology and archaeology show without doubt
that our primitive ancestors – going back a million years and more – lived
on a diet of flesh foods and fats together with whatever fibre-rich vegetables, herbs, seeds, roots and berries were available. Scientists estimate
that between 60 and 90 percent of the calories early men and women
took in came in the form of large and small game animals, eggs, birds,
reptiles and insects. Starchy vegetables like the modern potato and starchy
grains like our modern day rice did not exist. Examination of the remains
of these hunter-gatherers show that early man had superb bone structure,
flawless teeth and heavy musculature. And, whether our political and religious leanings like it or not, this protein-oriented flesh-based fare is the
diet on which our bodies appear to thrive. For it is on such a diet that
the forces of natural selection have refined and molded us to function
best. This is where our biological terrain was formed. To put it another
way, we have been genetically programmed to eat like this for at least ten
thousand centuries.

STONE AGE HEALTH NUTS

Our Paleolithic ancestors ate so well that today they might be accused of being food fanatics. Theirs was a diet far in excess of the official recommendations today for vitamins and minerals, essential fatty acids and high quality proteins. They had never seen or heard of refined carbohydrates such as sugar or flour – they did not exist. The odd bit of honey which they were able to steal from wild bees was all the sweet they knew. They never consumed milk products except at their mother's breast, they ate more than 200 different kinds of plants (we eat on average 18) and more protein than we get today: fish and shellfish, wild animals large and small, insects and grubs – all rich in omega-3 essential fatty acids. Their foods were fresh and most were eaten raw. Although they often died young from famine or cold or violence, they had great biological terrain, were tall, strong, and experienced no tooth decay or bone loss as we do now from an early age.

GO WILD, GO FREE

The physiology of the body has changed little over the millennia. We are still genetically adapted to wild foods and good protein – if eaten raw – not to the refined and processed stuff we now consume. Examining the skeletal remains of early hunter-gatherers, Paleopathologists – those who study the eating patterns of humans in relation to health and disease – have determined that pre-agricultural people were robust and about the same size as people are today. Their diet was three times higher in protein than ours and often – although not always – lower in fat. Not only was their protein to carbohydrate ratio much lower than ours, their fibre intake was much higher – around 100 grams a day compared to the 20 grams we eat today. The foods they ate were fibre-rich, unprocessed, unrefined non-starchy herbs and vegetables and non-sugary fruits.

PRIMITIVE MEANS HIGH FIBRE

There are many benefits to the high fibre foods our ancestors ate which we need for Age Power:

- ☐ They demand more chewing and slower eating.
- ☐ They satisfy your appetite and counter overeating.
- ☐ They buffer natural sugars preventing sharp increases in glucose and insulin associated with Syndrome X.
- ☐ They release glucose into the blood slowly.

Their calcium intake was higher than ours, even though dairy products did not exist and they got more potassium than we do. Early human vitamin C intake is estimated to have been 400 milligrams – several times higher than the government recommended daily requirement. And their intake of phyto-nutrients – the amazing plant factors from flavonoids to carotenoids with powerful anti-oxidant and immune-enhancing properties – was 300 times greater than ours. Even early man's polyunsaturated to saturated fat ratio was different. For the beasts they hunted, including small animals, birds, fish and insects were themselves high in polyunsaturated fats (especially omega-3s) – in marked contrast to the saturated fat meat from grain fed animals we eat now.

ALL CHANGE

Ten thousand years ago in the Middle East a massive change began to take place in man's diet. This was the beginning of the agricultural revolution. The spread of agriculture did not get into full swing until six thousand years later. A high degree of urbanisation occurred. Collect people together en-masse and you need to feed them from a small area. This meant relying heavily on carbohydrate foods, mostly in the form of starchy vegetables like potatoes and cereal crops like rice and wheat. Gradually cereals, fruits and starchy vegetables began to play a big part in human nutrition, and protein intake decreased dramatically. By then farmers had domesticated animals.

99.99 percent of our genes were formed before the development of agriculture.

Dr S Boyd Eaton, MD,
Medical Anthropologist

TOO FAST FOR HEALTH

Genes change slowly – over hundreds of thousands of years. The forces of natural selection have acted on us for millions of years, shaping and molding our genetic makeup and biochemical functioning. We have only been exposed to large volumes of high density carbohydrate foods like bread and rice for the last four thousand years.

Not only did agricultural man add grains, legumes and milk to his diet, the growth of farming meant he led a more sedentary lifestyle than his hunter-gatherer ancestors. It was all great for the development of civilisation. But not without cost: At that time the human body lost as much as six inches in stature and health began to deteriorate. There was also an upsurge in bone malformations, osteoporosis, tooth decay and cardio-vascular disease began to show up early on in people's lives.

SECRETS OF THE MAYANS

Anthropological studies carried out on the ancient Mayan Indians demonstrate just how costly, in terms of physique and health, the switch from a primarily meat-eating hunter-gatherer existence to an agricultural one, over-rich in cultivated grains and starchy vegetables, can be – especially for slaves and peasants who could not afford to eat scarce flesh foods. During the early Mayan civilisation meat was plentiful. At that time the average male skeleton was 165 centimetres tall. Later on, as the availability of meat became limited and agriculture developed, the height of the average lower class male – who now lived mostly on corn and beans – declined to 150 centimentres. Yet the stature of his ruling-class cousin, who could still afford to supplement his diet with animal protein, increased to 170 centimetres.

TWENTIETH CENTURY CHANGES

At the beginning of the twentieth century – when degenerative diseases like cardiovascular disease and diabetes were still uncommon – about 30 percent of the average Western diet came from dairy products, meat and eggs. Half of the population in North America lived on farms and raised domestic animals for food. These animals – chickens and pigs, cows and

---

DEGENERATION BEGINS

By the time the agricultural revolution was in full swing –
four thousand years ago – an enormous amount of degeneration had already taken place in the human body. Men and
women had shrunk in height. Dental decay and malformation
of the jaw had become widespread. Disease epidemics shortened human lifespan. This moment in history marks the
beginning of what we nowadays call the diseases of civilisation.

---

sheep – were neither given hormones nor chemicals to fatten them. They
were simply put out to pasture and let graze. The protein composition of
the diet of the people living then was not enormously different from that
of Paleolithic times except that their meats were not as lean and had a
lower level of the important omega-3 fatty acids. The other difference was
that twentieth-century man ate dairy products as well. Both groups of
people still fished the lakes and rivers and the sea and both hunted for
wild game.

IT GETS WORSE

Before long, however, meat farmers began to fatten their animals on soya
beans and corn – both of which are high in carbohydrates and in omega-
6 fatty acids – instead of letting them graze on natural grasses high in
omega-3s. Animals were not allowed to roam as widely. This combination
of a decrease in exercise and a cultivated grass and grain-based diet made them grow fat and significantly altered the quality of protein and the fatty acid profile of their meat. Men began to eat less fish and more beef and dairy products. Hormones and antibiotics were increasingly added to feeds to increase meat production. Herbicides and pesticides began to pollute the environment. Animals fed on crops treated with them ended up with pollutants in their flesh which we, in turn, take into our own bodies.

> The further we, as humans, have moved away from the Paleolithic diet, the more susceptible we have become to Syndrome X and other diet-dependant diseases. In a very real sense, the best anti-Syndrome X diet is the Paleolithic diet – or at least a more modern and convenient variation of it.
>
> Jack Challem,
> Burton Berkson MD,
> Melissa Diane Smith

A MODERN LOOK

In the nineteen thirties, when the American nutritional researcher and dentist Weston Price travelled the world searching out groups of people who remained largely untouched by civilisation, his travels took him from the mountains of Switzerland to the plains of Africa and the frozen tundra of the Eskimos. Everywhere isolated communities were living on primitive diets of natural, unrefined foods and were free of chronic disease. Although the diets of these people varied greatly from one area to another, they had certain things in common. Almost all of them contained liberal quantities of protein from seafood, game, meats and dairy products. And these people believed foods played an important part in their diet and were essential for good health. They also ate vegetables, legumes, nuts and seeds as well as whole grains – but in a fresh unrefined state. Also, every one of their diets boasted good quantities of raw foods – both of animal and vegetable origin.

Price reported that those who consumed a high protein diet showed virtually no dental decay and suffered little mental illness. Unlike twenty-first century man with his heart disease, diabetes, arthritis and gout, these were sturdy, strong people who produced healthy children generation after generation. Throughout his travels Price had many opportunities of comparing the bone structure, general health and longevity of these isolated peoples in relation to the kinds of natural foods they ate. Those whose diets consisted largely of legumes and grains, although much healthier than modern men in cities and developed areas, none-the-less had more dental problems, were smaller in stature and less healthy than those whose diets centered around protein foods such as fish and meat together with herbs and seeds and non-starchy vegetables.

> Our evolution over the eons has provided us with a digestive system which is based upon foods of the Paleolithic era and earlier. We can term our very genes Paleolithic, evolved to flourish from hunter-gatherer eating patterns. Only about 25 percent of mankind has adapted a body able to cope with the foods of the Age of Agriculture without obesity and all of its problems.
>
> *Richard L Heinrich*

> ## DO YOU HAVE THE THRIFTY GENE?
>
> The thrifty gene is a survival mechanism which enables the body to store energy long-term, and to make the most of any food that's eaten. It made it possible for ancient humans to live through times of famine, while those without it died off. In Paleolithic times, the thrifty gene was one of the greatest gifts a child could inherit from its parents. Now, in the face of an onslaught of convenience foods replete with refined carbohydrates, the thrifty gene people constantly struggle to get lean and stay that way.

SECRETS OF THE CAVE MAN

In the past two decades, Price's reports have been substantiated by studies of Paleopathologists who have examined the remains of pre-historic peoples in pre-agricultural times. They report that early human skulls were largely free of dental caries and abscesses – that is until the advent of agriculture when the levels of carbohydrates they ate went up. Such findings are helping scientists determine the 'ideal' diet for human health based on our biological inheritance and our genetic makeup. It is a diet higher in protein than the one we eat now and much lower in carbohydrate – a way of eating based on non-starchy low-glycaemic carbohydrates which do not readily cause insulin and blood sugar problems. It is also higher in vitamins and minerals, anti-oxidants and other phytonutrients, with a ratio of the essential fatty acids omega-3 and omega-6 very different to ours today.

ENTER FOOD MANUFACTURING

Carbohydrate foods are cheap to manufacture – they are also highly addictive. For more than half a century, food manufacturers intent on making a profit have been producing a great variety of palatable foods by fragmenting and reducing raw material foodstuffs – grains and seeds, fats and sugars, vegetables and legumes – to simple 'nuts and bolts'. These nuts and bolts are then whipped up into the manufactured convenience foods that we find on our supermarket shelves – from ready-to-eat meals in a minute, to chocolate bars, cakes, breads and cereals – in short, the stuff that makes up almost three quarters of what most people eat these

> An archaeologist is the best husband a woman can have; the older she gets, the more interested he is in her.
>
> *Agatha Christie*
> *(who was married to one)*

EAT FAT

In the nineteen fifties a British psychiatrist, Dr Richard Mackarness, revived interest in low-carbohydrate eating. His expertise lay in the field of food allergies and mental illness. He began to experiment with a low carbohydrate diet. Not only did it solve his own personal weight problem, it also cleared up many other ailments for which he had been unable to find a cure. Mackarness also discovered in the course of his psychiatric clinical work, that a low-carb and adequate protein diet exerted a significant improvement in the health of his mental patients too. In 1959 he wrote a book called *Eat Fat and Grow Slim* which became a best-seller. The diet he propounded, rich in protein, fresh non-starchy vegetables and essential fatty acids, worked wonders for his readers, yet his work was largely ignored by the medical community. Most doctors and government advisers on health still did not grasp the significance of what was going on: that the human body thrives on a low carbohydrate diet. That is because we are genetically programmed to thrive on such fare and not to handle massive doses of starchy, sugary carbs like muffins, bagels, pasta, breakfast cereals and sugar. Yet that is what we continue to eat. Why?

days. White flour and sugar-based convenience foods full of denatured fats have an ultra long shelf life. Yet these convenience foods are really junk foods, often devoid of any nutritional value other than calories. The processed fats they contain, along with the masses of artificial chemicals used as flavourings, colourings and preservatives, are far removed from the foods we need for health. It is little wonder many human beings today – even those in economically privileged countries – do little more than survive.

HERE COME THE CARBS

With the coming of agriculture, man shifted away from a high protein diet. As population grew, grains were necessary in order to survive. Once the agricultural revolution was in full swing, people began using grinding stones to grind their grains into flour. This was the beginning of food processing which made a big leap forward (or backward, depending on how you look at it) in the mid nineteenth century with the introduction of roller milling. Before that, only aristocrats ate fibre stripped white flour for it was very labour intensive to produce. After all, some peasant had to sit with a winnowing basket tossing the ground flour into the air to separate out the bran from the white stuff. As man consumed more carbohydrates and as these carbs were more processed, degenerative conditions such as heart disease and diabetes as well as obesity, once only known to the rich and royals, began to spread. With the introduction of roller milling, it became easier and cheaper to produce large quantities of white flour. The steel roller mill refined whole-wheat grains and sugar cane quickly and cheaply. The white products that were produced from refining held a fascination for the masses. They were not only pleasant to taste, they also carried a certain caché since it was only the rich and privileged who until then had been able to eat them.

As far back as the nineteen thirties, health professionals began to notice that people who used white bread as a staple in their diet tended to suffer from conditions related to nutritional deficiencies – especially deficiencies of vitamin B_1, B_2, B_3, calcium and iron. This led to governments insisting that white bread be 'enriched' – namely that some of the nutrients lost in refining flours had to be added back before bread was baked. Except the nutrients that were added back were vastly inferior to the nutrients lost in the processing. Calcium, for example, was added to white bread in the form of chalk, which the body does not absorb. The synergy of nutrients characteristic of natural unrefined foods – where the whole is greater than the sum of its nutrient parts – had also been destroyed. You cannot take one, two, three or four nutrients lost in processing and expect, by adding them back to a food whose intrinsic wholeness has been compromised, to restore nutritional value.

> The Food Pyramid, the icon the US government plasters on every flat surface in an effort to inspire Americans to eat less meat and fat, is badly in need of repair.
>
> *Loren Cordain PhD*

> Simply put, carbohydrate consumption has a direct effect on hormonal balance and, therefore, a direct effect on overall health. Yet most endocrinologists, those physicians who specialise in hormones, do not recognise the fact that carbohydrate consumption is that major dietary source of hormonal imbalance. Instead, multiple hormone supplements and various other drugs are prescribed to alleviate conditions that often can be resolved merely by a reduction of carbohydrates in the diet.
>
> *Christian B Allan PhD and Wolfgang Lutz MD*

SWEET AND NASTY

Take sugar – sugar is a highly refined substance which provides nothing but empty calories. We in the so-called civilised world eat between 22 and 88kg (50–200lbs) of the stuff per head per year. Both sugar and white flour are devoid of magnesium, chromium and zinc. These three minerals are absolutely essential for your body to be able to process carbohydrate foods properly. When you do not have adequate levels of these three, insulin resistance, premature ageing, obesity and degenerative diseases develop at an accelerated rate. The more industrialised and commercial in orientation our societies have become, the more processed carbohydrates have we eaten. The more processed carbohydrates we eat, the more our blood sugar and insulin levels get screwed up.

Tinned vegetables raise insulin and blood sugar more than fresh vegetables do. Concentrated fruit juices raise insulin and blood sugar more than fresh fruit does. Ever since Paleolithic times, our carbohydrates have become increasingly dense. This means that our foods have more and more grams of carbohydrate per serving in them and less and less fibre, as well as fewer nutrients such as chromium, important for blood sugar regulation. All of these changes have played a central role in the development of widespread obesity and the increasing incidence of Syndrome X. All of these issues need to be addressed if you are going to slow down the ageing process and improve your overall health.

RULE OF 20 YEARS

In the nineteen seventies, British surgeon Captain T. L. Cleave was hard at work charting dietary change as a director of medical research at the Institute of Naval Medicine. In 1974, he published a brilliant study called *The Saccharin Diseases* which is one of the most important books on health of the twentieth century. He carried out meticulous studies of hospital records of many of the world's nations, particularly in West Africa. He found that not one native experienced diseases common to Western cultures – obesity, colon cancer, gall-stones, diverticulitis, heart disease or diabetes. These diseases do not exist until refined high density carbohydrates enter a native diet. They appear almost exactly 20 years after introducing convenience foods. Within another 20 years, all of these diseases became widespread. Cleave dubbed this phenomena his 'Rule of 20 Years'. Recently Cleave's discourses have been validated by other studies of the Pima Indians in Arizona for instance, and in Saudi Arabia. The same phenomenon is taking place in India, Mexico, Japan and many other countries. However, Cleave's book is now out of print – another fine researcher whose work is still largely ignored to the detriment of human health throughout the world.

STEPS TOWARDS DEGENERATION

In the wake of Cleave's work, Dennis Burkitt and Hugh Trowell carried out their own extensive studies, taking things even further. They carefully documented the exact sequence of events which takes place when diet changes from primitive to convenience. Most of these changes revolve around shifts in the kind and ratio of carbohydrates that are being eaten.

Stage 1 – The primitive unprocessed diet of plant eaters complete with large quantities of unprocessed wild, low glycaemic carbohydrates and whole foods is eaten. There are very few examples of degenerative diseases.

Stage 2 – Western diet is introduced with refined carbohydrate and high glycaemic carbohydrates. Obesity and diabetes become common among privileged groups able to afford foods of commerce.

Stage 3 – Diet becomes moderately Westernised. Obesity becomes more widespread as do constipation, haemorrhoids, varicose veins and appendicitis.

Stage 4 – Western diet is now widespread. Being overweight and obesity are common in all social groups. So is heart disease, high blood pressure, diverticular disease, hiatus hernia, cancer and other Western diseases.

Q. What did the yogi say to the hot-dog vendor?

A. Make me one with everything.

Vogue magazine

Anthropologist Dr. Kathleen Gordon at the Smithsonian Institute in Washington D.C. puts it rather well when she says 'not only was the agricultural "revolution" not really so revolutionary at its inception, it has also come to represent something of a nutritional "devolution" for much of mankind'.

COMPARISON OF THE LATE PALEOLITHIC DIET AND THE CURRENT AMERICAN DIET

US Senate

	Late Paleolithic Diet*	Current American Diet
Total dietary energy (%)		
Protein	24	12
Carbohydrate	45	46
Fat	21	42
P:S ratio‡	1.41	0.44
Cholesterol (mg)	591	600
Fibre (g)	45.7	19.7±
Sodium (mg)	690	2300–6900
Calcium (mg)	1580	740§
Ascorbic acid (mg)	392.3	87.7§

* Assuming the diet contained 35 percent meat and 65 percent vegetables.

‡ P:S denotes polyunsaturated:saturated fats.

± British National Food Survey 1976.

§ U.S. Department of Agriculture Food Consumption Survey 1977-1978

Reprinted from 'Paleolithic Nutrition', Eaton & Konner, Jan. 31 1985, *New England Journal of Medicine and Surgery*. Copyright, 1985, Massachusetts Medical Society, All Rights Reserved.

AMERICANS GO FIRST

The United States led the way to the low-fat-high-carbs revolution in 1988 when in a wave of enthusiasm the U.S. Surgeon General officially directed all Americans to cut their consumption of fat – especially saturated fat – and increase the number of carbohydrates that they eat. The rationale was simple: Reduce fat intake to almost zero and you will leave behind heart disease, diabetes, obesity and most of the degenerative conditions plaguing modern man. It was based on studies which looked at animals and people who – for limited periods – were put on low-fat diets. These groups showed better cholesterol levels, weight loss and improved health. Sadly, the study had two major flaws: 1. Carry on eating such a diet for months or years and you develop fatty acid deficiencies to seriously undermine hormones, energy levels, skin and good health. 2. Virtually no-one – unless you happen to be a rat confined to a cage with no access to foods other than those provided – can live on such a diet long-term. People get hungry and crave sugar and carbohydrate. Some even develop food sensitivities or food allergies. And they begin to age, rapidly, and the rest of us just get fatter by the year. The now famous USDA Food Pyramid, still recommended by most English-speaking governments, is best avoided as a guide to how to eat well.

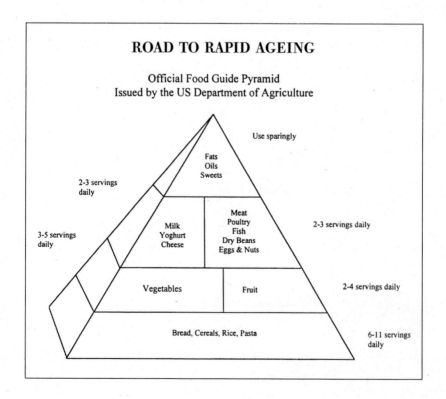

ROAD TO RAPID AGEING

Official Food Guide Pyramid
Issued by the US Department of Agriculture

Use sparingly

Fats
Oils
Sweets

2-3 servings
daily

Milk
Yoghurt
Cheese

Meat
Poultry
Fish
Dry Beans
Eggs & Nuts

2-3 servings daily

3-5 servings
daily

Vegetables

Fruit

2-4 servings daily

Bread, Cereals, Rice, Pasta

6-11 servings
daily

HOW TO AGE FAST

The twentieth century high carbohydrate, low fat, low protein diet is not good for long-term health. Here are some of the negative effects of living on it:

- ❏ Raised serum insulin levels causing insulin resistance, resulting in metabolic distortions which undermine health and vitality.
- ❏ Lowered basal metabolic rate leading to weight gain and low energy.
- ❏ Increases adipose tissue growth and reduction in lean muscle tissue.
- ❏ Acceleration of biological ageing.
- ❏ Development of common food allergies or sensitivities to grains and dairy food.
- ❏ Development of over-active immune system and eventual immune failure.
- ❏ Soaring incidence of degenerative diseases including heart disease, obesity and cancer.

Americans, like the rest of us, embraced the advice wholeheartedly. We have been munching our way through a low-fat-high-carbs universe ever since. Meanwhile, health statistics get worse. In the 10 years following the U.S. Attorney General's dietary directives, obesity in the United States tripled. Adult onset diabetes, otherwise known as Type II diabetes, soared while other degenerative diseases continued to mount. In fact so far, the only people who have benefited from the low-fat-high-carbs revolution are the food manufacturers. They whip up cheap and tasty no-fat products by adding lots of sugar and salt to cheap foodstuffs like flour and junk fats, then sell them – often at inflated prices – under the guise of 'healthy' foods. As we try to halt the march of degeneration in our bodies we buy more and more of their concoctions thinking they will do us good, all to no avail.

Gaining a little weight aren't you honey?

You're no cream puff yourself, dearie.

Two performing elephants, Dumbo

TIME TO QUIT

It is time to face facts: The high-carbohydrate-low-fat diet has proven itself a failure. It does not reduce cholesterol significantly as we have been told, unless it is followed in extremis – that is at the same time lowering the level of calories to something like 1000 to 1200 a day – a level impossible for the average person to maintain for more than a few weeks (and one which long-term can create deficiencies in essential nutrients). Such a diet causes problems with blood sugar levels and causes endless suffering to people with diabetes. It does not reduce high blood pressure either. That is unless you are consuming very little food. People who lose weight on a low-fat-high-carbs diet cannot keep it off. Yet the myth persists. We are stuck in a frustrating circle of mis-information and temptation. We need to strip away the myths and misap-prehensions and get 'back to basics'.

END TO MADNESS

At last we are beginning to emerge from low-fat-high-carbs junk food madness. A burgeoning body of medical research reveals startling information about the part just one hormone – insulin – plays in premature ageing and degenerative disease. Scientific research into Syndrome X and its impli-cations continues to uncover mistakes we have made over thousands of years in understanding our physical require-ments. To find out what our bodies really need we will have to turn back time to see how our ancestors responded to the basic human challenge – feeding life.

In recent years volumes of information and articles have appeared in books and on the net on largely-raw diets which include raw animal foods like fish and meat as well as raw plant products. Proponents claim that such a way of eating:

☐ Helps recovery from degenerative conditions
☐ Brings rapid healing from illness
☐ Increases vitality

It is important that students bring a certain ragamuffin barefoot irreverence to their studies; they are not here to worship what is known, but to question it.

J Bronowski

THE WAY FORWARD

It is time to go back to the future to get out of the mess we are in. We need to make major shifts in both the ratio of proteins to carbohydrates and fats that we are taking, as well as the kinds of foods that we are eating. It is not practical for us to try and live on a diet of only 1800 calories a day or to try and precisely measure every nutrient we eat. There is a better way – Age Power's Insulin Balance.

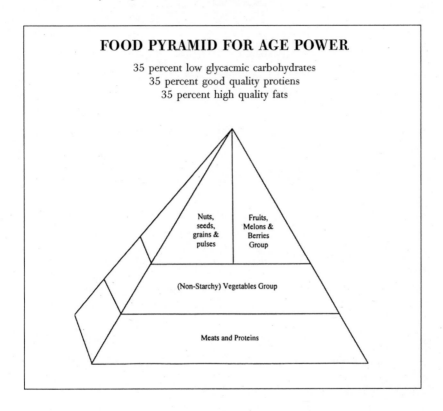

FOOD PYRAMID FOR AGE POWER

35 percent low glycacmic carbohydrates
35 percent good quality protiens
35 percent high quality fats

Nuts, seeds, grains & pulses

Fruits, Melons & Berries Group

(Non-Starchy) Vegetables Group

Meats and Proteins

GARBAGE IN, GARBAGE OUT

Why is it that lemon pie filling and lemonade are made with
'artificial lemon flavouring', but dish soap and furniture
polish are made with fresh lemon juice?

Bruce Johnson

There is a well-known saying about computers: 'garbage in, garbage out.' The same can be said of your body. It is no use thinking of food as if it were dead, indifferent fuel. Lots of people do. They assume so long as you get the 'right' quantity of calories, protein, and fats, plus a few vitamins, that's all you need to worry about. It is a deadly inaccurate assumption.

Feed yourself on highly processed convenience foods grown on chemically-treated soils and not only will you age quickly, you will feel only half alive. Feed yourself on foods rich in the ineffable power of life from fresh foods and you rejuvenate. It's 'Life in Life out' that matters for Age Power. Every day, a report appears in the scientific or the popular press linking junk fats with arteriosclerosis. Another stresses the importance of fresh, non-starchy vegetables like broccoli and greens as well as fruits and fibre in protecting yourself from stroke and cancer, diabetes and early ageing. By now, both the medical profession and general public are beginning to be more aware that there is a lot wrong with the average diet. But what few people are yet aware of is that the *state* and *quality* of the foods you eat is the single most important issue in determining how slowly or rapidly you age. Is it fresh? Was it grown in healthy soil? Has it been processed? Is it raw or has it been cooked? And if so, how?

One of the problems people face in reversing Syndrome X is perceptual: the long-held belief that food has relatively little to do with the development and progression of disease and the maintenance of health. In contrast, we believe – and are supported with overwhelming scientific evidence – that the quality of our foods has a direct and fundamental bearing on the quality of our health, more so even than the genes we inherit.

Jack Challem, Burton Berkson MD, Melissa Diane Smith

THE TYRANNY OF COMMERCE

Why then do we continue to eat the foods we do? It is partly because we have lost track of common sense and partly because we are bombarded by propaganda from nutritional food manufacturers who sell us foods that may be great for their bottom line but are an absolute disaster for *our* bottom line. A lot has happened to our foods in the last century. First, food is *grown* differently from the way our ancestors for thousands of years grew theirs. We grow it in chemically fertilised soils in which the organic matter has been degraded or destroyed. Eating foods grown in this way leads to a depletion and imbalance in the minerals and trace elements available to our bodies – both of which we need in good quantities to support the complex metabolic processes on which a long and healthy life depends. These are not the foods we as human beings have been genetically programmed to thrive on over a million years of evolution. Therefore they do not produce the highest genetic expression nor support optimal well-being. Second, our foods are now highly *processed.* Raw foodstuffs, instead of being made into meals in home kitchens as they used to be, are now sent to food manufacturers where they are fragmented then put through complex processes which alter them out of all recognition. Third, our foods are shipped over long distances and stored for long periods of time, both of which dramatically degrades nutritional value.

These practices destroy a food's *wholesomeness* – a property hard to measure except in terms of the degenerative effects that eating such foods has on our bodies, yet vitally important for Age Power. Destroy a food's wholesomeness and you destroy its ability to support the highest levels of health year after year. Once the health-giving integrity of any food has gone, it has gone for good.

> Your nutrition can determine how you look, act and feel; whether you are grouchy or cheerful, homely or beautiful, physiologically and even psychologically young or old; whether you think clearly or are confused, enjoy your work or make it a drudgery, increase your earning power or stay in an economic rut. The foods you eat make the difference between your day ending with freshness which lets you enjoy a delightful evening or with exhaustion which forces you to bed with the chickens.
>
> *Adelle Davis*

DEGENERATE NOW

The typical Western diet is based on 'foods of commerce' –
the type of food you can buy at the local corner shop and in
run-of-the-mill supermarkets. These foods are very different
from the simple foods that our bodies have become genetically adapted to over thousands of years. Modern convenience
foods are high in fat and depleted of natural fibre. They
consist of highly refined carbohydrates like white bread and
packaged cereals spiked with lots of sugar and junk fats –
oils which have been separated out from their source food
and chemically altered by solvents and heat processing. We
also swallow a kaleidoscope of chemical colourants, flavourings, additives and 'enhancers', not to mention pesticides,
herbicides and fungicides which our ancestors could not have
imagined in their wildest dreams. Our bodies are not genetically equipped to handle them.

GROUND ZERO

How did we get into this mess? Early on in the twentieth century a few
scientists – mostly in Germany – experimented with chemicals as a means
of fertilising food crops. They found that a mixture of nitrogen, phosphorus and potassium (NPK) would grow big-yield crops of good-looking
vegetables, grains, legumes and fruits. Nobody paid much attention to
their discoveries until the end of the Second World War. At that time
most foods were still grown pretty much as they had always been – by
farmers who manured, mulched and rotated crops to keep soils rich and
in good condition. To put it another way, most food was grown organically. When the war ended, big commercial conglomerates who had been
involved in the manufacture of phosphates and nitrates as war material
found themselves stuck with huge stockpiles. They went looking for new
markets.

Aware of the early research into chemical fertilising, they turned towards
unsuspecting farmers and began to sell them artificial NPK fertilisers at
costs low enough to make it all look very
attractive. The purveyors of chemicals also
spread the false belief that NPK was all
you needed to grow healthy crops. There
were unfortunately two important facts that

> In ancient times they had
> no statistics so they had to
> fall back on lies.
>
> *Stephen Leacock*

got left out, probably because they were not understood. The first is that although plants grow *big* on artificial fertilisers they do not *grow resistant to disease.* The second is that neither do people eating food grown this way become resistant to age degeneration.

CHEMICAL HAWKERS

Plants grown only on NPK are deprived of essential minerals and other micro-substances they need to synthesise natural complexes in roots and leaves which ward off attack by insects, weeds and animals. Before long, the new artificially fertilised vegetables and fruits began to develop diseases. The chemical hawkers were quick to come to the rescue – with more chemicals. This is how pesticides, herbicides, nemacides and fungicides came into being. They provided chemical companies with yet another exciting business opportunity – especially since the longer you fertilise chemically the more depleted in organic matter your soils become – so that even if minerals and trace elements are there, they are not available to the plants because they are unable to synthesise natural protective complexes during growth – so more and more pesticides and other chemicals were sold. Yet, before long, another important fact became apparent. Like plants, human beings need a lot more than nitrogen, phosphorus and potassium from the foods they eat to maintain health.

The landmark 1989 Kellogg Report stated: 'There are over 1,000 newly synthesised compounds introduced each year, which amounts to three new chemicals a day.' But many of these chemicals, we are now learning, are not just ordinary chemicals. They are petrochemicals found in pesticides, plastics, household cleaners, automobile exhaust, and even makeup, hair dyes and every day beauty products like fingernail polish and polish remover. Petrochemicals are known as xenobiotics or xenoestrogens, which function as hormone disrupters. And xenoestrogens include such exotic substances as bisphenol-A, found in the lining of the inside of tin cans, phitates, contained in plastic wrappings that leach into foods; and pesticides.

Anne Louise Gittleman

THREE STEPS TO DEGENERATION

The processing of food can be divided into three phases, every one of which undermines Age Power.

1. Grains and animal products are refined to obtain proteins, fats and starches.
2. Refined products are treated by chemical procedures that change their molecular structure.
3. These artificial constructs are made into your final products.

SOIL POWER

The organic matter in healthy soil is nature's factory for biological activity. It is built up as a result of the break down of vegetable and animal matter by the soil's natural 'residents' – worms, bacteria and micro-organisms. In the right type and quantity they give rise to physical, chemical and biological properties that create fertility in our soils and make plants grown on them highly resistant to disease.

The minerals and trace elements we need to take in to trigger the metabolic processes on which health and age retardation depend must be in an organic form – that is taken from living things – plant or animal foods. Destroy the soil's organic matter through chemical farming and slowly but inexorably you destroy the health of those living on foods grown on it.

Your body has a remarkable ability to compensate for a mineral or trace element missing from your food. But, as a result of many years of eating nutritionally depleted foods, multiple deficiencies have become widespread. According to large-scale studies, few people in the West still receive all the minerals they need to ensure that metabolic processes work adequately. These deficiencies cannot be easily corrected, and popping a multi-vitamin and mineral pill will not do it. A balance of

> Scientists involved with the Human Genome Project, and affiliated research, are learning that such age related diseases as heart disease, adult onset diabetes, arthritis, digestive disorders, loss of mental acuity and certain forms of cancer are not inevitable consequences of ageing. They are...the result of a poor match between the genetic needs of the individual and the choices he or she makes regarding overall diet, specific nutrient intake, lifestyle and environment.
>
> *Jeffrey Bland*

bio-available minerals and trace elements is infinitely more complex than the vitamin fanatics would have us believe.

FRAGMENT AND DESTROY

Like our soils, the industrially prepared foods of commerce have been taken to pieces. To create a variety of palatable foods from raw materials you first have to reduce the foodstuffs – grains and seeds, vegetables and legumes – to simple factors that lend themselves to manipulation but bear no relation to the foods our bodies need and crave. From milk to meat to garden peas – whatever food is involved – processing destroys nutrients. Nutrients are also lost during other phases of food handling. Store asparagus for a week and it loses 90 percent of its vitamin C. Keep grapes for a week and they shed 30 percent of their B vitamins. Freeze meats and they lose as much as 50 per cent of two important B vitamins – riboflavin and thiamine. The list is endless.

The multinational food industry, which covers the packaging of its products with 'nutritional information', would have you believe that any goodness lost in processing can be made up for by 'enriching' – adding a few vitamins and minerals in synthetic form. It is categorically impossible to restore the health-giving power of wholeness to any food that has been fragmented. Foods that have been chemically grown, sprayed, treated and highly manipulated not only do not support our health, they don't even satisfy our hunger because they are nutritionally inadequate and chemically distorted.

ORGANIC MATTERS

You may feel that enough has been said over the past twenty years about organic foods and why we should eat them. But it goes deeper than that. There are unquantifiable benefits to eating healthy foods grown on nutrient rich soils that science is only just beginning to grasp.

THE VITAL MESENCHYME

The state and quality of what you eat also determines the health of your capillaries and the condition of the *mesenchyme* – connective tissue, blood and blood system, and the smooth muscles through which nutrients and oxygen must pass to nurture cells, genes, glands and organs.

This microscopic tissue element – the mesenchyme – carries the 'nutritional stream' to all parts of your body. The Swiss expert in the use of nutrition for healing and for retarding degeneration, Max Bircher-Benner, referred to it as 'vegetatives Betriebsstuek' – the *seedbed*. Giving it this name is an excellent way of understanding its importance. If the seedbed of the body is right, if it facilitates an easy passage of oxygen and nutrients and the rapid elimination of cellular wastes, then your cells' metabolic processes are carried out as they should be: *efficiently and cleanly*. Then you also get a high degree of protection from oxystress and free radical damage. If not, then the foods you eat – no matter how 'good for you' – can slowly and persistently increase the rate at which you age.

MODERN NUTRITION – WHAT'S MISSING?

Like much of modern science, most nutrition tends to be highly reductionist. Reductionism is the world view which asserts that an effective understanding of any complex system can be gained by investigating the properties of its isolated parts. This is a spot-on description of what has happened to our attitude to food. The standard science of nutrition is based on the notion that the function of a vitamin or mineral or protein is encapsulated in its chemical structure. It assumes that man needs certain quantities of these nutrients as well as some protein, fat and carbohydrate in order to avoid gross nutritional deficiencies such as beriberi, pellagra and scurvy and it doesn't concern itself greatly with how he gets them. But it gives little thought to the importance of the complexity of how these elements are combined in natural fresh foods, or to how important this complexity is to the highest expression of our genes and the preservation of our DNA.

In truth, the function of a vitamin or protein or any other nutrient can only be expressed by its interaction with its biochemical and physiological milieu. And unless you are reasonably knowledgeable about this milieu, its function cannot be understood. The body's biochemical milieu, like fresh foods grown on healthy soils, is highly complex. It includes vitamins, minerals, phytonutrients and other accessory factors such as negatively charged hydrogen atoms. There is much evidence that a shortage or an excess of one vitamin and a dearth of phytonutrients interferes with utilization of others. Once you split off a nutrient from the milieu in which it occurs, even if later you combine it again with all of the known factors with which it was originally linked, you undermine its health enhancing power. Many pill-popping health nuts make this mistake when they assume they can eat anything they like so long as they take massive quantities of anti-oxidant nutrients. The whole really is greater than the sum of its parts in living systems. Our genes and DNA express themselves best when we are exposed to the wholeness of healthy fresh foods.

CYBERNETIC AGE POWER

As Russian biochemist I. I. Brekhman, winner of the Lenin Prize for Science would say, when we significantly alter the *structural information* which comes to us from the natural foods to which our bodies have become accustomed through our evolution, we vastly undermine the potential of our gene expression.

Brekhman uses the term structural information to describe that it is not only nutrients – vitamins, minerals, protein and so forth – which are important for health. So is the complexity of the way they and as yet other unidentified factors are combined in a particular food as well as the quality of energy the food carries. Food processing degrades the structural information delivered to an organism, and thus its health supporting properties. Fresh foods contain more structural information than cooked or processed foods. They are in effect more biologically active.

In experiments Brekhman has shown that foods high in structural information, such as organically grown fresh non-starchy vegetables, enable animals to carry out physical tasks for significantly longer periods that processed foods, which are low in structural information. Even when the foods compared are equal in calories and therefore, by orthodox biochemical standards, supplying an organism with the same amount of energy. Brekhman has shown that drugs or highly processed foods, which are relatively simple both in their chemical structure and in the low level of structural information they impart, have little to offer in helping your body maintain homeostasis – the system by which an organism maintains metabolic equilibrium by compensating for disruptive changes. This is particularly important in preventing early ageing. But vegetables and fruits – particularly when they are eaten fresh and raw – as well as a few pulses and grains, are complex natural compounds which carry a high degree of biological information necessary for health in the living organism. This kind of biological information is essential if we are to maintain a high degree of *order* necessary to resist degeneration.

> Sometimes I lie awake at night, and I ask, 'Where have I gone wrong?' Then a voice says too me, 'This is going to take more than one night.'
>
> *Charlie Brown*

Yet this is something of which most nutritionists and food techno-logists are still ignorant. Over eighty percent of the foods we eat in Europe and North America continue to be factory processed. Manufacturers routinely add almost two hundred chemicals to bolster the texture, taste, and appearance of foods engineered from modified starches, proteins, carbohydrates and fats, and there are several thousand more chemicals close at hand which can be thrown in for special purposes and this does not even take into account the pesticides and herbicides sprayed on the foods we eat.

TROPHICS FOR YOUTH

The American biochemist Roger Williams emphasises our need for structural information when he says that the body extracts *trophic factors* from the molecular balances of the entire food and insists that this complexity of information is essential for maintaining high-level health and for restoring it when it has become lost. We have great need of the trophic factors in natural fresh foods – the quality of structural information they contain. Only a diet rich in structural information provides the right kind of seedbed for our cells and organs to live well into ripe old age.

EUROPEAN SECRETS

To my knowledge most of the study of what kind of diet can do this comes out of Austria, Germany, Switzerland and Scandinavia. This is probably why the topic is so little understood in English-speaking countries. In Europe there is a long tradition of natural healing and age-retardation using foods – a high degree of them uncooked. European scientists have also carried out elaborate clinical and laboratory studies to determine how, on a cellular level, fresh foods are able to work wonders for the health of human beings. Let's look at how and why.

> I remember when people used to step outside a moment for a breath of fresh air. Now sometimes you have to step outside for days before you get it.
>
> *Victor Borge*

> Wholeness might be defined as health restored. Here the internal environment of the body is stabilised and in perfect balance. This is balance at all levels, from the whole to each system, to each organ, to each cell, to each chemical reaction in the cells.
>
> *James F Balch MD*

LIFE IN LIFE OUT

... you too must learn to defy conventional wisdom in order to defy age.

Robert Atkins MD

It is time to think differently: Nutrition is not only chemistry. The state and quality of living energy – *sunlight quanta* – which a food carries, plays an enormous role in determining the health of your capillaries and cells, your organs and tissues – your life as a whole. Now this is hot stuff. So far ahead of most nutritional thinking that it makes heads spin. Yet it is a truth known for centuries to experts in natural healing. This is where raw foods come in.

Most of the study of what a high raw diet can do to detoxify, restore homeostasis – the natural order of your body – and rejuvenate the body, comes out of Austria, Germany, Switzerland and Scandinavia. This may be why we know so little about it in English-speaking countries like Britain and the United States. In Europe there is a long tradition of healing and age retardation using organic foods – a high percentage of them uncooked. For more than half a century, European scientists have carried out elaborate clinical and laboratory studies to determine how, on a cellular level, fresh foods are able to work wonders for the health of human beings. Their clinical experience and their laboratory findings contributes a lot to Age Power. Many of their findings – such as the way raw foods increase the microelectrical potentials of your cells enabling good cellular nourishment and efficient elimination of wastes – are directly relevant to the growing awareness of the body as a *negentropic open system* of *free energy*. Even electromagnetic phenomena from exposure to the effects of TVs, electric blankets and mobile phones play a part in how your body grows, regenerates or becomes damaged.

RAW FOODS AND IMMUNITY

European scientists such as Paul Kouchakoff at the Institute of Clinical Chemistry in Lausanne, discovered that there are significant differences in the way the body responds to cooked foods and to raw foods. Kouchakoff discovered that a phenomenon known as *digestive leucocytosis,* which was long believed to take place whenever we eat food, doesn't actually occur when the food is eaten raw. Digestive leucocytosis happens like this: When some kind of message triggers the release of leucocytes – white blood cells into the gut – these cells swarm out to the intestine walls, especially to the colon, as if to defend a front-line attack on the body. This was assumed to be a normal physiological phenomenon until Kouchakoff's discovery. He also found that it does not occur even if you only *begin* your meal with something raw. Raw foods not only don't challenge the immune reactions in the way cooked foods do, they leave immune functions free to deal with day-to-day biochemical housekeeping instead. This is perhaps not surprising considering that most of what Paleolithic man ate was raw.

POWER HEALING

The tradition of using natural foods for healing is a long and fascinating one, involving the use of organically grown foods – fruits and vegetables, seeds, fish and other protein foods. Only healthy soil imparts the right kind of biological information to the plants grown in it – information we use for our own bodies to thrive when we eat them. Many of these foods have been used in their uncooked state to bring about a reversal in serious chronic illness from cancer and arthritis to high blood pressure, arteriosclerosis, migraine and diabetes. For more than a century in the finest European clinics for natural healing, a diet of such foods has been combined with exercise, good stress management and simple treatments using air, water and sunlight. It has also been used to treat emotional disturbances, resistant obesity and addictions. The story of how the tradition developed, its phenomenal success and how it is now being used is also fascinating, but far too

> We can easily forgive a child who is afraid of the dark; the real tragedy of life is when men are afraid of the light.
>
> *Plato*

long to tell here. My daughter Susannah and I have explored it in some depth in another book *The New Raw Energy*. But there are a couple of aspects of it which are particularly important to Age Power.

RAW ENERGY WORKS

The proportion of cooked to uncooked foods in a person's diet, which are traditionally used in natural healing, are proportional to the seriousness of the illness being treated. The more serious, the greater the proportion of foods will be raw. An all-raw diet is often used for a specific period of time to detoxify in the treatment of cancer and other chronic conditions. As a patient improves, the physician gradually reduces the quantity of uncooked foods to somewhere between 50 to 75 percent. Once a high level of well-being is restored to a patient, he is encouraged to maintain himself permanently on a diet where at least 50 percent of the foods eaten are raw. Such a way of eating is a powerful tool for Age Power. It helps create a seedbed of the highest order for good gene expression and cell integrity as well as improving the efficiency with which your cells use oxygen. It also strengthens cell walls and improves metabolism. Finally, it protects your body from a build up of toxic wastes which can cause the molecular damage of ageing.

The first, most obvious reason is that fresh uncooked foods are higher in almost all of the anti-oxidant vitamins and minerals as well as the immune-enhancing phytonutrients. Storing, heating and processing destroy vitamins and cause mineral loss. But this only scratches the surface of the high-raw phenomena. More about this in a moment.

PROCESS AND DESTROY

Four kinds of damage to amino acids occur as a result of heating and processing protein foods:

❑ Under high heat some proteins become resistant to digestion so that the bio-availability of the amino acids they contained is reduced.

❑ Lysine (one of the essential amino acids) can be lost when you heat proteins especially in the presence of reducing sugars – as in the pasteurisation of milk.

❑ When protein is exposed to treatment with alkali, as it is in many food manufacturing processes, lysine and cysteine (a natural anti-oxidant and another essential amino acid) residues can not easily be eliminated from your body and toxic amino products can be formed.

❑ When oxidising chemicals like sodium dioxide are used in food processing, methionine from the protein can be lost. Methionine is another of the natural anti-oxidant amino acids, important as a protection against cross-linkage and oxidation damage to the cells and in methylation-fueled detoxification.

Fats – particularly unsaturated oils such as those we cook with – have also been shown to change during heating and processing. Not only is much of their nutritional value lost, they too can produce mutagenic and carcinogenic compounds. Other important substances such as essential oils in plants, the chlorophyll, the flavenoids, carotenoids and other phyto-nutrients with health-enhancing properties – these too can be changed or destroyed by heat. Such substances are part of the structural information biologically necessary to support our best genetic expression and to slow degeneration.

OUTDATED THINKING

Many experts on the use of a high-raw diet believe that the reason why orthodox nutrition has not yet twigged to the value of fresh foods is precisely because of the reductionist nature of twentieth century nutritional science. Ralph Bircher – late biochemist son of physician Max Bircher-Benner – spent fifty years compiling laboratory and clinical research on this subject. He edited a scientific journal in Europe for more than a generation and wrote almost a dozen technical books on the subject. He says: 'It is not the vitamins, nor the mineral salts in raw vegetable foods which do it, nor chlorophyll, nor the quality of the proteins, nor the essential oils, nor excess of alkalines, nor fibre, nor the fact that this diet is low in sodium. The problem is complex and much more interesting than that. Heating and even wilting destroys many qualities, the significance of which is not yet known, and mankind will possibly never know it completely. But new analytic work of recent years has given interesting insight.'

ENZYMES MATTER

Raw foods are rich in natural enzymes. These are destroyed when a food is cooked. Orthodox nutrition stills pays little attention to these enzymes in the belief that they are wiped out by digestive processes and therefore can have no beneficial effects. But researchers such as Kaspar Tropp in Wurzburg and Nobel laureate Artturi Ilmari Virtanen in Finland have shown this is simply not true. Virtanen – the teacher of Finnish chemist Johan Bjorksten, one of the most famous researchers in the world – discovered that although many of the enzymes in raw fruits and vegetables are broken down in the mouth as a result of chewing, their substrates react chemically with substances in saliva to produce new chemical compounds beneficial to the health of animals and man.

Kaspar Tropp discovered that the human body knows how to protect many of these enzymes and escort them through the digestive tract to reach the colon intact. There they attract and bind with whatever oxygen may be present, thus removing the aerobic condition which can result in putrefaction, fermentations, intestinal toxaemia and dysbacteria or dysbiosis – the importance of which is only beginning to be acknowledged so far in Britain and North America. It can have far reaching consequences for human health including encouraging an overgrowth of Candida albicans.

I've been in the twilight of my career longer than most people have had their career.

Martina Navratilova

BUGS – GOOD BAD AND UGLY

Dysbacteria or dysbiosis means 'colonic dysfunction as a result of altered flora.' Your colon contains a colony of flora consisting of many forms of bacteria including various strains of friendly-guy bacteria such as *Lactobacillus acidophilis* and *Bifidobacterium bifidum lactobacilli*. In the large intestine, too, are smaller quantities of yeast such as Candida albicans and many bacteria which, unlike the friendly groups, can cause the following:

- ❑ Leaky gut syndrome
- ❑ Vitamin deficiencies
- ❑ Predisposition to colon cancer
- ❑ Skin problems like cystic acne, eczema and psoriasis
- ❑ Chronic fatigue
- ❑ Irritable bowel syndrome
- ❑ Symptoms mistakenly diagnosed as other diseases including mood disorders, arthritis, rheumatic disorders and a myriad other chronic conditions.

Enzymes present in raw foods encourage the production of the protective bacterial flora and help protect from Candida overgrowth.

Abnormal flora are a common cause of so-called food allergies. When flora are abnormal, the gastrointestinal mucous membrane becomes abnormally permeable, allowing the absorption of toxins from the bowel. These wastes enter circulation and can be carried throughout the body causing toxic effects. The widespread incidence of high colon concentrations of Candida albicans yeast is associated with a number of common illnesses.

GOOD SELECTIVE CAPACITY

Even more interesting are the effects which raw foods have on the body's circulatory system, the mesenchyme and the cells themselves. A central issue in protecting your body from degeneration is making sure that there is a constant interchange of energy substance and information between the capillaries – the very ends of the circulatory system – and the tissue cells. This takes place simultaneously, at something like a billion points in your body. Its efficiency depends to a large degree on the electrobiological energy which make exchange possible. Professor Hans Eppinger at the University of Vienna discovered that a diet high in raw foods significantly improves intra-extra cellular exchange, micro-circulation and waste elimination.

Cellulite in women is one of the consequences which develops from such a marsh.

FREEWAY TO ENERGY

Unless your metabolic pathways are kept open, your biochemical processes become sluggish and toxic, intermediate products such as AGES and acetyldehide build up to a point where they cause damage. Making sure you get plenty of raw vegetables and fruit helps protect from this happening. This is another reason a high raw way of eating can be so helpful to Age Power. It restores the selective capacity of your cells and ensures that nutrients carried through the bloodstream via the capillaries are available for clean and efficient use. A substantial intake of raw foods was the only thing that Hans Eppinger and his co-workers found which could do this in people whose bodies were already undergoing degeneration. Again, in Ralph Bircher's words, 'Under the influence of a raw vegetable diet the life-giving antagonistic tensions grew and capillaries were slowly restored to their vigorous efficient state. You saw how raw vegetable foods work. It is an unspecific, general treatment, tending to restore the organising centre in every cell in the organism.'

> Throughout your life the most profound influences on your health, vitality and function are not the doctors that you have visited or the drugs, surgery or other therapies that you have undertaken, the most profound influences are the accumulative effects of decisions you have made about your diet and lifestyle on the expression of your genes.
>
> *Jeffrey Bland MD*

SUNLIGHT QUANTA

The discoveries concerning raw foods and their regenerative power and ability to restore order as well as to encourage clean and efficient metabolic processes still can't fully explain precisely how and why this happens. This stuff is so new and revolutionary that we can only begin to penetrate the mysteries. It is of absolute importance in the Age Power programme that you understand that things cannot be measures purely in chemical terms. Science in this area is wrestling with the nature of life itself.

Max Bircher-Benner said that 'fresh foods are the sine qua non of natural health and healing' because they carry to the organism eating them 'complex sunlight energies which have been stored in the vegetable kingdom during its construction of living matter, in the form of *sunlight quanta*. Our blood, our organs, our tissues, and our central nervous system are not only being nourished by calories and nutrients which can be chemically measured alone, but highly charged energy waves which show their rich diversity in the colours of the rainbow.'

ELECTRON CLOUDS

In the thirties, what Bircher-Benner referred to as sunlight quanta – which he claimed we acquired through the electronic nature of living material – couldn't be measured in the way that one can measure calorie energy from combustion. He realised that the nature of sunlight quanta was not understood by the somewhat blinkered approach to nutritional science intent on devising tables of vitamins. He was a brilliant Swiss physician and was often accused of 'mysticism' despite the quite exceptional healing and regeneration that application of his theories brought to patients.

> An electron going around is a little current. What drives life is . . . a little electric current kept up by sunshine. All the complex-ities of intermediary metab-olism are but lacework around this basic fact.
>
> *Albert Szent-Györgyi*

As the twenty-first century begins, thanks to developments in submolecular biology and quantum physics, what once appeared 'mysticism' has become, at least partly, explainable in scientific terms. The handful of scientists who from one point of view or another have tried to penetrate

the mystery of life energy and how it is maintained within a living system
– many of them Nobel laureates such as Erwin Schrödinger and Albert
Szent-Györgyi – have come up with descriptions of non-chemical energy
exchange in living systems which lend credence to Bircher-Benner's own
analysis of how the energies in raw foods support high level health.

While a classic chemical reaction in a living system – known as *biva-
lent oxido-reduction* which is what chemistry concerns itself with – involves
a rearrangement of the molecular structure, there also exist energy
exchanges associated with *monovalent* electron transfers. These involve elec-

NEGATIVE POWER

Raw foods from plant or animal sources carry a high level of
a powerful, primordial anti-oxidant in the form of a hydrogen
ion. This is another reason why a high raw diet of fresh
foods can be so powerfully regenerating and rejuvenating to
the body. In its normal state, the hydrogen atom holds only
one proton and one electron. The smallest and the most
primary element in the universe, hydrogen appeared fifteen
billion light years ago with the Big Bang later giving birth to
helium and the other elements from which the universe is
made. Hydrogen plays a central role in the biochemistry of
life. It is a primary donor of an electron, a pair of electrons
or a proton to make biochemical reactions in the body
possible. In fact, most electron exchanges in biochemical
pathways within your cells take place in the presence of some
form of hydrogen. Hydrogen ions are carried by or react with
enzymes. They are also carried by co-factor vitamins such as
nicotinamide which empower enzyme reactions. H-molecules
even take part in energy producing reactions initiated by
coenzyme A in the mitochondria which create ATP.

trons going it alone. They do not necessarily bring about rearrangements.
Yet they are equally important. They belong to the world which Robert
O. Becker, twice nominated for a Nobel prize, and other scientists working
in the field of electrobiology have been working to unravel, and to Patrick
Flanagan's breakthrough in harnessing the power of hydrogen molecules.

MASTER DONOR

Hydrogen, a highly unstable molecule, is a powerful donor of electrons especially when in the form known as a hybrid ion (H-ion) where it carries an extra electron. In this form, found in vast quantities in live foods and destroyed the minute you heat or process them, it has the distinction of being the most powerful antioxidant in the world. For it readily donates an extra electron to quench free radicals as they flare up thereby protecting the body from oxidation damage. Our human ancestors who ate most of their foods raw going back a million years or more got high levels of H-ion in their diet and therefore a high level of protection against free radical damage. Nowadays we get low levels by contrast although we need the protection they offer more than at any time throughout human history. For we now live in an environment riddled with ionising radiation and chemical pollution both of which create high levels of free radicals. Eating a high raw diet of fresh foods helps to counter this to some degree. Until recently this was just about the only way we had of making use of what H-ion has to offer. For, although many scientists tried, until five years ago no-one had succeeded in making the powerful anti-oxidant properties of the hydrogen ion available in supplement form. Hydrogen is just too unstable an element.

GLACIAL WATER POWER

For many years geologists have known that water derived from melting glaciers such as the Ultar glacier in Pakistan appears to benefit health. It may even – as in the case of the Hunza peoples – help prolong life. For generations health researchers, writers and cardiologists have joined geologists in an attempt to decipher what made this water special. One major factor appears to be that – like raw, fresh, organic fruits and vege-tables and the juices made from them, long celebrated for their health enhancing powers – this water is rich in H-ion molecules (the scientific name of which is *hydride*). Most nutritionists and physicians have as yet no knowledge of them. Yet life itself depends upon their existence. So does the health of the human body. It now appears that hydrogen is at least as important as oxygen in the role it plays in fuelling life and protecting us from premature ageing.

SUPER ANTI-OXIDANT

Thanks to the trailblazing work of eccentric American scientist Patrick Flanagan the negative hydrogen ion has been tamed and captured and is now available as an anti-oxidant supplement called Microhydrin™. A powerful one it is too. It was first given to me in Dublin a year ago. I had been up since 3a.m. travelling from London, had worked all day and was about to give a talk to several hundred people in the early evening. My response to taking it with a big glass of spring water was almost immediate. I felt as though I could go on for hours more working from a place of centered calm and clarity. It has become part of my own Age Power way of life ever since.

After decades of experiments in which he attempted to stabilise the negatively charged hydrogen molecule, he finally succeeded. He had some years before been singled out by *Life* magazine – at the tender age of 17 – when they insisted that he was the young genius to watch. Microhydrin™ is not derived from any plant or animal source in nature; instead Flanagan created it in the laboratory in the form of a white powder. It is sold in capsules which can be opened and added to pure water, turning your bottle of Volvic into a powerful anti-oxidant to sip throughout the day. It also comes in tablet form which you swallow with a large glass of water. The supplement consists of stabilised negatively charged hydrogen atoms, which carry an extra electron creating high level anti-oxidant properties – encased within a 'cage' of silicate minerals. Rather like Nicholaos Skouras's matrices, Flanagan's silicon cage acts as an active transport system enabling it to be absorbed through the walls of the gut and delivered to the body's tissues. A recent double-blind cross over study found that four capsules of Microhydrin™ taken 30 minutes before strenuous exercise increases the body's ability to use oxygen so well that there was a reduction of blood lactate levels by almost 50 percent during a 40 kilometer cycling exercise. Microhydrin's™ antioxidant abilities are a boon to anyone wanting to calm inflammation, increase vitality or detoxify the body.

ELECTRON POWER

Like hydrogen ions, Bircher-Benner's 'sunlight quanta' – an important healing force behind the high-raw phenomenon which is lost when foods are heated – are also likely to be proven and seen to be part of this world. Single electrons cascading and giving up their energy, as Szent-Gyorgyi says, 'can do anything but cannot be expressed in classical chemical terms. A wandering electron belongs to the changing shapes...of those electron clouds which belong to the submolecular, dominated by quantum mechanics.' This is a realm about which orthodox nutrition remains generally ignorant. It may be years before it is charted. But you needn't wait to make use of the remarkable age-retarding benefits of high-raw foods in Age Power's Insulin Balance eating programme. The proof of the pudding (sugar-free, of course) is in the eating. And the best eating of all comes in the form of a nutrient-rich calorie-poor foodstyle.

EAT UP AND AGE FAST

Eating more than your body actually needs is a major cause of oxy-stress – free radical damage and cross-linking. When animals are both underfed *and* provided with optimum quantities of *all* the essential nutrients they need for excellent health, they not only live longer, they tend to remain free of chronic infections and degenerative diseases including cancer, arteriosclerosis and arthritis. So do we. There is now every indication that if you gradually decrease the amount you eat while increasing the quality of your diet, you can dramatically *decelerate* the rate at which you are ageing. This doesn't mean holding your breath and putting yourself in starvation mode. Far from it.

LEAN, MEAN,
AND ENERGETIC

Man lives on one quarter of what he eats. On the other three quarters his doctor lives.

Carving on Egyptian pyramid

Chisel this 5000 year old piece of advice into your brain and you will take a big step towards Age Power. Eat less and you will live longer is the most potent piece of advice you can follow – provided of course that what you eat delivers first rate nutrition to your cells and bathes your genes in wholesome substances which promote their optimal expression.

Thanks to expanded research – with humans and animals – into what has come to be called *nutrient-rich-calorie-poor nutrition*, it is highly likely that when you eat this way, you will not only live longer, it will be a largely disease-free life.

ASK ANY RAT

More than half a century ago, a researcher called Clive McCay at Cornell University severely restricted calories in rats while supplying them with vitamin and mineral supplements from the time of weaning. These animals lived up to two times as long as his control group which were allowed to eat as much as they wanted. Their lives were also far healthier. Not only was their lifespan increased, the rate at which they aged was slowed. Researchers determined this by measuring specific biomarkers of ageing in their animals.

Researchers testing calorie-restricted animals find that, by virtually all known biomarkers, these animals are significantly younger than their chronological age indicates they should be. Restricting calorie intake while enhancing nutritional supplementation is demonstrating how one can alter gene expression and slow ageing in animals. Richard Weindruch, professor of medicine at University of Wisconsin, one of the most well respected scientists working in the

Numerous studies have shown that high-carbohydrate low-fat diets lead to high triglycerides, elevated serum insulin levels, lower HDL cholesterol levels, and other factors known to raise the risk of coronary heart disease.

Metabolism 1993

area of calorie restriction, calls this phenomenon 'nutri-modulation of gene expression'.

ENTER THE HUMAN

In the late seventies, E. D. Schienker heading a research team at Michigan State University published the surprising results of an investigation into a group of ninety-seven women, middle-aged and older, whose histories he had followed for 25 years. At the beginning of the 25 year study, each woman provided the research team with a list of foods and quantities eaten during one day as well as a health and nutritional history. At that time all these women were rated in good, fair or poor health, following the qualitative index of ageing, set out by the *American Journal of Public Health*. After a quarter of a century of monitoring these women, those still living were again examined. Researchers found that women who looked younger than their years ate fewer calories. Also, fewer of their calories came from fats and they managed to consume substantially more vitamins B_1, A and C than their older-looking counterparts. Since then a number of other experiments have been carried out which support the advice that if you want to look better, live longer and feel great, you need to decrease the amount of food you take in while vastly improving its nutritional quality.

WHAT ABOUT US?

For a long time animal experiments seemed to have little relevance in retarding human ageing. For most research projects restricted calories in animals from the time they were weaned. And such a practice is hardly something we can carry out acceptably on our children. For one thing, a small percentage of these calorie-restricted animals die very early. No one would be willing to take such a risk with a human baby. Second there is always the fear that calorie-restriction might cause some kind of brain damage in a developing child. This is why, for many years, McCay's findings and those of other researchers working in the same way were relegated to that place on the bookshelves of science which holds the curiosities of laboratory research. Then a dynamic American age-researcher at the UCLA Medical School in California began to play about with calorie-restricted diets, and to design his own laboratory experiments which were variations on the McCay theme. His name is Roy Walford. He was, and still is, a hard-headed sceptical research scientist of the highest order, with an all-encompassing fascination with finding means, not only of halting premature ageing, but of increasing *maximum lifespan*.

> The optimistic belief that we are in control, capable and competent to make changes, is critical to health.
>
> *Robert Ornstein PhD, and David Sobel MD*

WHISPERS FROM THE RATS

Roy Walford, who has worked extensively with Richard Weindruch, reasoned that if you could restrict calories, not from weaning, but from middle age – all the while replacing any nutrients lost through supplements – then perhaps you could avoid the undesirable 'side-effects' of trying to do it from birth, yet still extend life. When Walford began to explore calorie restriction as a possibility for de-ageing humans, nobody had yet been able to do this by restricting calories in adult animals. Walford reasoned that this may be because they had always made the changeover from normal diet to restricted one too rapidly. Together with his colleague Richard Weindruch he decided to try it more gradually. It worked. Walford and Weindruch were not only able to retard the ageing rate of animals and to lengthen their *maximum* lifespan, they were even able to bring about some degree of immunological rejuvenation.

IMMUNE ENHANCEMENT

This particularly intrigued Walford since immune response is a major issue in biological (as opposed to chronological) ageing. He wrote, 'One good indicator is the response of critical agents of the immune system – white blood cells or lymphocytes – to a substance called phyto-hemagglutinin (PHA for short). PHA causes a lymphocyte to produce fresh DNA (the hereditary gene material in each cell) and divide into two new cells. The ability to respond to PHA declines with age. Dr Weindruch and I found that the lymphocytes of 16-month-old mice, who had been restricted since 12 months of age, responded to PHA at the same level as 6-8 month-old mice. (Natural lifespan in mice is 2 to 3 years, so 12 months is well into young adulthood.)'

JAPANESE CONNECTIONS

Inhabitants of the island of Okinawa in Japan eat between 17 to 40 percent fewer calories than do their brothers and sisters in the rest of Japan. At the same time research shows that Okinawans experience only 59 percent as much heart disease, 59 percent stroke and 60 percent cancer as the rest of the Japanese. Okinawa also boasts five to 40 times as many centenarians as elsewhere in Japan. So impressive has the Okinawa way of eating become in scientific circles, that there are whole books written about how it can prevent and reverse degeneration and slow ageing.

DREAM COME TRUE

Walford and Weindruch's mice put on calorie restriction later in life, showed significant resistance to illness and degeneration. About 50 percent of the fully fed mice developed cancer while only 13 per cent of the restricted mice did. The incidence of kidney disease, vascular disease and heart disease at 800 days old among the fully fed group was 100 percent, 63 percent and 96 percent respectively while in their leaner counterparts the figures were a mere 25, 10 and 26 percent. The restricted animals did not develop increased blood cholesterol as they got older. Their fat cells remained significantly more responsive to hormones (a decrease in responsiveness to hormones also tends to occur with age) and the auto-antibodies which are believed to be an underlying cause of senile dementia were greatly reduced. The findings of these two scientists have by now been well substantiated by other researchers such as those working at the Gerontology Research Centre in Baltimore, Maryland. For a long time debate raged over whether or not experiments such as these could be extrapolated to human beings. It appears that they can.

THE TEMPERATE BOWL

Animals on a nutrient-rich-calorie-poor regime are more active and more energetic. They retain sexual interest and energy long after their fully fed brothers have fallen by the wayside. Let the last word on the subject be left to Walford himself: 'Appropriate dietary restriction will give you better vision, hearing, mental function, an improved sense of physical well-being, retained sexuality and increased disease resistance in relation to your chronological or birthday age.' Here he quotes the Greek poet Hesiod who, some 2700 years ago, wrote: 'Fools not to know that half exceeds the whole, How blest the sparing meal and temperate bowl.'

There's one thing about children – they never go around showing snapshots of their grandparents.

Ed Wynn

Similarly, scientists who have studied the long-lived peoples of the world such as the Hunzas, the Georgians of Russia and the Vilcabamba Indians in South America, discovered that all of them lived on a low calorie, nutrient-rich diet, high in fresh, organically-grown uncooked foods. They also drank pure, clean glacial water rich in hydrogen ions – minute molecules of this element carrying a negative charge thanks to an extra electron. Raw, organic foods are also riddled with these health-enhancing hydrogen ions which now appear to be the most powerful anti-oxidants in the world. American scientist, Patrick Flanagan, has recently harnessed the ion molecule and created a nutritional supplement which is a great adjunct to any anti-ageing lifestyle (see page 171). All these long-lived peoples experience very few of the degenerative patterns that we do in the West surviving on our convenience foods.

REVERSES BIOMARKER

The results in terms of rejuvenation were remarkable. All participants registered decreased changes in blood pressure, cholesterol and trigylcerides, paralleling the rejuvenating changes already witnessed in animal studies. During the first six months the men had an average weight loss of 18 percent, their body fat stabilising at between 6 to 10 percent, while the women experienced a weight loss of 10 percent, with body fat stabilising at 10 to 15 percent. Fasting blood sugar levels dropped on average 20 percent, cholesterol levels 38 percent and blood pressure 30 percent – all stabilising themselves at more youthful levels. As Walford himself says, 'no other long-term sustainable diet has ever been shown to produce changes as dramatic as these . . . You will live longer, you will need less sleep, you'll have a sharper mind, you'll feel better, you'll get fewer colds, flu, and be generally less susceptible to other diseases.'

In Spain researchers carried out an interesting experiment in rejuvenation on two groups of elderly people living in a nursing home. They fed one group their normal diet. To the other group they gave a calorie-restricted diet that was, however, rich in essential macro- and micro-nutrients. After three years of study, scientists confirmed that those living on the calorie-restricted, nutrient-rich diet had only half the rate of illness and half the rate of death of those who had been left free to eat whatever they wanted.

LESSONS FROM BIOSPHERE II

One of the most interesting and exciting human research projects into the effect of a nutrient-dense-calorie-poor nutrition was carried out by Roy Walford, almost by accident. Walford had himself lived on such a diet for many years. A few years ago, he and seven of his colleagues sealed themselves inside a closed environment for two years – Biosphere II – in the Arizona desert, which was intended to duplicate the earth's environment. There, these eight participants followed a nutritious diet that was low in calories and consisted of fresh vegetables and fruits, grains, goats milk, yoghurt, meat, fish and eggs.

GO FRESH

Syndrome X contributes to ageing, and from a growing awareness of how many of us are developing insulin resistance from eating a high carbohydrate diet, many experts in natural medicine insist that we need fewer grains and fruits and more fresh vegetables and protein foods – in short a way of eating akin to that our Paleolithic ancestors followed. By necessity, a low-calorie-nutrient-dense way of eating regime needs to be rich in fresh vegetables – many eaten raw to preserve as many of their nutrients as possible and as much as their life-enhancing power as possible.

UNDER NUTRITION WITHOUT MALNUTRITION

Another fascinating thing about the Biosphere experiment is that the participants who took part did not feel particularly hungry. The nutrient-rich, fibre-filled, low-calorie way of eating, both fills your stomach and satisfies your hunger.

... evidence that low-fat diets are by and large ineffective and possibly even dangerous continues to accumulate in some of the world's most prestigious medical journals.

Dean Esmay

Walford is quick to point out that living in a nutrient-rich-calorie-poor way has nothing whatever to do with going on slimming diets. Far from it. Neither is what he recommends some kind of crankiness, as it might seem to the uninformed. *Undernutrition* is not *malnutrition*. It is a way of nourishing your body on fewer

HIGH NUTRIENT INSURANCE

An absolutely essential ingredient in this new approach to nutrient-rich-calorie-poor eating is a good supply of extra nutrients from nutritional supplements – of vitamins and minerals, essential fatty acids and perhaps a protein source of ultra-high biological value such as microfiltered or ion exchange whey (see Resources). The anti-oxidant nutrients are particularly important: vitamins C and E, the mineral selenium as well as the sulphur amino acids cysteine and methionine because they act as free radical scavengers. So are the phytonutrients whose anti-oxidant potentials are even greater than most vitamins and minerals.

calories, yet ensuring you get a full supply of essential vitamins, minerals and plant factors, fatty acids and fibre. In practical terms we *gradually* restrict our calorie intake to about 60 percent of what we would eat if, like his mice, we let ourselves eat as much as we wanted. Such nutrient-rich caloric restriction, Walford believes, should be achieved slowly over a period of five to seven years.

SUPREMELY NOURISHING FOODS

To achieve 'under nutrition without malnutrition', you need to choose your foods the Age Power way – carefully and eliminating all over-processed, nutritionally 'empty' convenience foods from your kitchen. These still make up the greater part of most people's menus – from white sugar and white flour to breakfast cereals and margarines containing hydrogenated oils, including soft drinks and potato crisps.

Dieting is a national obsession. Sixty million adult Americans are trying to lose weight. More than half of these people are not overweight.

Robert Ornstein PhD, and David Sobel MD

Walford refers to free radicals as 'great white sharks in the biochemical sea' because of their ability to do untold damage on a cellular level. Taken together, the health-enhancing effects of a combination of anti-oxidants is always greater than the sum of its parts. You could not ask for better protection from these sharks than the sulphurophane in broccoli, the lycopene in tomatoes, and the flavonoids and carotenoids which make bright coloured vegetables powerhouses for well-being. Other vitamins and minerals are important also. All essential nutrients are synergistic – they work best together. Because of the complexity of the web of metabolic pathways in our bodies, a nutrient without all its related nutrients is of little use in combating age-degeneration. Do we need nutritional supplements? Almost certainly we do. Computer analyses of attempts to establish whole food diets without taking nutritional supplements continually show up common human deficiencies. They include: zinc, vitamin E, copper, magnesium, iron, niacin, vitamin B_{12}, pantothenic acid, calcium, riboflavin, folic acid, vitamin A, vitamin B_6, thiamine and vitamin C. Many studies have shown that four of these nutrients are almost always deficient in the average Western diet – vitamin C, vitamin A, folic acid, calcium and iron while zinc, chromium, manganese and potassium follow close behind them.

SHUKUBEN AGES YOU

The concept of shukuben – stagnated faeces in the colon and uneliminated waste – is still difficult for the average doctor to grasp. Trained in symptomatic drug treatment and interventionalist medicine, he or she still views illness visited upon the body an accident of fate, or the direct result of exposure to micro-organisms as in colds and flu. The natural approach to medicine has long insisted that, by contrast, neither premature ageing and degenerative illness nor infectious diseases will take seed in a body that is not burdened with toxicity. This approach is very much in line with current age research.

JAPANESE CONNECTIONS

In Osaka, Japan, Dr Mitsuo Koda has introduced some six thousand people over the last forty years to nutrient-rich-calorie-poor eating. Tucked away amidst the twists and turns of Osaka's narrow streets, you will find his simple, yet remarkable, clinic. People from all over the world come to learn the art of self-cure and rejuvenation under Koda's guidance. Born in 1924, Koda graduated from Osaka University Medical School. For the past forty years this lean and vital clinician has been treating people with a wide variety of illness from atopic eczema and collagen diseases to cancer, vascular disease – even AIDS – using changes in diet, simple exercises, hypnotherapy and prayer.

Like almost every great healer cum medical doctor in previous generations who worked in natural health – from Max Bircher-Benner in Switzerland to Max Gerson in Germany and Francis Pottenger in the United States – Koda came to his healing as a result of wrestling with his own serious illness after finding that orthodox medicine could do nothing to help him. He began to study natural approaches and to test them out, first on himself and then on others, with excellent results. Koda was not interested in rejuvenating the body or prolonging life but specifically in providing optimal conditions for the bodies of ailing people – many of them very ill – to heal themselves. In the process, Koda learned that eating lightly rejuvenates the person and delays ageing. His assertions have been clinically confirmed by a growing number of Japanese doctors and scientists who have assessed the results of the Koda treatment. Koda discovered for himself two important things: First, he found that the methods of naturecure – the aim of which is to help the body heal itself by natural means – are based upon the same principles throughout the world going back many generations. Second, he found that what all the great nature doctors have taught is true: the fundamental cause of degeneration and most chronic illness is toxicity – a build up of uneliminated waste – *shukuben* in Japanese.

Koda aims to reduce and control the food intake of a person at about 60 percent of normal calorie intake. By using a very high level of raw foods and green foods, he has shown that you can avoid the accumulation of toxic waste in the body. Shukaben is a major cause of free radical damage. Raw foods help detoxify the body and eliminate the accumulation of shukaben in the colon which most of us carry around for decades, despite the fact that we may be having so-called normal bowel movements every day. Koda and his colleagues insist that nutrient-rich-calorie-poor eating also protects the body from accumulating further wastes. Once the accumulation of shukaben is halted, says Koda, you are highly protected against premature degeneration and disease, both acute and chronic. Age power eating has absolutely nothing to do with going onto a low calorie slimming regime. Far from it. One has to be extremely choosy about the quality of food you eat in order to make light eating work for you. It is especially important to eat plenty of fresh vegetables, as many as possible in their raw state.

This is where raw vegetables and super green foods become so important. They contain nutritional elements that are not found to the same degree or quality as in other foods. They are also rich in hydrogen ions – the most potent anti-oxidants as yet identified (see page 170). Vitamins, minerals and trace elements, as well as proteins and fatty acids come to us in raw vegetables in a quantity and balance that is *qualitively* different than the same foods when they are heated.

BENEVOLENCE TOWARDS LIFE

Koda loves to quote an old Japanese saying which translates roughly as 'Eat light to maintain your might.' He also points out that: 'Food is life. Food is not merely a thing, as many people assume. Human beings and all living creatures receive our lives from the "life" of food. Eating lightly is, to this extent, killing as little life as possible . . . a concrete demonstration of love and benevolence to the life on this planet.' One could also add to ourselves, as human beings, as well.

We find greatest joy, not in getting, but in expressing what we are . . . Men do not really live for honors or for pay; their gladness is not the taking and holding, but in doing, the striving, the building, the living. It is a higher joy to teach than to be taught. It is good to get justice, but better to do it, fun to have things but more to make them. The happy man is he who lives the life of love, not for the honors it may bring, but for the life itself.

R.J. Baughan

WHAT'S IT LIKE?

To most people the idea of restricting the number of calories they consume and leaving the sticky buns and chocolate out of their lives seems like some kind of terrible deprivation – an action which can only be carried out by a gargantuan effort of the will. In fact, the calorie restrictors tell us this is only the view of someone who has not yet experienced the enormous rewards that come with dietary temperance.

EAT FOR AGE POWER

The work of Weindruch, Walford, Koda and others, like that of the great pioneers in natural health and healing promises – for those who want to make use of what they can teach us – the possibility of regenerating energy and rejuvenating life to a degree that until recently has only been dreamed of. If you want to make a nutrient-rich-calorie-poor diet – undernutrition without malnutrition – begin by sorting out first principles. Gradually come to eat only the kind of foods your body thrives on. They will form

---

HOFFER'S BIG FOUR

Canadian expert on the orthomolecular approach, Dr Abram Hoffer has been treating people with anti-oxidant nutrients for several generations. Before he ever gives a patient nutritional supplements, he insists that they get themselves into a new way of eating – a way of eating based on four principles:

❑ Eat foods whole – not convenience foods which have been refined.

❑ Eat foods as fresh as possible and in as close to their living state as possible, so they have little or no time to deteriorate through oxidation. When you cook any foods, do so as lightly as possible. Cooking destroys many nutrients, distorts essential fatty acids and denatures some proteins, as well as increasing the carcinogenic properties of certain foods. It also destroys much of the life energy present which can not be measured in physical or chemical terms.

❑ Eat only non-toxic foods which do not contain synthetic flavours, colours, preservatives or other additives used by food manufacturers to enhance a food's cosmetic aspects.

❑ Vary your diet by eating lots of fresh herbs and low-starch vegetables, herbs and spices. For down through evolution the human body has adapted to a wide range of foods which offer a broad spectrum of nutrients.

❑ Then and only then, is it time to add supplementation. Explore what nutritional supplements you can benefit from using, to ensure your diet is nutrient-rich and geared to your own unique genetic and biochemical needs, including vitamins and minerals.

---

the foundation on which to build with anti-oxidant nutrients and other substances for Age Power.

Once these things become established and your body begins to thrive, then slowly and gradually, if you wish, decrease the level of the calories you are taking in, preferably checking with a doctor or health practitioner to monitor progress. How low in calories you go depends on whether you are male or female and on how high a level of strenuous physical activity you have in your life. A top athlete will need many more calories than an office worker. People exploring nutrient-rich calorie-poor eating aim to eat somewhere between 1800 and 2000 calories a day. In my opinion, for most of us, this is highly impractical and just a bit too tough. One great thing about Age Power's Insulin Balance is that it quite naturally decreases the amount most people eat by restoring insulin sensitivity, banishing cravings and improving overall metabolism greatly.

AUTOMATIC APPETITE CONTROL

So many people have difficulty controlling the amount they eat. They have cravings for carbohydrate foods such as muffins or pasta, fatty foods such as fried fish and potatoes or sugary foods like chocolate. We have been taught that these cravings need to be controlled with will power. This is just not the case. Where there are cravings there is always some imbalance. The most common culprit is Syndrome X which is becoming more and more widespread. High fasting insulin levels roller coaster blood sugar which goes up and down, dragging your energy and moods with it and result in insulin resistance at a cellular level. As a result the energy from your food does not get into the mitochondria of your muscle cells where it can be turned into ATP, the body's energy currency. You grow increasingly tired, eat more, but find that you still feel 'hungry'.

SET YOURSELF FREE

I have seen great numbers of people who have changed their way of eating away from the low-fat-high-carbohydrate diet, cutting out sugar and sweet things, convenience foods based on refined flours and grains, and starchy vegetables, lose their cravings within a week or two at the most. This feels to them like being set free from prison: Their appetite drops, their blood sugar levels stabilise and their life transforms. Providing they are drinking enough water – for thirst is often misinterpreted as hunger by the body – they quite naturally eat far less. Before long people on Age Power's Insulin

You still have your hourglass figure, my dear, but most of the sand has gone to the bottom.

Bob Hope, The Lemon Drop Kid

Balance eating feel uncomfortable when they eat more than their body actually needs. For them the transition from an ordinary good quality diet to nutrient-rich-calorie-poor eating becomes a graceful natural experience. They report that they have never felt better, while their friends and family tell them they look wonderful. I would never have believed this if it had not happened to me. You will only know it for yourself by experimenting with Age Power's Insulin Balance and seeing where it will take you.

This is a way of eating which automatically provides you with anti-ageing nutrition of the highest order – a way of eating which is high in fibre and non-starchy vegetables – rich in a full complement of natural anti-oxidant plant compounds. It is a diet rich in the structural information necessary to maintain a high degree of order or negative entropy in your body, to help protect you from degeneration. If your foods are fresh enough, and you choose to eat between 25 to 75 percent of them raw, this way of eating will also carry with it as yet undefined life properties – what Bircher-Benner called 'sunlight quanta' – which give fresh foods their ability to retard degeneration and promote a high level of health in living systems. You will create for yourself an anti-ageing lifestyle that would be hard to beat.

At the very core of natural health and healing you find the belief that when you provide the body with a diet and lifestyle to which it has been genetically adapted, you give it what it needs to re-balance whatever is not in balance and restore healthy form and harmony. This is what Age Power's Insulin Balance Programme will do for you – not by popping a pill – but by shifting the way you eat and live. Nothing else will work. A shift in both the kind and ratio of three fundamental nutrients – protein, carbohydrates and fats – plus increased physical activity, will transform your body, slow age degeneration and help you reach levels of energy and vitality you may have only dreamed of – until now.

PART FOUR:
THE
PROGRAMME

GET SAVVY

Life is a banquet, and most poor suckers are starving to death.

Rosalind Russell, Auntie Mame

Age Power's Insulin Balance Programme goes to the source and origins of life to gather power. This way of eating not only makes use of an optimal balance between the best quality proteins, carbohydrates and fats based upon as much as science now knows about our genetic inheritance, it also calls on an abundance of immune supporting, energy enhancing, anti-ageing phytonutrients from fruits and vegetables.

Such foods are not stuffed full of anti-oxidant enhancers, they carry masses of life energy – especially when you eat them raw. Let's look at what the *best* of these foods are like.

THE DOPE ON CARBS

In the scientific context, carbohydrates are just organic compounds made of carbon, hydrogen and oxygen. When carbohydrates are eaten by a healthy body, they turn into glucose to supply fuel for metabolism and vitality. But throughout the history of human civilisation, as we've seen, carbohydrates have been manipulated, used and abused in a number of ways, most of them pointing down a road that ends in premature ageing, physical degeneration and obesity.

Nutritionists divide carbohydrates into two categories – simple and complex. Yet all carbohydrates are made up of simple sugars called *monosaccharides*: fructose, glucose and galactose. Monosaccharides, in turn, link together into chains of two – *disaccharides* – and then into longer chains called *polysaccharides* or simple starches. These can be hundreds of thousands of glucose molecules all connected up.

The scale of Syndrome X (and its underlying insulin resistance) as a public-health problem sinks in when you consider that glucose intolerance and insulin resistance affect more than half the population . . . Because of the aggressive marketing and sale of highly processed and refined foods around the world, these conditions are becoming very common in other nations.

Jack Challem, Burton Berkson MD, Melissa Diane Smith

COMPLEXITIES AND REFINEMENTS

Simple carbohydrates are also called 'refined' carbohydrates. These include not only sugar, honey and other obviously sweet foods, but snack foods like breads which, digested and assimilated quickly, lead to a rapid increase in insulin and glucose in the blood. Complex carbohydrates, in contrast, are made up of more complicated sugars and starches as well as various types of fibre. It takes us longer to digest them. These include whole-grains, brown rice and some vegetables, beans and legumes as well as certain fruits like apples and berries. Complex carbohydrates are richer in fibre than their simple cousins, so your body assimilates them more slowly. They cause a more moderate insulin and glucose response and – provided you do not eat too many of them – help protect from high insulin levels, energy swings and from Syndrome X and age-related degeneration.

BLOOD SUGAR SECRETS

Simple or complex, all ingested carbohydrates get into your blood stream as glucose and raise blood glucose levels. Each gram of dietary carbohydrate from your foods shows up in your blood stream as one gram of glucose. Once there, this glucose can either be burned right away for energy, or, if your body is vital and healthy, it can choose instead to store it as glycogen in your muscles or liver for use later. If you eat more carbs-rich foods than your metabolism can use as energy, the glucose in your blood may be converted into fat in your liver or shunted directly into the fat cells to make you fatter. It can also lead to brain chemistry distortions or the furring up of veins and arteries and all the distortions in biomarkers that accompany glucose overload.

BACK TO THE FUTURE

Paleolithic man's carbohydrates came from uncultivated herbs and vege-tables which he gathered by foraging. These plants bear little resem-blance to the highly cultivated starchy vegetables and sugary fruits we eat today. In fact, our ancestors ate little or no fruit. The plants they did eat had much more fibre than our modern plants do. The average diet today contains a meagre 20 grams of fibre. In Paleolithic times man ate

100 grams of fibre or more each day. These are just a few of the ways that carbohydrate foods we now eat have deviated a long way from what our bodies need for the very best genetic expression essential for Age Power.

Fibre refers to the components in plant cells and cell walls which are not broken down by digestive enzymes. Fibre is by no means one single substance. It has many different components – cellulose and hemicellulose, pectin, lignins, gums and mucillages for instance, as well as the polysaccharides found in algae and seaweeds. Except for lignins, all the components of fibre are polymers of carbohydrate. But these are carbohydrates which pass through your body without yielding energy. Good quantities of fibre in your diet improves your insulin and glucose responses – helping to protect you from age degeneration and improving blood glucose control. Soluble fibres such as the lignins, gums and mucillages act favourably on blood insulin concentrations. This is not only because they slow down the rate at which the stomach empties and therefore the rate at which glucose is absorbed, they also inhibit the degradation of starch in the small intestine.

The more industrialised and commercial our societies have become, the more processed carbohydrates have we eaten. The more processed carbohydrates we eat, the more our blood sugar and insulin levels get screwed up. Keep that chocolate cake smothered in whipped cream for twice a year celebrations. If you value your life, mental clarity and personal power, toss out any foods containing sugar from your pantry.

MEET GLYCAEMICS

To make matters even more complicated, carbohydrates are not only separated into complex and simple, they are also categorised according to their *glycaemic index* (GI). The glycaemic index is a measure of just how much a specific carbohydrate food will raise your blood glucose level and also how fast. The glycaemic index is a major ally in eliminating from your life the early ageing and insulin resistance which accompany Syndrome X, not to mention ridding your body of Candida overgrowth. A food's glycaemic rating will tell you whether it will cause a sharp rise in blood sugar and insulin levels or whether it will enter into your blood stream more gradually.

What might surprise you is that foods high on the glycaemic index – those you want to avoid – not only include honey and table sugar but all sorts of snack foods

We cannot put off living until we are ready.

Jose Ortega Y Gasset

In a very real sense we are the authors of our own life.

Mandy Aftel

like corn chips, breakfast cereals and most grain products such as bread and pasta – but both whole-wheat bread and the refined white varieties. Good glycaemic control reduces your serum cholesterol reversing biomarkers, improves your overall health and increases your energy. It also decreases the formation of cross-linking collagen in the skin which amongst other things causes wrinkling and discourages free radical damage, so that you age more slowly. Finally, to make it even more complicated, it is not only the *kind* of carbohydrates we consume that affects insulin and blood sugar, it is also how much fibre we take in and how much protein we eat at the same meal. The more fibre you eat, especially together with good quality protein at a meal, the slower will glucose rise and the less insulin your pancreas needs to secrete to control it. Coffee is something you want to avoid (or at the very least cut down to only one cup a day) while you are restoring your insulin sensitivity and reversing your biomarkers. Caffeine causes a major rise in blood sugar which in turn calls forth massive secretions of insulin.

All of these things need to be considered when you eat for Age Power. Taking them into account is not as complicated as you might imagine. We have already gone back to the first principles and asked the question: 'What did our ancestors eat?' Now we need to ask: 'How can we adjust our own diet to supply the *kind* of carbohydrates, in the *quantities* and *balance* to support our genetic inheritance and enhance our health?'

> The belief that caffeine provides energy is a myth: There is evidence that chronic caffeine intake may actually lead to chronic fatigue. While mice fed one dose of caffeine demonstrated significant increases in their swimming capacity, when the dose of caffeine was given for six weeks, the caffeine caused a significant decrease in swimming capacity.
>
> *Michael T Murray ND*

HEALTH BY NUMBERS

This is how the glycaemic index works. Different foods are given a numeric value ranging from 0 to as much as 150. This value indicates a healthy body's blood sugar response to eating these. There are two standard glycaemic indexes. One assigns a value to glucose of 100 on the glycaemic table. The other assigns a value of 100 to white bread. It doesn't matter very much which of the two standards of the glycaemic index you work with, for the measurements are only relative. It is their relative nature that makes them valuable (see chart opposite). For instance, where glucose is attributed a glycaemic index of 100, you can compare it to the glycaemic index of brown rice which is assigned the number 50. This means that eating brown rice produces only half the rise in your blood sugar that glucose does. The lower the glycaemic rating of a carbohydrate, the more desirable it will be for your body's glucose and insulin responses. Eating foods high on the index are more likely to create blood sugar problems and insulin resistance. To guard against premature ageing, always emphasise foods which are moderate or low on the index.

DON'T BE DECEIVED

When you first come upon the glycaemic index you might be inclined to conclude that all refined carbohydrates – simple carbohydrates – have a high glycaemic index, while complex carbohydrates – the so-called natural foods like whole-grain breads and rice – are low. This is not actually true. Some vegetables such as carrots and potatoes have an amazingly high glycaemic index. They can produce a more rapid rise in blood glucose than ordinary table sugar. Almost as surprising is the fact that certain simple sugars like fructose – fruit sugar – are lower on the glycaemic index than a number of common grains, vegetables and legumes. That doesn't mean that you should eat masses of fructose. Although fructose is low on the index, it encourages fat storage. Consuming a great deal of fructose has also been shown to have a number of other degenerative effects on the body, including an increase in oxidation damage, the cross-linking of collagen and the formation of AGE's (see pages 83–4).

I am not afraid of dying. I just don't want to be there when it happens.

Woody Allen.

Low glycaemic foods form the basis of Age Power's Insulin Balance eating. These include all of the non-starchy vegetables and fruits like broccoli, cauliflower, courgettes, tomatoes, sprouts, spinach and other leafy greens and celery. Foods which are fundamentally protein foods, or fundamentally fats such as butter and meat or fish are not even rated on the glycaemic index as they are virtually devoid of carbohydrate. As such they too are excellent foods for Age Power's Insulin Balance.

If ever you find yourself eating foods that are too high on the glycaemic index you can, in part, mitigate their effect on insulin and blood sugar by eating them only in small amounts and by making sure that you eat them at the same meal with proteins, fats and plenty of fibre. These three help buffer their glucose-elevating effect to some degree.

GLYCAEMIC INDEX OF COMMON FOODS USING GLUCOSE AS THE STANDARD OF COMPARISON

Food	GI
Maltose	110
Glucose	100
Baked potato	98
Cooked carrots	92
Instant white rice	91
Honey	87
Cornflakes	80
White bread	72
White rice	72
Bagels	72
Mashed potatoes	70
Whole-wheat bread	69
Shredded wheat	67
Brown rice	66
Raisins	64
Beetroot	64
Rye bread	63
Banana	62
Sucrose	59
Sweet corn	59
Pitta bread	57
Popcorn	55
Buckwheat	54

Potato crisps	51
Green peas	51
Spaghetti	50
Ice-cream	50
Oatmeal	49
Sweet potato	48
Whole-grain cereal	48
Pasta	41
Orange	40
Apples	38
Plain yoghurt	36
Chickpeas	36
Skimmed milk	32
Strawberries	32
Kidney beans	29
Lentils	29
Tomatoes	28
Peaches	26
Pearl barley	25
Cherries	24
Fructose	20
Soya beans	15
Peanuts	13

PROTEIN FOR POWER

When it comes to slowing down the ageing process and enhancing overall health, no food is more important than protein. Every molecule of muscle in your body is made from the proteins you eat. Muscle is the engine which turns food calories into energy and burns fat. Enhance the quality of your muscle and you enhance the vitality of your whole body. You also enhance your sex hormones, improve your skin and gain strength and power. Protein foods help *ground* you – so much so that they can even play an important part in living out your dreams and help make your spirituality a day-to-day part of ordinary life, rather than something rarefied that can't influence your goals and paths.

> But our health, our happiness, and future depend upon understanding and reversing this deep-rooted cultural denial of pleasure and leisure. Sensuality and spirituality need not conflict.
>
> *Robert Ornstein, PhD, and David Sobel, MD*

One half of the dry weight of your body – that is when water is removed – is protein. Of this, one third of your body's protein is in your muscles, one fifth in bone and cartilage, one tenth in skin and the rest in your blood and tissue. Your brain cells, your genes and the haemoglobin which transports oxygen throughout your body are all made from protein. So are the thousands of enzymes which orchestrate your body's metabolic functions – from the growth of nails and hair to the digestion and assimilation of the foods you eat. No protein structures in your body are fixed. Each is constantly being broken down and reshaped. In fact the whole structure of your body is being rebuilt day by day, entirely from the proteins you eat. Ninety eight percent of your body's molecules, including your teeth and bones, your organs and your muscles, are replaced each year. Within the last month, your skin has completely rebuilt itself. Within the last 3 months you have received a whole new blood supply. Within the last 6 months just about every molecule of protein in your muscle has been replaced. What is exciting about all this is that, when you shift for the better both the quantity and the quality of proteins you eat, you can completely transform, regenerate and rejuvenate not only the way your body functions, but also the way you look.

UNIQUE STUFF

Unlike fats and carbohydrates, the chemical structure of protein not only includes the elements carbon, hydrogen and oxygen, but it also nitrogen. In fact nitrogen is the key element in determining the crude protein content of foods. Experts calculate protein content by multiplying the number of nitrogen atoms in a food by 6.25. This figure is based on an average nitrogen content in protein of 16 percent.

Protein is a kind of umbrella term used to describe the 22 biological compounds called amino acids. Because your body has the ability to synthesise 13 of these amino acids, those eight remaining are generally considered *essential proteins*. This is why we are told that we must obtain them from dietary sources. The eight essential amino acids, *isoleucine, leucine, lysine, methionine, phenylalanine, threonine, tryptophan* and *valine* are those amino acids which we are told we must eat each day, either by taking animal source foods all of which contain them or, by mixing together vegetable foods, each of which contributes some of the essential amino acids, so the entire spectrum of essential amino acids are present in our bodies to be able to build new proteins. When it comes to babies and animals, two more amino acids, *arginine* and *histidine*, are also considered essential. In truth, we adults also need these two regularly through our foods if we are not just to *survive* but to *thrive*.

PROTEIN FOR STRONG IMMUNITY

Having said all this, it is time to lay aside the notion of *essential* and *non-essential* amino acids. For, although your body does indeed have the capacity to turn non-essential amino acids into essential amino acids, it can do so only if there is *sufficient quantity* of the specific amino acids needed. High quality proteins – the kind of proteins you need to create a lean, powerful body – are found in foods which offer not only the essential amino acids but good quantities of the rest as well. Your body cannot build a strong immune system, blood, skin and muscle if you are not supplying it with proteins of the very highest biological value. The older you get chronologically, the more important this becomes.

The amount of protein eaten by our distant ancestors varied with the season and geographic location, but the average amount consumed was almost three times what the average person eats today. Much of the protein consumed during Paleolithic times came from what we now call game meat – wild animals that were hunted, not bred. Because wild animals moved about freely (in contrast to animals kept in a pen) their meat was higher in protein (muscle) and significantly lower in total fat and saturated fat than most commercial meats sold today. The meat found in the Paleolithic diet had other beneficial properties as well. It was rich in omega-3 fats (often called 'fatty acids'), a family of healthy dietary fats that help prevent insulin resistance, Syndrome X.

Jack Challem, Burton Berkson MD and Melissa Diane Smith

OUT OF DATE NONSENSE

Most books and government guidelines about protein quality are based on an obsolete science which depends on how much protein you *eat*, rather than the amount of protein you *absorb*. The only real measure of protein quality is known as Biological Value (BV). This measure determines the amount of protein that is actually *retained* within your body per gram of protein you absorb. The BV measurement was developed a long time ago when eggs were still believed to be the highest biologically assimilable protein in the world. They were therefore rated at 100 percent. Within the last 20 years, thanks to some pretty remarkable developments in food technology – the unusual kind of food technology which actually produces foods that enhance health instead of exploiting it – a number of micro-filtered whey, ionised whey products and whey peptide blends have appeared on the market with biological values much higher than a whole egg. They are a brilliant addition to an Age Power way of eating.

In truth, the development of microfiltered whey proteins has rendered the whole concept of BV percentages meaningless. However, the biological value measurements still work. Considering the biological value of a whole egg as '100' the biological value of lactalbumin (also used in sports supplements) would be 104 and the biological value of the microfiltered whey protein and ionised whey powders varies from 110 to 159. Here is a chart of the biological value of common dietary proteins:

BIOLOGICAL VALUE (BV) OF COMMON PROTEINS

Whey peptide blends, whey isolates, microfiltered whey and ionised whey	110–159
Lactalbumin (whey protein concentrate)	104
Egg	100
Cow's milk	91
Egg white (albumin)	88
Fish	83
Meat	80
Chicken	79
Soya	74
Rice	59
Beans	49

HEAT DENATURES

It may surprise you to see that meat and fish, which we've always been told are the top quality proteins – are rated much lower on the biological value scale than many other protein sources. There are a number of reasons for this. First of all, the biological value of proteins when it comes to meat, fish and other common foods, is measured from these foods after they have been *cooked*. When proteins are heated, some of their amino acids become so *denatured* – changed in their molecular structure – as to render them useless. For the digestive enzymes in the gut have difficulty processing them onwards.

A few amino acids can even be destroyed by cooking. Grill a steak at 239° Fahrenheit, and the amino acids cystine and lysine are lost. Glutamine, one of the important amino acids in the prevention of arthritis and the regulation of appetite, can also be destroyed by heat. There is evidence that cooked milk proteins as well as cooked meat, poultry and egg proteins can chemically bind with vital nutrients too, making them unavailable for use by the body in building the new protein molecules it needs. Most of the meat, game, small insects and animals that Paleolithic men ate came in their natural uncooked form. The biological value of their proteins was therefore much higher – probably close to the BV of microfiltered whey protein – than are the animal sources of protein we eat now.

Whey protein concentrate brings other health and beauty benefits as well. There is growing evidence that it can increase the activity of osteoblasts. These are the cells responsible for building new bone. There is every indication that glutathione plays an important role in increasing bone density as well as in improving the quality of collagen in the connective tissue and skin. There is even some evidence that it may prevent or reverse the cross-linking of collagen that comes with ageing.

END TO FOOD ALLERGIES

Another great thing about whey protein concentrate is that many people with food sensitivities, once they eliminate high carbohydrates from their diet and add good quantities of whey protein concentrate, find they are no longer troubled by them. Whey protein concentrates also work well even for many people with a known milk allergy. For the fractions of milk which tend to cause food sensitivities are usually eliminated in the processing.

AGE-SLOWING IMMUNE POWER

Microfiltered whey is the best and easiest way to take quality protein. Use it to make a great snack or quick liquid meal by mixing it with pure water and maybe a handful of berries. Use it regularly and it is a superb way to help bring about cell renewal and new tissue growth. It improves skin, strengthens arteries and restructures the musculature of your whole body. Whey protein does wonderful things for the immune system, too, thanks to some of its active ingredients known as *subfractions*. These subfractions, as well as other ingredients, mean that whey protein has the remarkable ability to increase your body's level of age-slowing *glutathione* – by providing your body with the building blocks it needs to produce glutathione itself. This is hot stuff when it comes to preventing and reversing ageing as well as protecting you from illness. Glutathione is an anti-oxidant. It neutralises toxicity in the body from pesticides and herbicides in our environment, from cancer-causing substances and from heavy metals and peroxides. It helps protect many physiological processes related to immune functions. It also enhances enzyme activities and protein synthesis and protects your DNA. Using microfiltered whey protein enables you to increase the levels of glutathione and therefore your protection from free radicals in a manner that's virtually impossible any other way. You cannot rely on taking oral supplements of glutathione since your body breaks it down before it can be used.

AMAZING OESTROGEN PARADOX

Soya isoflavones, like so many health-enhancing phytonutrients help restore some of the balance in a living system where it has been lost. Many of soya's protective and health enhancing influences have to do with its oestrogen-like activity. Isoflavones – weak oestrogen-like plant chemicals – bind together with the body's oestrogen receptors and help protect it from damage. And here lies a paradox. Although isoflavones are oestrogen-like themselves, they are very weak in their oestrogenic activity. When they hook up with your body's oestrogen receptor sites these plant chemicals actually exert an *anti-oestrogenic* affect which is beneficial. One of the ways they do this is that, in binding with your oestrogen receptor sites, they block the uptake of the dangerous oestrogen-like chemicals in our environment. Known as *xenoestrogens*, they reach us through herbicides and pesticides in our foods, as well as taking oestrogen drugs, all of which have been linked with the development of cancers. Post-menopausal Japanese women who eat soya foods regularly, rarely suffer menopausal symptoms and nor do they often use hormone replacement.

Eating a little soya protein can also help strengthen your bones. In one placebo controlled double-blind cross-over study a mere 45 mg of soya isofavone increased the bone density of post-menopausal women in only 24 weeks. Studies carried out on older Asian women who eat soya foods over a lifetime suggest that isoflavones not only improve bone integrity but protect against bone loss and reduce our risk of osteoporosis and fractures.

Nowadays, more and more women, urged by their doctors or the media to take synthetic hormone replacement on the assumption that it may help protect them from osteoporosis, decide that the benefits promised are not off-set by the risks implicit in subjecting their bodies to long-term drug treatment. Many are turning to soya as a safe alternative. Isoflavones improve bone mass because, like whey protein, they trigger activity in the osteoblasts – cells responsible for the formation of new bone tissue. They probably also increase your body's ability to absorb and retain calcium from the foods you eat.

Bill's 32. He looks 32. He looked it 5 years ago. He'll look it 20 years from now. I hate men.

Bette Davis, All about Eve

Food allergies have been implicated as a causative factor in a wide range of conditions; no part of the human body is immune from being a target cell or organ.

Michael T Murray ND

BUY THE BEST

When choosing whey proteins go for those that have been produced without heat or acid extraction. For both of these methods destroy bonds between the di-peptides and tri-peptides which your body needs to be able to trigger its protein-building functions. Otherwise, what you're putting in your body is simply not going to be used. The chemical keys that come from di-peptide and tri-peptide bonds are recognized by your cell's receptor sites (locks) so they can make use of them in a way that they cannot absorb single amino acids. This enables your body to hold onto and make use of twice the protein you would get from high quality ordinary protein foods like meat and fish. The best wheys are 'micro-filtered' and 'ion-exchange'. Denatured whey proteins are simply no good. Only buy from companies who have built a solid reputation in nutrition. (See Resources)

HELP FROM SOYA

Although soya protein is much lower in biological value than many other proteins, what makes it a useful food is the fact that, as numerous cross-cultural scientific studies reveal, the humble soya bean has other anti-ageing and anti-disease properties. If you are not using some soya foods in your life, you are definitely missing out on something. Eating even small quantities of soya – a mere 25 grams of soya protein a day (about half a cup of tofu) – reduces your risk of heart disease, lowers cholesterol levels, helps alleviate Syndrome X, helps prevent osteoporosis, decreases PMS and menopausal symptoms and reduces your risks of many types of cancer.

Much of soya's health-enhancing power comes from a group of phyto-chemical compounds it contains called *isoflavones*. These phytonutrients include *genistein diadzein* and *glycitein*. Each has its own unique benefits, but they also act together in synergy. This is probably why soya can be beneficial in reversing insulin resistance, obesity and Syndrome X. Isoflavons decrease insulin levels. In doing so, they bring about

> . . . cells of the body are not harmed by an excess of quality amino acid molecules floating in the cell fluid. The cell can take in what it requires of each amino acid and leave what it does not need. Lack of quality proteins is serious, a state that the functioning of the body will not long endure before showing deficiency symptoms.
>
> *Abram Hoffer MD PhD*

beneficial changes in blood lipid profiles and a decrease in arteriosclerosis. Soya has been shown to significantly reduce total cholesterol, low density lipoproteins (LDL) or 'bad' cholesterol and triglycerides, although it only minimally affects the high density lipoproteins (HDL) or 'good' cholesterol.

DOWN SIDE

Not all soya is worth using – far from it. Almost 95 percent of the soya beans grown now come from Genetically Modified Organism seeds. In the opinion of many well-informed scientists, eating such foods is like drawing a wild card in poker. You quite frankly do not know what you are getting. Rather than gamble with the unknown, I choose soya products that are made only from organic soya bean. In most – not all – countries this is a guarantee that they contain no GMO's. By weight, soya beans are 42 percent protein, 33 percent carbohydrate, 20 percent fat and five percent fibre. Products made from them include soya protein isolate, which is about 90 percent protein. When buying soya protein isolate make sure that it says 'water processed' on the label. This practice leaves most of the valuable isoflavones intact for your body to use. Other soya foods include tempeh, miso, tofu, lecithin, textured vegetable protein and soya milk.

THROW OUT THE JUNK

Fat-free and low-fat diets cause your body to age prematurely. They create sub-clinical fatty acid deficiencies. So do diets high in junk fats – margarines, ready-made salad dressings and sauces, convenience foods and the golden vegetable oils you see lined up on supermarket shelves which many still claim are supposed to be good for us. On a typical Western diet, where 45 percent of our calories come from fats, fatty acid deficiencies are rampant. Why? Because your body can not make use of the trans fatty acids – or 'junk fats' – in the foods they are eating. Here are only a few of the conditions that result from a fatty acid deficiency: premature ageing, heart disease,

SOYA FOODS

- ❏ Help reverse Syndrome X.
- ❏ Reduce the risk of some cancers.
- ❏ Rebalance sex hormones.
- ❏ Help prevent osteoporosis.
- ❏ Lower LDL ('bad' cholesterol).
- ❏ Build strong bones.

suppressed immunity, PMS, arthritis, dry skin, raised cholesterol levels and emotional and behavioural problems.

WHAT IS A FAT?

Fat is a macronutrient which exerts little effect on your insulin levels, but which strongly decreases your appetite. Provided you are getting the right kind of fats in your diet, they can rejuvenate and balance your hormone levels and re-orient how you look and feel, thanks to their effects on important regulatory chemicals called prostaglandins. Organic compounds scientifically known as triglycerides, all fats are composed of a glycerol molecule with fatty acids connected to it. Chemically, a fatty acid consists of a chain of carbon and hydrogen atoms to which one oxygen atom is attached. A molecule of fat differs from a molecule of carbohydrate (which is also made of carbon, hydrogen and oxygen) because the fat molecule contains a lot less oxygen. This is what makes fat highly concentrated and why there are

---

FORGET FAT FREE

For generations we have been told fat is unhealthy. Don't you believe it. Many false beliefs surround fats. Your body's tissues, hormones and all of its cells are dependent for their health on a good supply of essential fats. If you don't get enough of these (and almost nobody does on a low-fat regime), your overall health is compromised and you age more rapidly.

---

nine calories to each gram of fat you eat, while only four calories to each gram of carbohydrate or protein. Incidentally, we tend to think that a 'calorie' is a bad thing. A calorie is just the measurement used to describe the energy-producing value of foods.

Scientists divide fats roughly into two groups – saturated and unsaturated. A saturated fat is a fatty acid with a molecule in which each carbon atom is connected to a hydrogen atom. This means there are no empty *spaces* to allow one or more of its carbons to reach out and join together with molecules of other substances. Because of this, saturated fats – found in meat, dairy products like cheese, ice cream, milk and

> Despite the fact that the world is forging ahead with the latest technology, your fingertips are cracking, your nails are breaking too easily, and your skin is often covered with rashes, bumps, blackheads and pimples. Why? It's simple. You're living in a chemical world.
>
> *Anne Louise Gittleman*

tropical oils like palm kernel oil and coconut oil – are stable, relatively inactive and virtually inert in your body. There are exceptions to this however which we will look at in a minute. The raison d'être for most saturated fats is to provide energy which can be stored in your body's fat cells, especially in times of famine, to be used later.

NECESSARY AND POWERFUL

The second group of fats, the unsaturates, are very different. They are mostly found in foods of vegetable origin like nuts and seeds, grains and avocados, although some of the most important omega-3 oils are also found in fish and game. Unlike saturated fats, such as butter, which are solid, unsaturated fats come in liquid form. According to classical nutrition, only two unsaturated fatty acids are necessary for human health – linoleic and alpha linolenic acids. Out of these two, your body is supposed to be able to make all of the other fatty acids it needs. The trouble is that many people, having lived for years on commercial foods, lose their ability to make conversions. They need to get their fatty acids in a more direct way

---

EXTRA VIRGIN

Rich in omega-9 fats, olive oil contains oleic acid, a mono-unsaturated oil that is more resistant to the denaturing effects of heat and light than polyunsaturated oils. While omega-9 fats are not essential to the body, olive oil has many health-enhancing properties. Use it often in your salads and for wok frying foods.

Essential fatty acids are essential because they are the fundamental nuts and bolts that your body uses to structure the brain, eyes, ears, reproductive organs and cell membranes that surround and protect every cell in your body. Without them you would not be able to move a muscle. You could not think, see or hear. Essential fatty acids are also needed for your body to make hormone-like chemicals called prostaglandins. Critical to cellular functioning in the body, a good balance of prostaglandins helps your body resist illness – from arthritis and ulcers to migraines and cancer. It also supports the functions of your immune system, reproductive system, central nervous system and heart. Finally, prostaglandins regulate your brain chemicals – neuro-transmitters – themselves created out of essential fatty acids. When their balance is good you thrive and are protected from inflammatory conditions including rheumatic problems as well as a trigger happy immune system.

MEET THE OMEGAS

The omega-3 group of fats and the omega-6 group make up the essential fatty acid group of fats. Head of the omega-3 family is alpha-linolenic acid. Head of the omega-6 family is linoleic acid. Paleopathologists have determined that our distant ancestors consumed these essential fats in a ratio of between 1:1 and 3:1 omega-6 to omega-3. In other words, these essential fats were eaten in relatively equal quantities compared to the balance we get now. This, scientists now believe, is an ideal balance.

OUT OF BALANCE

In modern times the balance between our omega-6 and omega-3s has become completely screwed up. We now consume omega-6 and omega-3 in a ratio of about 22:1 compared to our Paleolithic ancestors – far too high for optimal health.

NATURAL APPETITE CONTROL

The omega-3 fats are particularly good satiety nutrients. These natural appetite suppressants work in an interesting way. They release a hormone called *cholecystokinin* or CCK from the stomach when you eat them. This hormone signals to your brain letting it know that you feel satisfied. When you reduce the level of fat in a meal, your brain does not receive the same message and – although you may be filled with food – you still want to eat more. This is a common experience of people who sit down to a meal and, no matter how much they eat, still crave food at the end of it. This can lead to eating disorders and a real mistrust of your body and yourself where you feel you have to watch yourself carefully lest your eating get out of hand. Add enough good quality essential fatty acids – especially the omega-3 fish oils – to your diet and you gradually begin to feel full and satisfied. You also learn that you can trust your body's messages.

ESSENTIAL FATTY ACIDS PREVENT RAPID AGEING. THEY:

- Ensure insulin sensitivity and good blood glucose control.
- Reduce excessive inflammation.
- Regulate cholesterol levels, triglyceride levels and blood pressure.
- Maintain cellular hydration.
- Build good semi-permeable cell walls for beautiful, well-hydrated skin and healthy arteries.
- Enhance good prostaglandin production.
- Protect the myelin sheaths around nerve cells in the brain.

PROTECT YOURSELF FROM INFLAMMATION

Essential fatty acids help protect from inflammation that occurs in some people as a result of omega-6 oils being turned into *arachidonic acid* in the body. Arachidonic acid is a precursor to the inflammatory prostaglandins. You don't want too much of it. Since omega-6 vegetable oils are readily available in the modern diet, we don't need to add more omega-6 to the Age Power's Insulin Balance. Omega-3s can be harder to come by. Using cold-processed flaxseed oil on salads and supplements of omega-3 fish oils DHA and EPA can be a great asset to your health. This helps redress the balance. Studies which show the benefits of the omega-3 fats from DHA and EPA – rich fish oils – now number in the thousands. We know now that adequate omega-3s decrease insulin resistance, improve cardiovascular health, counter both chronic and acute inflammatory conditions from arthritis to a hyper-active immune system and help protect your body from degeneration.

FAT SHEDDING FATS

Omega-6 and omega-3 essential fatty acids – in the right balance – can help your body shed fat stores in at least three different ways.

- ❏ They increase metabolic rate and fat metabolism so more of your stored fat can be burnt as energy.
- ❏ They enhance the production of helpful prostaglandins – hormone-like compounds which regulate vital biological functions – in subtle but powerful ways favourable to fat burning.
- ❏ They increase insulin sensitivity and help counter Syndrome X.

SUPER PROTECTORS

There is no better way of enhancing your health than with phytonutrient-rich foods – lots of them. These are powerful anti-oxidant and immune-enhancing plant chemicals which nobody can afford to be without. Our Paleolithic ancestors took in as much as 300 times the phytonutrients that we do today. So we have some catching up to do. These powerful plant chemicals help decrease your risk of various kinds of cancers including colon cancer, breast cancer and skin cancer, as well as slow down the growth of cancerous cells. They are even being heralded as ways of being able to help prevent macular degeneration – the kind of changes that take place in mid-life where suddenly you have to put the menu on the floor to be able to read it.

Fruits, vegetables and herbs are not only storehouses for vitamins and minerals, but boast high levels of *phytochemicals*. These powerhouses for health, energy and fat loss, also known as *phytonutrients* or *nutriceuticals*, are not nutrients like vitamins and minerals. There is no research to show that if we do not get them we will die. Neither are there known 'deficiency symptoms' associated with our not getting them in our diet. Yet these colourful plant factors play a vital health and anti-ageing role. A good supply of phytonutrients minimises your risk of cancer and heart disease and brings protection from other degenerative conditions associated with ageing, such as inflammation of the joints, loss of memory and concentration. Many now believe they help slow the ageing process altogether.

SURE PROTECTION

Many phytochemicals interfere with, or block, specific disease processes. They do this either by acting as anti-oxidants and preventing free radical damage, or by inhibiting enzymes which allow the development of diseases like cancer to occur. Some plant factors clear our cells of toxins and other damaging substances such as herbicides and pesticides. Others such as berries, grapeseeds and cherries, as well as citrus fruits are excellent sources of water-soluble phytochemicals known as flavonoids. Flavonoids guard the integrity of collagen within your body. They work synergistically with vitamin C and other vitamins and minerals to enhance the positive effects of antioxidants in the body. They improve the function and the integrity of the tiny blood vessels known as capillaries, which deliver nutrients and oxygen to your cells. This not only helps raise overall energy, it also helps create smooth and elastic skin, protects against bruising, enhances memory and improves eyesight. Many phytonutrients carry weird names like *catechin, quercetin* and *hesperidin.* Among the more than 20,000 known, hesperidin, rutin, quercetin, catechin and pycnogenol are especially important. Catechin reduces allergic reactions by calming histamine release in your body. Rutin helps guard the integrity and health of capillaries, veins and arteries as well as your skin itself. Vegetables can be a good source of *flavonoids* too: green peppers, tomatoes, red and yellow onions and cucumbers. Even yams and buckwheat contain good quantities. They help protect and rebuild collagen damaged by age.

SECRETS OF SULPHUR

By now practically everybody has heard how powerful broccoli is. This dark green vegetable is a locus of nutrients including anti-tumour phytochemicals like sulforaphane, which encourages the formation of enzymes that have the ability to process and remove cancer-causing substances from your cells. Cauliflower, Brussels sprouts, collard greens and kale, as well as other green vegetables, are all rich in sulforaphane.

Cabbage also boasts a bounty of phytonutrients – each of which can improve your health and good looks in its own unique way. Take the *isothiocynates*. They inhibit the production of a group of highly destructive enzymes in the body known as Phase 1 enzymes which can change non-dangerous chemical compounds into cancer-causing ones. The isothiocynates throw a monkey wrench in the works, minimising the formation of cancer-causing compounds. Their presence also increases another group of enzymes, known as Phase 2, which helps lower the level of cancer-causing chemicals in your body altogether.

Another main group of players in the plant factor symphony is the carotenoids. You find these pigments in the protein complexes of bright

COLOUR HAS CLOUT

Many of these amazing plant factors are found in common foods, from berries, citrus fruits and grapes to broccoli, cabbage, spinach, carrots, soya beans, onions, garlic and tomatoes. They occur in spices and herbs – from red pepper to basil, oregano, parsley and mint as well. You will find lots of phytochemicals tucked inside the red, yellow, orange, green and blue colours of the vegetables our ancestors ate. But in the average Western diet of manufactured convenience foods they are scarce as hen's teeth. It is these rainbow-coloured plant factors which give autumn leaves and spring flowers their colour as well as imparting the wonderful fragrances to fresh, organically grown fruits and vegetables. Phytonutrients come packed together in groups within the same plant, to impact the body at deep physiological and biochemical levels. And they are always best gleaned not from supplements, but rather eaten from whole foods that contain them.

coloured fruits and vegetables. Carotenoids live in green plant tissues as well, but in this case they tend to be covered by chlorophyll so that their presence is only evident after the green pigment has degraded as it does when you cook the vegetable, or when it begins to die in the autumn.

A number of epidemiological studies have shown that the more fresh fruit and vegetables rich in carotenoids we eat, the more our risk of cancer is diminished. Part of this is due to the carotenoid's powerful anti-oxidant activity. They help protect the body from oxidative free radical damage associated with the development of degenerative conditions such as arthritis and coronary heart disease. Carotenoids, like vitamin A, vitamin C and vitamin E, are able to quench free radicals and de-activate them. Scientists estimate that there are probably more than 600 naturally-occurring carotenoids in our foods. These are certainly the most widespread pigments found in nature. The most well known include *lutein, lycopene, alpha carotene, zeaxanthin* and *beta-carotene.*

Age Power's Insulin Balance can take you to places of energy, radiant health and well-being that you may have longed for but not known how to achieve. So read on.

AGE POWER'S INSULIN BALANCE PRINCIPLES

❑ Eliminate both refined and high glycaemic carbohydrates, including flour, starchy vegetables like potatoes, white rice, sugar and other sweeteners.

❑ Choose natural, fresh unprocessed foods.

❑ Eat as many as possible of these raw foods.

❑ Go for non-starchy vegetables.

❑ Avoid soft drinks, fruit juices and alcohol.

❑ Eliminate omega-6 rich vegetable oils from your diet and use cold-pressed extra virgin olive oil instead.

❑ Enrich your diet with omega-3 fats from fish oils and flaxseed oil.

❑ Refuse all trans-fatty acids found in deep-fried foods, margarine and foods containing partially hydrogenated oils.

❑ Eat protein foods at every meal and snack.

CAROTENOID CARE

Here are just a few of the beneficial effects of carotenoids:

❑ They improve the flow of electrical or life energy from cell to cell in the body, enhancing what is known as *gap junction communication*. This means that small molecules bringing nutrients to the cells can pass between the cytoplasm of two cells with much greater ease.

❑ They carry anti-tumour activity, helping to protect you from cancer and other degenerative illnesses as well.

❑ In your body they act very much as they do in plant cells from which they come. They offer protection as a cellular screen against photo-oxidative damage from the sun as well as from other kinds of free radical damage. They help protect your skin from ageing.

❑ A high intake of both beta-carotene and the other carotenoids is associated with a significantly reduced rate of skin cancer, lung cancer and cervix cancer probably because beta-carotene helps improve the integrity of epithelial cells.

❑ They intensify the health-protective properties of interferon, a protein that we make in our body, one purpose of which is to inhibit the replication of viruses.

AGE POWER'S
INSULIN BALANCE

You already have the precious mixture that will make you well. Use it.

Rumi

Age Power is designed to transform your body by maximising insulin sensitivity, increasing lean-body-mass-to-fat ratio, detoxifying the body and heightening overall energy. It makes use of what is currently known about ageing – the biomarkers – and how they can be reversed. It offers you a practical way to go about changing your life permanently for the better, beginning right here and right now.

Age Power's Insulin Balance is a way of eating that honours our genetic makeup stretching back more than a million years of human evolution and fosters the highest expression of our genes through the whole of our lives. In short, it helps you week after week, year after year, to live out more of your potential for energy, joy, creativity and personal power.

THE NITTY GRITTY

The programme is rich in anti-oxidants from foods containing beneficial phytochemicals, thanks to its emphasis on natural, fresh – preferably organic – unprocessed foods. It eliminates refined and high glycaemic carbohydrates including flour and all the junk foods made from it including most breakfast cereals, starchy vegetables like potatoes as well as white rice. It gets rid of excessive sweetening of foods from sugar, malt extract, corn syrup, honey and most chemical sweeteners. It suggests that you eat as many of your vegetables and fruits raw if you can, to get the benefits of the non-chemical, yet very important, energies for health and healing which these foods carry. It asks you to reject soft drinks including diet colas as well as most fruit juices and other highly processed drinks. It also eliminates highly processed vegetable oils and all those ready made salad dressings that grace the inner sanctum of supermarkets, and suggests you go for extra virgin olive oil instead for your salads and wok fries. It leaves out the margarines too, as well as all those convenience foods replete with partially hydrogenated oils, refined flour and sugar. As far as alcohol is concerned it suggests you eliminate it, or limit your intake of it to one glass of wine a day, if you want to reach your full potential for vitality, mental clarity and autonomy.

RAW POWER FOR REJUVENATION

Age Power's Insulin Balance asks that you aim to eat at least 50 percent of your foods in their natural raw state. From sashimi to strawberries clean, wholesome foods eaten raw have remarkable health-enhancing, anti-ageing properties. This is why they are used throughout the world at the most famous natural clinics and spas for rejuvenation and healing of both chronic and acute illness. Uncooked foods improve cellular functioning. Making a high percentage of what you eat raw increases overall energy and stamina, supplies a high level of negantropic structural information to counter ageing and brings the best natural anti-oxidant support.

DELICIOUS FARE

The programme is rich in precious vegetable fibres – from aubergines, lettuces, spinach, leeks, asparagus – eaten together with good quality protein at every meal. It is a way of eating and living which can be an absolute pleasure to follow, once you work out how to reorganise your life to make it happen for you. The foods you will be eating are not just good for you, they are absolutely delicious whether or not, like me, you are committed to simplicity – ready in ten minute meals – or to the delights of true gourmet fare. Although the basis of this way of eating is food alone, the programme also asks you to look at the possibility that nutritional supplements can help get you going on an Age Power track faster and more efficiently than food alone. Let's look specifically at the nuts and bolts of how to put it all together. Then we will be learning what Age Power menus look like.

NICE WORK IF YOU CAN GET IT

❑ Use Co-enzyme A to enhance your body's production of ATP and catalyse your body's major anti-ageing processes (see chapter 8).

❑ Take a good quality multiple vitamin plus a plant factor anti-oxidant such as flavonoids, pygnogenol and alpha-lipoic acid daily.

❑ Supplement your diet with a good quality fish oil rich in EPA and DHA omega-3 fats.

❑ Take extra magnesium – 230 mg of chelated magnesium one to three times a day.

Age Power's Insulin Balance reduces insulin levels by encouraging you to be selective about the kind of carbohydrate foods you eat. It is a life-long food style great for any age. It is most certainly *not* a slimming diet although you are likely to find you lose fat. In fact, making use of this way of eating puts an end to a need for slimming diets forever. It also puts an end to the heartache, fatigue and subclinical nutritional deficiencies they cause. Calorie controlled slimming diets age your body rapidly. They raise insulin levels which in turn encourage your body to lay down more fat stores. Meanwhile, insufficient good quality protein on most slimming diets brings about the loss of precious muscle tissue from your body, causing sarcopenia and undermining your health and increasing your biological age by negatively affecting your biomarkers.

Age Power's Insulin Balance takes you so far along the road to healthy living and healing, it can be nothing short of amazing. Even though it places little emphasis on the number of calories you eat, the programme is an effective fat loss tool. It works beautifully for women whose body is less than 35 percent fat and men who carry less than 22 percent fat. For women who carry more that 35 percent fat and for men whose body fat is above 22 percent, the Ketogenics Diet explained in my book *The X Factor Diet* is appropriate (see Further Reading). It works faster and goes deeper.

MAKE THE SWITCH

Age Power's Insulin Balance shifts the ratio of carbohydrates, fats and proteins so that:

- ☐ Thirty-five percent of your calories are low glycaemic carbohydrates.
- ☐ Thirty-five percent of your calories are good quality proteins.
- ☐ Thirty percent of your calories are high quality fats.
- ☐ Twenty-five to 75 percent of your foods are eaten raw.

FAST TRACK TO ENERGY

Age Power's Insulin Balance works hand-in-glove with Age Power's exercise programme to increase your body's insulin sensitivity and glucose tolerance and to slow down your risk of degeneration. The exercise programme consists of simple weight training for half an hour, four days a week at home and daily half-hour walks (see chapters 18 and 19). How long it takes to start reaping the benefits of the programme varies from one person to another. Most people start to see changes very quickly. Within a few days they have more energy. Carbohydrate and sweet cravings disappear in five to seven days. Digestion works better. Tummies quickly flatten. Insulin sensitivity is quickly enhanced. Blood sugar levels stabilise. Almost right away you feel more alert and have more energy to keep you going, hour after hour, day in day out. By all accounts it should take three months or longer before you get decreases in blood pressure and shifts in cholesterol. However, most people experience significant measurable positive change in their biomarkers in as little as four or five weeks.

FOOD CHOOSING

- ❑ Your foods should, as much as possible, be whole-foods, not fractions of foods as a result of refining and processing.
- ❑ Your foods need to be as fresh as possible and eaten as close to a living state as possible. They should be allowed little time for the deterioration which occurs as a result of oxidation.
- ❑ When cooked, your vegetables are best steamed, boiled or wok fried and cooked as lightly as possible.
- ❑ All the foods you eat should be non-toxic and non-polluting to your body. They should contain no synthetic flavours, colours, preservatives or other additives used to cosmetically 'enhance' the foods.
- ❑ Your diet should be varied, for down through evolution the human body has adapted to a wide range of foods which offer a broad spectrum of nutrients.

THE PROTEIN QUESTION

On Insulin Balance you may be eating somewhat more protein than you have been used to. This is important. The single most widespread deficiency of macronutrients as people get older is as a result of eating too little protein. Scientists once believed (I used to believe it myself) that we had to be careful not to eat too much protein. Any excess, they thought, would leach calcium from bones and make us prone to osteoporosis. Several large scale studies have recently proved this wrong. It is a *lack* of sufficient protein that predisposes us to bone thinning. As we get older we often eat less and less meat, fish, eggs and other protein foods. Yet these are exactly the kind of foods we need to support the immune system and keep hormone levels from flagging, not to mention enhancing lean body mass and keeping skin youthful.

HOW MUCH PROTEIN DO YOU NEED ?

Just how much protein food you need is relatively easy to figure. First, calculate your lean body mass by working out the percentage of body fat that you carry (see pages 267 and 268).

Multiply your weight in kilos times your percentage of body fat. This gives your total body fat weight. For example, an 82 kilo man with 21 percent body fat:

82		0.21		17.2
Weight	x	% of body fat	=	Total body fat weight

Once you know the weight of your total body fat, subtract this from your total weight. What you get is your lean body mass. Your lean body mass measurement is the total weight of all of the non-fat tissues in your body. You'll need this measurement to work out your ideal level of protein each day. This in turn will enable you, by comparison, to work out how much carbohydrate foods to balance with it. Our 82 kilo man then has:

Total weight	82	
(Minus) Total body fat	17.2	
=	64.8	Lean body mass

Now we have to take into account how much physical activity you get, because the more you exercise, the higher your need for protein will be. Here is a chart to help you make that calculation.

Activity	Protein Requirements (grams)	Adjustments (if any apply add to your Physical Activity Factor)	
Sedentary	0.5	Significantly overweight	increase by 0.1
Light (i.e. walking)	0.6	Pregnancy	increase by 0.2
Moderate (30 mins daily, 3 times per week)	0.7	Lactation	increase by 0.1
Active (1 hour daily, 5 times per week)	0.8	Caring for young children	increase by 0.2
Very active (2 hours daily, 5 times per week)	0.9	Body Building	increase by 0.1
Heavy weight training or twice-a-day exersise (5 days per week)	1.0	(30% for males) (40% for females)	

NOW YOU CAN WORK OUT YOUR DAILY PROTEIN REQUIREMENT.

Here's how:

Your Lean Body Mass x 2.2 x Physical Activity Factor = Your Total Daily Protein Requirement

For instance: An 82-kilo male has 21 percent body fat and is sedentary
Weight of Body Fat: 82 x 0.21 = 17.2 kilos body fat
Lean Body Mass: 82 – 17.2 kilos body fat = 64.8 kilos lean body mass
Physical Activity Factor (sedentary): is 0.5

Daily Protein Requirement: 64.8 x 2.2 x 0.5 = 71.3g of protein per day

Or: A 59-kilo female has 34 percent body fat and is active
Weight of Body Fat: 59 x 0.34 = 20 kilos
Lean Body Mass: 59 kilos – 20 kilos body fat = 39 kilos
Physical Activity Factor (active): is 0.8

Daily Protein Requirement: 39 x 2.2 x 0.8 = 68.6g of protein per day

It's vital to note that this is NOT the weight of meat or fish, but the weight in grams of the *protein* it contains. Most meats and fish, for instance, are only 20 to 30 percent protein.

MAKE IT EASY

How do you figure out the protein content of food, on a practical, day-by-day basis? Of course, you could spend hours mulling over long lists of the protein, fat and carbohydrate contents of every food that you eat. In my opinion, this does little more than make people neurotic. Happily, there is another way. Called the 'palm' method, it's a technique frequently used by doctors, nutritionists and other practitioners trained in functional medicine. Once you grasp the general idea behind it, the answer to how much protein you have to eat literally lies in the palm of your hand. It's great to use this as a general rule, but let your appetite be the best guide.

The size of the palm of your hand, including its thickness and excluding your fingers and thumb, is about the same as the volume of protein food you will need to eat at each Insulin Balance meal. It may be a little more or a little less, depending on your lean body mass. In any case, the ratio of how many palms of protein make a good balance with carbohydrate remains constant (see page 221). For snacks, a third of a palm of protein food is excellent. If you get a great deal of exercise, or are pregnant, you will need to add an extra third of a palm to each meal.

There is one way in which the palm method breaks down: It is when you are having a meal or a snack based on microfiltered whey protein. This doesn't matter much, however, since the exact protein content of a specific amount of whey protein – a scoop or a tablespoon, for example – is given on the package. You will need to judge your whey protein by grams of protein content rather than using the palm method. If you have a snack of microfiltered whey protein it should contain between 10g and 15g of pure protein. A meal replacement should contain 15g to 30g.

HOW MANY CARBS

Use the same method to find out how much carbohydrate to eat – except that here, things become slightly more complicated. On Age Power's Insulin Balance you will need *at least* two palms of good 'best choice' carbohydrates – that is low glycaemics such as steamed broccoli, spinach, cauliflower, green beans and salad vegetables – for every 'palm' of protein. Occasionally, you might go for one palm of medium-to-high glycaemic carbohydrates. Or you can combine best-choice carbohydrates and higher glycaemic carbohydrates by having at least one palm of the best choice and half a palm of the higher glycaemics.

MAKE GOOD USE OF GLYCAEMICS

Developed over many years, the glycaemic index is a system of rating carbohydrates. It enables you to choose foods that offer a gradual conversion of carbohydrate into glucose. By doing so, you help your body release insulin more slowly and keep your levels of insulin lower. The benefits are enormous. Once you improve insulin control using the glycaemic index in GET SAVVY, you help burn away body fat, reduce serum cholesterol, prevent and even reverse hypertension, improve your overall health and increase your energy. Good glycaemic control also decreases the formation of cross-linking collagen in the skin and discourages free radical damage so that you age more slowly.

QUICK CHECK GLYCAEMIC INDEX FOR FRUITS AND VEGETABLES

VEGETABLES

LOW GLYCAEMIC	MEDIUM GLYCAEMIC		HIGH GLYCAEMIC	
	(low-medium)	(high-medium)	(high)	(very high)
asparagus	aubergine	artichokes	beans, dried	sweet potato
bean sprouts	beans, string	oyster plant	beans, lima	yams
beet greens	beets	parsnips	corn	
broccoli	Brussels sprouts	peas, green	potato, white	
cabbage	chives	squash		
cauliflower	collards	carrots		
celery	dandelion greens			
chard, swiss	kale			
cucumber	kohlrabi			
endive	leeks			
lettuce	okra			
mustard greens	onions			
radishes	parsley			
spinach	peppers, red			
watercress	pimento			
	pumpkin			
	rutabagas			
	turnips			

FRUITS

LOW GLYCAEMIC	MEDIUM GLYCAEMIC		HIGH GLYCAEMIC
cantaloupe	apricots, fresh	apples	bananas
rhubarb	blackberries	blueberries	figs
strawberries	cranberries	cherries	prunes
watermelon	grapefruit	grapes	or any dried nuts
melons	guava melons	kumquats	
tomatoes	lemons	loganberries	
	limes	mangoes	
	oranges	mulberries	
	plums	pears	
	raspberries	pineapples, fresh	
	papayas	pomegranates	
	tangerines		
	peaches		
	kiwifruits		

GAUGING THE FATS

The amount of fat you need at each meal is a total of about one table-spoon of the best: extra-virgin olive oil, flaxseed oil, coconut oil or the fats in foods such as avocados, olives, fish or game, macadamia nuts, almonds or tahini. This amount of fat usually doesn't cause deficiency. From the point of view of the palm method, you will be eating a smallest finger-full of fat at a meal.

ALPHA LIPOIC ACID – A GREAT HELPER

Supplements of ALA offer great support to the biomarker-reversing powers of Insulin Balance eating. Consider taking ALA as a supplement. It is 400 times stronger than vitamins C and E and raises the levels of these two vitamins in your body. It also counters inflammatory reactions. Take 100–200mg a day with meals. ALA:

❑ Reduces insulin balance
❑ Improves insulin sensitivity
❑ Lowers glucose levels
❑ Reduces the formation of AGEs
❑ Neutralises free radicals.

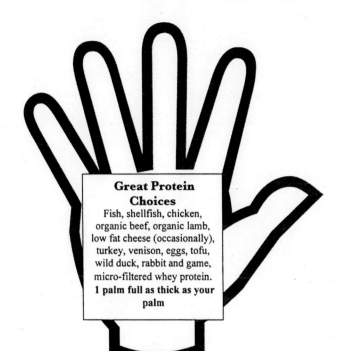

Great Protein Choices
Fish, shellfish, chicken, organic beef, organic lamb, low fat cheese (occasionally), turkey, venison, eggs, tofu, wild duck, rabbit and game, micro-filtered whey protein.
1 palm full as thick as your palm

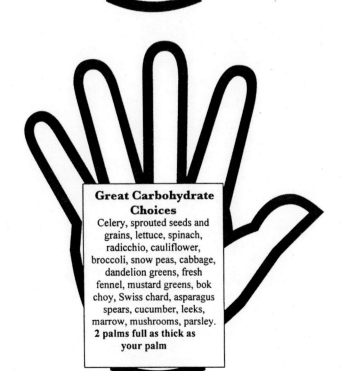

Great Carbohydrate Choices
Celery, sprouted seeds and grains, lettuce, spinach, radicchio, cauliflower, broccoli, snow peas, cabbage, dandelion greens, fresh fennel, mustard greens, bok choy, Swiss chard, asparagus spears, cucumber, leeks, marrow, mushrooms, parsley.
2 palms full as thick as your palm

The palm method is an easy way to go about getting the right balance between top-quality proteins, good carbohydrates and good fats when you start on Insulin Balance Programme.

PROTEINS

GOOD CHOICE PROTEINS	POOR CHOICE PROTEINS

Meat and Poultry

Beef, lean – organic	Bacon
Beef, minced – organic	Beef, fatty cuts
(less than 15% fat)	Liver, chicken
Micro-filtered whey protein	Pepperoni
Chicken breast, skinless –	Salami
free range, organic	Sausage – pork, beef,
Liver, lamb – organic	turkey or chicken
Turkey breast	
Eggs	
Egg whites	

Fish and Seafood

Bass
Bluefish
Calamari
Clams
Cod*
Crab
Groper
Haddock
Halibut
Lobster
Mackerel*
Prawns
Salmon*
Sardines*
Scallops
Snapper
Swordfish
Taraki
Trout*
Tuna, canned in water
Tuna, steak*

Protein-Rich Dairy Foods (only occasionally)

Cheese, fat free
Cottage cheese, low fat 1%
Cottage cheese, no fat
Parmesan

*rich in Omega-3 essential fatty acids

CARBOHYDRATES
GOOD CHOICE CARBOHYDRATES

Salad Stuff Raw/ Cooked	Vegetables Cooked	Fresh Fruit
Alfalfa Sprouts	Artichoke	Apple
Avocados	Asparagus	Apricots
Bamboo shoots	Aubergine	Blueberries
Beans, string	Beans, green	Boysenberries
Beetroot	Bok choy	Cantaloupe
Broccoli	Broccoli	Cherries
Cabbage	Brussels sprouts	Grapefruit
Capsicum	Cabbage	Honeydew melon
Cauliflower	Cauliflower	Kiwifruit
Celery	Chick peas	Lemon
Cucumber	Collard greens	Lime
Endive	Courgette	Mandarin
Escarole	Kale	Nectarine
Fennel	Leeks	Orange
Lamb's Lettuce	Lentils	Peach
Lettuce	Mushrooms, boiled	Pear
Mushrooms	Okra	Plum
Onions	Onions, boiled	Pineapple
Radishes	Sauerkraut	Raspberries
Rocket	Silver beet	Strawberries
Salsa	Spinach	Tangerine
Snow peas	Turnip	Watermelon
Spinach	Yellow squash	
Tomato		

Grains
Barley
Steel Cut Oatmeal

CARBOHYDRATES
POOR CHOICE CARBOHYDRATES

Vegetables Cooked	Grains, Cereals, Breads
Acorn squash	Bagel
Baked beans	Biscuits
Beetroot	Breadcrumbs
Butternut squash	Bread, whole-grain or white
Carrot	Breadsticks
Lima beans	Buckwheat

Parsnips
Peas
Pinto beans
Potato, baked
Potato, boiled
Potato, chips
Potato, mashed
Re-fried beans
Sweetcorn
Sweet potato, baked

Condiments and Treats
Barbecue sauce
Cocktail sauce
Honey
Ice-cream
Jam or jelly
Molasses
Plum sauce
Relish, pickle
Sugar
Sugar, icing
Sweets
Syrup, Golden
Syrup, Maple
Teriyaki sauce
Tomato sauce

Bulgar wheat
Cereal
Cornflour
Couscous, dry
Crackers
Croissant
Croûton
Doughnut
Muffin/Cake
Granola
Melba toast
Millet

Alcohol
Beer
Spirits
Wine

FAT

GOOD CHOICE FATS

Almond butter
Almonds
Avocado
Butter (in moderation)
Coconut oil
Guacamole
Macadamia butter
Macadamia nuts
Olive oil
Olives
Tahini

POOR CHOICE FATS

Bacon bits
Cream
Cream cheese
Lard
Margarine
Sour cream
Cooking oils

START RAW

Try to start your meals with something raw. This helps avoid something called *digestive leucocytosis* which challenges the immune system. You could have a piece of low-glycaemic fruit like melon, a raw salad or some crudités. It can even be raw oysters.

SPICE IT UP

Make good use of the wonderful culinary herbs available: caraway, fennel, dill, chervil, parsley, lovage – the Umberiferae; summer savory, marjoram, the mints, rosemary and thyme – the Labiates which have a strong aroma and are particularly useful for seasoning; the Liliaceae such as garlic, onions, chives and leeks. These three are my favourites: basil, tarragon and horseradish.

Herbs have a special role to play in Age Power. They contain pharmacologically active substances such as volatile oils, tannins, bitter factors, secretins, balsams, resins, mucilages, glycosides and organic vegetable acids, each of which can contribute to overall health in a different way. The tannins, for instance, which occur in many common kitchen herbs, are astringent and have an anti-inflammatory action on the digestive system. They help inhibit fermentation and decomposition. The secretins stimulate the secretion of pancreatic enzymes – particularly important for the complete breakdown of proteins in foods to make them available for bodily use. Organic acids have an antibiotic action and are helpful in the digestion of fats. So do the bitter factors which are found in good quality rosemary, marjoram and fennel. They also act as a tonic to the smooth muscles of the gut and boost secretion of digestive enzymes. Use herbs lavishly in your meals and you will find you can create the most remarkable combinations of subtle flavours and aromas.

GO FOR COLOUR

The more vibrant and beautiful the colours of your vegetables and fruits are, the greater the immune-enhancing and anti-oxidant phytonutrient energy they carry. Bright blueberries or strawberries, deep green leafy vegetables such as spinach and rocket, tell us that the food we are about to eat is brimming with polyphenols, helpful in preventing diseases including cancer and heart disease, as well as countering Syndrome X.

DRINK YOURSELF YOUNGER

Coffee, although not completely forbidden, is not something to drink often. The occasional cup after dinner is not likely to do much harm. More than that and you are really undermining your potential for age-retardation. Coffee not only contains mutagenic and carcinogenic compounds to cause free radical damage, drinking it regularly encourages a build up of cadmium in your body and can interfere with proper pancreatic functioning. It also leeches calcium from the bones. Besides, coffee drinking raises blood sugar and triggers yet more insulin release, both of which you want to avoid to protect from or counter Syndrome X. Black tea is OK in moderation – a cup or two a day. There are plenty of other drinks which are not only good for you, they can be highly enjoyable as well.

COOL THE BOOZE

Alcohol is another substance you want to go easy on. Not only is it high in empty calories yet worthless in terms of nutrients, it causes your liver to produce one of the most potent cross-linkers known – acetaldehyde (see pages 116–8). The more acetaldehyde in your body, the faster it ages. Hard liquor like whisky, gin and vodka – raises insulin levels and is best avoided. A glass of dry white or red wine with one of your meals does most people no harm. It may even have a beneficial effect. A number of studies indicate that red wine, in particular, increases the body's sensitivity to insulin. This is one of the main goals of Age Power's Insulin Balance, so adding a glass of wine to lunch or dinner may further enhance the process. If you do, make sure it is good wine. The run of the mill *vin de table* is full of toxic substances which your cells can do without.

DRINK UP

You'll find some delicious mixtures of herbs in ready-made tea bags if you comb through a few delicatessens and healthfood stores. Some of my favourites have names like Cinnamon, Rose, Almond Sunset, Creamy French Vanilla and Red Zinger. They are great to drink for pleasure and refreshment, the way most people drink coffee and ordinary tea. But there are others which are quite wonderful because they affect the body in specific ways. Lemon Verbena, for instance, is a refreshing sedative, chamomile soothes the digestive tract and both horsetail and solidago (goldenrod) are excellent natural diuretics. The teas I like best just before bed are orange blossom – which you make by boiling a few fresh, frozen or dried blossoms for two to three minutes in two cups of water – red bergamot and lemon peel, all of which are natural sedatives. This last tea comes from an Italian tradition. You make it by peeling the outer yellow skin off an unwaxed, pesticide-free lemon (which has been washed well) with a potato peeler. Pour boiling water over this and let it steep for five minutes. Then strain and drink.

You may be in the habit of drinking fruit juice. But it doesn't fit well into Age Power's Insulin Balance way of life. If you feel you must have a glass of apple juice or orange juice every now and then, try diluting it – one-third juice to two-thirds water. Fruit juices are very high on the glycaemic index. Your body soaks them up like pure sugar and absorbs them very rapidly. Sugar-free colas and soft drinks are another category of drinks you will want to avoid. Fruit-flavoured mineral waters are fine provided they contain no carbohydrates and no artificial sweeteners (check the labels). By far the best drink of all is water. Drink at least eight big glasses every day even if you have to carry a bottle of water around with you to remind you to get your quota (see page 231).

BETTER AND BETTER

Following these guidelines will automatically provide you with anti-ageing nutrition of the highest order. It is a diet rich in the structural information necessary to maintain a high degree of order or negative entropy in your body and therefore to protect it from degeneration. Provided your foods are fresh enough, and provided you eat at least half of them raw, you will also benefit from a high degree of order-enhancing energy – what Bircher-Benner called 'sunlight quanta' – which gives fresh foods an ability to retard degeneration and promote a high level of vitality.

EATING FOR AGE POWER

There is no need to stick rigidly to a menu plan or to count calories, carbs, fats and proteins for you to reap the benefits of Age Power. Within a couple of weeks, when your body cleanses itself and your energy rises, you will begin to sense intuitively which foods work best for you. Insulin Balance is a great way to move towards nutrient-rich calorie-poor eating. You will become familiar with how your appetite diminishes gradually and quite naturally as the nutrient-rich foods you will be eating nourish you better than ever before.

The easiest way to begin is to follow the principles outlined above and check out some meal suggestions below. Remember the best way to cook your foods is to grill, steam, wok fry or sauté them. Check out how well you get on with red meat. Some people, especially as they get older, find they don't handle red meat well but get on very well with fish.

AGE POWER MEAL SUGGESTIONS

Let's look at some typical meals for breakfast, lunch and dinner and some good Insulin Balance snacks. The menus that follow are designed to get you started. They will help you grasp what Age Power eating is all about. You might like to change your eating habits over gradually. If so, start by adding a new meal choice to your normal diet every day or two. You will create for yourself a whole new way of eating and thinking about food. If, like me, you like to jump into things feet first, spend a day or two cleaning out your cupboards and refilling the fridge with Age Power foods (shopping hints are in the next chapter) and launch into it with un-bridled passion. Balance things so you get good quality proteins, fats and low glycaemic carbs at every meal. It's fun and you will be delighted with the changes you experience.

Breakfasts:

- **Instant Omelette** with fresh vegetables. Cook your omelette in olive oil and toss in chopped tomatoes, peppers, spinach – what-have-you. Serve with a slice of rock melon or honeydew. Herb tea or green tea if you wish.
- **Grilled Fish** – salmon is especially good with garlic and sweet onions plus a small bowl of mixed berries. Herb tea or green tea.
- **Unsweetened Yoghurt** or soya yoghurt sprinkled with slivered almonds. Herb tea or green tea.
- **Quick Shake** made with 20 to 30 grams of microfiltered whey protein powder, a teaspoon of flaxseed oil, an apple, pear or a handful of berries blended with a few ice cubes. Herb tea or green tea.
- **Slow Cooked Oatmeal** (not instant) with a grated fresh apple or fresh or frozen blueberries added when cooked. Top with cinnamon or nutmeg and a dab of butter (if desired). Herb tea or green tea.

Lunches:

- **Fresh Spinach Salad** with slivers of white meat – chicken or turkey – slices of yellow, red and green peppers, sweet red onions and sliced fresh mushrooms topped with grated hard-boiled eggs. Toss with olive oil and Dijon mustard dressing.

- **Chicken Kebabs** skewered with onion pieces, crunchy vegetables dipped in olive oil and seasoned with herbs and fresh lemon juice.
- **Fresh Grilled Tuna** on a bed of rocket, with black olives and herbs. Tossed mixed salad dressed with olive oil, balsamic vinegar and garlic dressing.
- **Big Greek Salad** with left-over chicken or lamb made with lettuce, cucumber, tomato wedges, sprinkled with sunflower seeds and a teaspoon of pumpkin seeds, Greek olives and two teaspoons of feta cheese – olive oil and lemon dressing.
- **Low-fat Cottage Cheese** on cos lettuce served with slices of fresh peaches, apricots and/or oranges.

Dinners:

- **Herb Salad** topped with shaved Parmesan (just for fun, occasionally). **Sautéed Sea Bass** with garlic, steamed broccoli and courgettes with slivered almonds. Strawberries with fresh lemon juice and mint. Sliced oranges with shaved coconut.
- **Slivered Raw Beetroot and Apple Salad** dressed with fresh orange juice and curry powder. **Bunless Turkey Burger:** Combine minced turkey with finely chopped green onions or scallions and red pepper. Grill with courgettes, onion slices and a Portobello mushroom or two. Fresh Strawberries dipped in finely ground almonds.
- **Crudités:** Cucumbers, tomatoes, celery and crunchy lettuce with fresh home-made avocado dip. **Grilled Wild Tuna** seasoned with fresh ground pepper and capers. Serve with green beans and spinach spiked with lemon juice.
- **Rocket Salad** with Greek olives. **Grilled Prawns** served with aioli. Fresh blackberries and raspberries.
- **Red Cabbage Coleslaw** with onions, garlic and an apple dressed with homemade mayonnaise. **Stir Fried Chicken** with bok choy, bean sprouts, ginger, green onions, garlic, water chestnuts cooked in coconut oil with a coconut cream sauce sprinkled with toasted sesame seeds. Watermelon balls with ginger.

Snacks:

Eat snacks only if you feel the need. If you do, decrease the amount you are eating at meals. Most people find they feel better simply eating only three meals a day. If you love snacks, here are some suggestions.

HOW ABOUT SNACKS

Judge for yourself whether or not snacks work for you. For some people they are terrific, for others eating more often than every 4 to 5 hours increases insulin resistance and leads to food cravings. You need to play it by ear and find out which works best. Here are some suggestions for good quality snacks:

❑ Half a chicken breast
❑ An apple, an orange, a pear or a few strawberries
❑ Half a cup of unsalted cashews, almonds, brazils or hazel nuts
❑ A few crudités splashed with vinegar, soya sauce and a bit of olive oil
❑ 25g of sunflower seeds, walnuts, macadamias, almonds
❑ A hard boiled egg
❑ Smoothie made with 10 to 15g of microfiltered whey and half an apple with cinnamon or a handful of berries
❑ A cup of low fat cottage cheese

DIGEST IT WELL

If you have been eating irregularly, or more than your body needs, or rely on lots of processed foods, your appetite and digestive system may be less than perfect. The digestive system of a person who has been eating a lot of refined foods or who chronically overeats does not function normally. It remains in a state of persistent stimulation. As a result, good digestion is impaired and nutritional deficiencies occur. Many people in this state go on to experience chronic fatigue and what are commonly known as 'food allergies' as their body calls out for adequate supplies of essential vitamins and minerals, yet doesn't get them. Another consequence of poor eating habits is metabolic slowdown – triggered again by poor digestion. When this happens, your energy levels sink and you gain weight easily. You might need to check out your own digestion and consider taking a good digestive enzyme supplement (see Resources) at the end of each meal.

WHAT CAUSES POOR DIGESTION

❑ Drinking too little water between meals
❑ Eating too much
❑ Eating before previous meal is completely digested
❑ Drinking iced drinks often (especially before or during meals)
❑ Too much alcohol
❑ Eating 'on the run'
❑ Eating at irregular times
❑ Eating heavy meals at night
❑ Infections from yeasts or parasites or bacteria
❑ Dysbiosis (low levels of Lactobacillus acidophilus and Bifidobacteria adolescentis)
❑ Food allergies or sensitivities
❑ Nutrient deficiencies (eg. iron, zinc, vitamin A)
❑ Low stomach acid
❑ On-going physical, emotional or mental stress
❑ Medications: antibiotics (even when used for as little as one day) and non-steroidal anti-inflammatory drugs (NSAIDs) in particular
❑ A low protein diet
❑ Increased demand for protein owing to trauma, surgery, excessive exercise, illness or fasting
❑ Too little fibre

WATER POWER

Water plays a major part in digesting your food and absorbing nutrients thanks to its role in helping your body create enzymes needed for digestion. When you fail to drink enough water between meals your mouth becomes low in saliva and digestion suffers. Water is also the medium through which wastes are eliminated from your body. Each time you exhale, you release highly humidified air – about two big glasses worth a day – and carried on it, metabolic wastes. Your kidneys and intestines eliminate another six or so glasses of water and waste every 24 hours, while another two glasses worth are released through the pores in your skin. That makes 10 glasses a day – and this is on a cool day. When it gets hot, when you are exercising, or when you are working hard, the usual 10 glasses lost in this way can triple.

On average, in a temperate climate – when you are not sweating from exertion or heat – we need about 3.5 litres or six pints a day for optimal health, although few of us consume as much as one third of that. The important thing to remember is that how thirsty you are is *not* a reliable indication of how much water you need to drink. If you want to grow lean and stay that way, you need to do as French women have done for decades. Keep a large bottle or two of pure, fresh, mineral water within easy reach and make sure you consume your quota of this clear, delicious health-giving drink.

CHECK OUT YOUR NEED FOR WATER

Here's how to figure it:

Divide your current weight in kilos by 8. If you weigh 58 kilos then 58 divided by 8 equals 7.25 big glasses (at least 200 ml). Then round the figure upwards to the next glass and there you have it: 8 glasses a day. But remember that this is only a base calculation on a cold day. You will need alot more during exercise or on a hot day

---

Provided you do not suffer from a kidney or liver disease, drinking eight big glasses of water a day not only helps you detoxify and rejuvenate your body, it improves the functioning of your whole body and heightens energy.

MAKE WAY FOR A NEW LIFESTYLE

Eating for Age Power leads you into a whole new way of living. You become more alert and more active. You may even sleep less – yet far better than before. This is because your whole system becomes clearer of toxicity than before so you need less time for tissue repair. You become able to deal with stress better than ever. Age Power eating provides you with high levels of potassium, rapidly restoring an excellent sodium-potassium balance. This leads to increased resistance to fatigue and a greater feeling of calm and stability, day in day out. Age Power eating may also set you slightly apart from your gravy-eating, hard-drinking friends and may even have them feeling slightly suspicious of you in the beginning. But as soon as they find you are not trying to sell them anything –

thanks to your live and let live attitude – they show a similar respect for your new lifestyle. In fact, the people around us who were once the most resistant to our changing lifestyle and the most opinionated to start with, are often the first to become intrigued about what an Age Power lifestyle can offer them. And thanks to their strong independent streak they are usually the ones with the energy and interest to try it for themselves.

GRAZE AT THE EDGE

I can see you now, bending over a hot stove ...
Only I can't see the hot stove.
Groucho Marx

You'll find the healthiest, freshest and the most natural foods for Age Power's Insulin Balance at the outside edges of your local supermarket. These include crunchy fresh vegetables and fruit, fresh game and meats, seafoods and eggs as well as the odd low-fat cheese. Skirt the edges, steer clear of the middle and you've got the secret to hunting and gathering.

Natural wholesome foods are perishable. They have to be replaced often, unlike the ready in a minute, pre-made stuff that you find in the inner isles. You will be shopping 'at the edge' in another way too: You'll be looking for foods as close as possible to those that our ancestors ate with a wide variety of crunchy, living vegetables – especially bright coloured ones – which are low or moderate on the glycaemic index.

GRAZE FOR AGE POWER

A good general rule when choosing healthy food is this: Foods with a long shelf life don't belong in your body. Processed high-carb foods often have a very long shelf life. This makes them great sales material for food manufacturers and retailers since they can sit on the shelves for a long time, and are cheap to produce with high profit margins. But most of them are whipped up out of white flour and white sugar plus a lot of junk fats, chemical additives and salt. Avoid them.

READ LABELS

Once you leave the perimeters of a supermarket and move into the inner circle, you need to be particularly savvy about what you're buying. Most of the products you find in the inner sanctum of a foodstore are made from junk fats, refined sugar, refined flour and partially hydrogenated oils. If you're in the market for low-carbohydrate whole-grain crackers, read each label carefully. If you don't find what you are looking for in the supermarket – say crispbreads or crackers with less than 5g and preferably 2 or 3g of carbohydrate per cracker – then look in natural food emporiums or gourmet food shops where you are more likely to find them.

The most important foods you will be buying regularly are low glycaemic carbohydrate fruits and vegetables, plus proteins like meat, seafood, eggs and game, and maybe soya proteins like tofu. You might find that most stuff in a supermarket is not worth eating.

ORGANIC IF YOU CAN AFFORD IT

Whenever possible, go organic. Not only do organic vegetables taste better, the organic matter in healthy soil is nature's factory for biological activity that, when you eat them fresh, is communicated to you. Organic vegetables supply us with an excellent balance of minerals, trace elements and vitamins. The organic matter in soil is built up as a result of the break-down of vegetable and animal matter by its natural residents – worms, bacteria and other micro-organisms. The presence of these creatures in the right quantity and type, which you never find in factory farming, gives rise to physical, chemical and biological properties which create fertility in our soils and make plants grown on them highly resistant to disease. This resistance to illness and degeneration is then passed on to us when we eat the foods. Destroy the soil's organic matter through chemical farming and slowly but inexorably, you destroy the health of the people and animals living on foods grown on it.

GO ORGANIC

Organic methods of farming help protect against significant distortions in mineral balance, such as an increase in one or more mineral elements which can alter the availability of others. Conventionally grown fruits and vegetables are sprayed with pesticides – petrochemically derived compounds which behave like low dose synthetic oestrogens in the body. Many are also treated with fungicides or wax. Each one of these chemicals contributes to the toxic overload which ages your body rapidly, putting pressure on your liver, encouraging free radical damage. When it comes to maintaining good insulin balance, you especially do not want this to happen. A stressed liver has trouble managing glucose levels and controls insulin poorly. Shop as often as you can in stores which offer organic produce and untreated food.

FISHY MATTERS

Add fish to your diet – two or three times a week – if you can. Fish is rich in 'pre-formed' omega-3 fatty acids – DHA and EPA. Omega-3 fatty acids are known to reduce the levels of triglycerides in the body – the blood fats characteristic of syndrome X which put you at risk of heart disease. Omega-3 fatty acids also help lower blood pressure and improve overall heart function.

Flaxseed oil is also a rich source of some of the omega-3 fatty acids. It contains plenty of linolenic acid, precursor to EPA. However, omega-3 from flax oil is a shorter chain omega-3 fatty acid than those you find in fish. Some people change these shorter fatty acid chains into arachidonic acid which can cause inflammation in excess. EPA and DHA in fish oils do not convert to *arachidonic acid*. (see page 207).

Did you ever see the customers in health food stores? They are pale, skinny people who look half dead. In a steak house, you see robust, ruddy people. They're dying, of course, but they look terrific.

Bill Cosby

BE DISCERNING

Just because you buy something in a healthfood store or natural food emporium does not mean that it will foster Age Power. These stores are chock-a-block with high carbohydrate treats, full of sugar, too. And organic sugar and organic flour can still upset the insulin/glucagon apple cart. Although they may look great in their packages, most of these 'treat' foods are the last thing you want to promote good insulin balance. Read labels carefully here, too.

When selecting meats, fish and eggs, there are two major considerations: Make sure they are *fresh* and as *unprocessed* as possible. Buy fresh fish and seafood instead of processed forms such as smoked fish, crab cakes and breaded fish to avoid encouraging AGE's. The more a fish is processed the less quality it brings you in terms of high level health.

GET IT FRESH

Always ask the person serving you which fish is the freshest and what days of the week different kinds of fish arrive in the shop, then choose accordingly. You can tell a lot about the freshness of fish just by its smell and look. Ultra fresh fish does not smell like fish at all. It smells more like the salty bite of a sea breeze. If it's a whole fish you are looking at, pull back the gills. They should be bright red. The moment they go pink or grey you know the fish has been sitting in the shop too long. Try poking the flesh of the fish with your finger too. If it springs back instead of forming an indentation then you're likely to have a piece of fresh fish on the end of your finger. Finally, check out the eye of the fish. It should be dome-shaped and clear and not sunken and murky. Because I live a fair way from the centre of the city where I can buy my fish, I always protect it by taking a chilly box with me when I buy it in quantity so that it stays ultra fresh until I can get it home, bag it and freeze whatever I am not going to use for later.

ON THE GAME

The meats we get today are a far cry from those our Paleolithic ancestors ate. Probably the closest you can come to them is wild boar, rabbit, buffalo, venison or kangaroo. These meats are higher in protein. The beef, lamb and pork you buy in the supermarket is six times as fatty and only about three quarters as rich in protein as that of game meat. Where a piece of meat from wild game boasts about 22 grams of protein in each 100 gram portion,

> Quit worrying about your health . . . It will go away.
>
> *Harry Allen*

domestic meat contains as little as 15 or 16 grams. 'Wild' meat is also lower in fat. On average, there are only four grams of fat in the same 100 gram portion compared with almost 30 grams in domesticated meat. That being said, all organic red meat is an excellent source of zinc – a mineral that's enormously important not only for insulin balance but also for skin and the reproductive system. Free-range and organic meat are a better choice than factory farmed in every way. Whatever meat you buy, always choose the leanest cuts you can find. Organic meats are guaranteed to be free of antibiotics, steroids, herbicides and pesticides too.

AT THE DAIRY

When choosing dairy food, it is good to remember that butter, although it is not a source of essential fatty acids, is a perfectly respectable fat – far better than any margarines, no matter how fancy or how sophisticated their formulation. When buying other dairy foods, try to go low fat. Look for low-fat cottage cheese, ricotta, mascapone and unsweetened yoghurt. Stay away from flavoured cottage cheeses, yoghurts and other dairy products which are almost always chock full of sugar or other kinds of sweeteners as well as questionable flavourings. Look for natural, unsweetened soya yoghurt as well. Some brands are delicious. Use dairy products sparingly, however – few people handle them well and little wonder: Our genetic inheritance enables us to make good use of human milk as babies, but that's about it.

HEALTH NUTS

When you're buying nuts and seeds, go for raw nuts which have not been roasted as often as you can, and always store them in the refrigerator.

FLAVOUR IS EVERYTHING

In my view you can't have too much seasoning! Fresh herbs are best. When I can't get them I use a wide variety of dried herbs. Buy organic whenever you can, since herbs and spices in a supermarket are often irradiated in order to give them a longer shelf life and you want to avoid irradiated foods whenever possible. Most canned foods are not worth bothering with. The exception to these are delicacies such as water chestnuts and bamboo shoots, which you can only get canned, water-packed tuna, water-packed anchovies or sardines, as well as sugar-free coconut cream. These are delicious and can be useful.

THE SURPRISING COCONUT

When it comes to sauces, you are better off making your own, although if you are a careful label reader you will probably find some are not riddled with trans-fatty acids and boast not more than three or four grams of carbohydrate per half cup serving. As far as oils are concerned, extra virgin olive oil is best for salads. You can also use it for wok frying. Coconut fat is good for this too, and for searing meat or fish, since being a saturated fat it is very stable. Coconut oil is rich in a certain kind of fat known as *medium chain triglyceride* (MCT). It is often used to feed race horses and has been shown to reverse arteriosclerosis, improve glucose metabolism, lower body fat and even lower serum and liver cholesterol, while raising HDL, the good cholesterol. Coconut oil is nature's richest natural source of MCT – over 50 percent of its fat is made up of MCT's.

NOT SO SWEET

Sugar replacers are not good alternatives to sugar. Take saccharin. Three hundred times sweeter than sugar, saccharin, which is stable in liquids and in cooking, has been shown in animal studies to bring about a significant increase in the incidence of bladder tumours. Of course the amount of the stuff fed to these test animals was major, much more than we would consume ourselves in the daily course of drinking saccharin-sweetened drinks and eating saccharin-sweetened foods. But saccharin, like most of the artificial sweeteners, is an *excitotoxin*. This means it is a substance which causes metabolic disruptions and can lead to neurological, mental and emotional shifts in some people which may be highly unpleasant and can even distort their perceptions of reality.

The other artificial sweeteners are not much better. Cyclamate was discovered in the United States in 1937 when a technician laid his cigarette near a pile of powdery residue and found when he put it back into his mouth that it tasted sweet. Recent studies exploring possible negative effects of this sweetener raise questions about its potential for causing cancers, as well as how safe it is for long-term use. Cyclamate was banned from the United States in 1970, but is still used in the United Kingdom and Canada as well as other countries throughout the world.

Aspartame, discovered by researchers at G. D. Searle & Co. while looking for a treatment for ulcers, is different in its chemical composition from the others. It's a molecule created by putting together two amino acids. In effect, it is a tiny protein fragment which can enter the blood intact and be carried throughout your body. Some scientists believe this artificial molecule can even invade delicate areas of the brain, passing through the blood-brain barrier. Once there it may stimulate the brain abnormally, resulting in the same kind of excitotoxicity that MSG (monosodium glutamate) can cause – the food additive used in cheap Chinese foods. Medical reports suggest that many people who eat a lot of foods containing aspartame end up with weird symptoms such as headaches, dizziness, loss of short-term memory, sleep disturbances and mood shifts.

BEWARE ARTIFICIAL SWEETENERS

Let's take a look at sugar-replacers. Many people tend to replace sugar with one of the chemical artificial sweeteners: *saccharine, cyclamate, acesulfame-K* or *aspartame*. Don't. The artificial sweeteners we have become used to in diet drinks, diabetic jams and 'sugar-free' foods are increasingly shown to be unsafe. Many make blood sugar rise and encourage insulin resistance thereby stimulating the pancreas to release yet more insulin. Most encourage a build-up of toxicity in your body and can interfere with brain function.

> You need to remove the mental, emotional and spiritual blocks that have been hindering your personal growth because, like toxins in your physical body, they too, can be reflected on your face in the form of frozen facial expressions of grief, depression and sadness.
>
> *Anne Louise Gittleman*

BETTER OPTION

There is a new sweetener called sucralose, which is the best alternative if you decide to use any kind of artificial sweetener. It is used more and more in proprietary foods and is now available in most countries on supermarket shelves. It sometimes comes in a sprinkle-on form called Splenda. This sweetener has been on the market in Canada for more than a decade. Sucralose is about 600 times sweeter than table sugar. It is derived from the sucrose molecule itself. What technicians have done is replace two of the parts of the sucrose molecules – the hydroxyl groups – with chlorine molecules. This manipulation of the sugar molecule not only enhances its sweetness dramatically, it also makes the molecule unrecognisable to your body's metabolic machinery. In other words, it is not broken down and absorbed as sugar is. So you perceive a sweet taste when you eat the stuff, but your body can't absorb it. Sucralose, unlike the other artificial sweeteners, doesn't cause a rise in blood sugar and insulin. Splenda is stable and works well in cooked food. You can measure it like sugar and it has no detectable after-taste. It also contains no calories. So far it is the most promising of 'artificial'. I doubt very much that it is perfect however. For if you are putting anything into the body which the body is unable to recognise, there is always the possibility that you may not have the enzymes to be able efficiently to eliminate this foreign substance with ease. The body's inability to eliminate foreign substances is what causes many drug side effects. Drugs are usually unique molecules that the body does not handle well. In fact, drugs have to be unique molecules otherwise pharmaceutical companies cannot patent them. At this point, no one has any real idea what the possible long-term side effects of sucralose or Splenda might be. So far, however, so good.

GREAT STUFF

A South American plant, *Stevia rebaudiana*, is incredibly sweet. Stevia has been used for generations, primarily as a natural sweetener. In its natural fresh or dried leaf form stevia tastes from 10 to 15 times sweeter than common table sugar – up to 300 times sweeter when you use it in an extracted form. Extracts of stevia are relatively stable during heat processing and have been widely used in Japan for decades. As far back as 1987 a total of 1700 metric tonnes of stevia leaves were harvested each year to yield almost 200 tonnes of stevioside extract. Before long, more than half of the sweetener market in Japan was filled with stevia. So stevia is hardly an 'untested element'. In the United States, in one of its many misguided attempts to 'protect' Americans (much more likely to protect the corporate giants which manufacture artificial sweeteners), the FDA refused to make stevia legal. After many years of public pressure, however, stevia began to be allowed to be sold as a 'herb'. This is the situation that Americans are in with it today. The FDA still does not permit stevia to be labelled as a 'sweetener'.

MANY OPTIONS

Stevia comes in many different forms. You can buy the plant and grow it yourself then use the leaves, either fresh or dried. You can buy stevia leaves dried and powdered. They sweeten powerfully. And, like cyclamate, saccharin and acesulfame-K, they can leave a bitter after-taste if you use too much of them. I use stevia leaves for sweetening in all its forms – fresh, ground powdered form, extracts and powders – for such things as hot drinks, shakes and smoothies and desserts. You can add dried stevia powder (10-20 times the sweetness of sugar) directly to your recipes. You can also make it into a syrup by dissolving a teaspoon into two cups of filtered water, bringing it to a boil, lowering the heat and simmering until it is reduced to a slightly thickened syrup. This you can store in the refrigerator in a small bottle for a week or two. (Be warned, however, in this form it will turn anything you add it to a greenish colour). For more serious cooking, most people prefer a water extract or even the white stevia or a clear liquid stevia extract. It is this white stevia powder that is mostly used in Japan. In contains about 85-95 percent of the sweet glycosides found in the plant, which makes it almost 300 times as sweet as sugar. In Japan you find powdered stevia in little packets on restaurant tables, served together with tea. The extracts and white powder have the least after-taste. Researchers in Canada are currently working on a new extraction process which completely eliminates any after-taste. It is important to be aware that not all brands of stevia products that you buy from health food stores – which is where they are mostly available at the moment – are the same.

DILUTE IT

Some stevia powders are so intensely sweet that I like to mix them with water and use them by the drop. Others have a flavour I don't care for. So shop around. Stevia also comes in a liquid concentrate. You can make the concentrate yourself by putting a couple of cups of filtered water in a saucepan, bring it to a boil, reduce the heat to a simmer and add half an ounce of crushed stevia leaves. Cover and allow to simmer for three minutes, then remove the pot from the heat and allow the liquid to steep. Once cool, strain it though a cheesecloth and refrigerate in a covered container. This form of stevia has been used for generations for its medicinal effects. It has anti-bacterial and anti-fungal properties and is used to treat burns and wounds and to strengthen the pancreas. When sweetening any recipe with stevia it is important to experiment. Everyone has a different threshold for sweetness. Some people like things very sweet. I, for one, am put off by anything that is too sweet. So when mixing up any recipe for a dessert or smoothie or anything else with stevia, put a little bit in and taste it to see if you want more. Remember it is very sweet, so go easy. You can always add more later.

THE TROUBLE WITH STEVIA

Although Stevia is readily available in most countries of the world including the United States, Canada, New Zealand and Australia, in the United Kingdom it is not. The European Commission looked at an application for its use a couple of years ago. The European Scientific Committee for Food, presented with somewhat bogus data, concluded that a test tube derivative of stevia known as steviol 'might produce adverse effects in the male reproductive system and damage DNA'. The EC Standing Committee on Foodstuffs ruled that stevia, the plants and leaves of the dried *Stevia rebaudiana*, should not be approved for sale due to 'lack of information supporting the safety of the product'. Since no adverse effects in people have *ever* been associated with stevia in its long history of use I am forced to conclude that this is yet another unjust attack on this natural non-caloric sweetener. Stevia poses no threat to human health. It does, however, pose a potentially big threat to corporate projects of companies producing artificial sweeteners. Thankfully stevia is easy to order by post for your own use in many different forms from the USA, Australia or New Zealand – especially if you have a friend there who is willing to send it to you as a 'gift' (see Resources).

OUT AND ABOUT

Navigating your way through the Age Power Insulin Balance when you're out and about is not as difficult as you might imagine. These are some of the ways you can steer a good course into your own Insulin Balance lifestyle.

STIR FRY IT

Success, even in small things, supports a feeling of self-confidence and comp-etence.

Robert Ornstein, PhD, and David Sobel MD

Stir-fries are good so long as you make sure the chef leaves out the monosodium glutamate and any sugar. Chinese chefs have a way of putting sugar in just about everything. But a good stir-fry based on snow peas and ginger, bean sprouts, bamboo shoots, broccoli, spring onions and garlic is great. Water chestnuts, bok choy and Chinese cabbage are also great low-carb vegetables to be used in hot dishes or in a salad. Chinese restaurants usually have a beautiful steamed fish on the menu which is also worth ordering. What you want to be careful of are things like noodles, mu shu pancake, egg rolls and anything deep-fried, since they tend to stuff their deep fried foods with sweet and sour sauces and sugar.

SOUTH OF THE BORDER

Mexican food tends to be a bit of a hodge podge, most of it high carbs. There are some excellent ways to go however. You can order a tostada or taco salad, but don't eat the shell beneath. Grilled fish, beef, pork medallions, chicken as well as shredded beef, chicken and pork are great, served with an insalata mista – a tossed salad. Mexican restaurants often have a good selection of fish served Vera Cruz-style, foods with tomatoes, peppers and onions. I adore red snapper prepared this way. Camarones al mojo-de ago, which is a sautéed dish made from prawns riddled with garlic, is another excellent low-carb main course. Stay away from high-fat cheeses, too much sour cream and ask for a salsa or a guacamole made from olive oil on the side – since many of the guacamole tends to be made with cheap vegetable oils. Gazpacho is a great soup to start.

FISH SOUP FRANÇAIS

French restaurants are easy too. You can always go for their gorgeous vegetables, spinach, cauliflower, asparagus and marrows, as well as grilled or poached fish or any kind of roasted game. Stay away from heavy cream sauces. They often contain a lot of carbohydrate from the flour used to make them. Avoid French bread and shun potatoes and rice. Some of my favourite dishes in French restaurants are poulet aux fines herbes and roast chicken smothered in herbs and bouillabaisse – my absolute overall favourite as it is a fish soup with everything high in protein and omega-3s: steamed mussels and poached salmon.

> The older I get, the greater power I seem to have to help the world; I am like a snowball – the further I am rolled the more I gain.
>
> *Susan B. Anthony*

> During one of our trips through Afghanistan, we lost our corkscrew. We had to live on food and water for several days.
>
> *W C Fields*

SOUVLAKI SPECIAL

Souvlaki – skewered lamb, beef, chicken or prawn kebabs with vegetables is great.

You can even get it in fast food shops, where it comes stuffed inside a piece of pitta bread. I throw the pitta bread away and eat the rest. What you have to be careful of in these restaurants are the pastries, breads and pastas and of course the honey-based sauces that garnish so many Middle Eastern and Greek dishes. Their salads are wonderful, particularly those full of feta cheese with olive oil and red wine vinegar dressing. And their tzatziki sauce, which they pour on top, is delicious.

WHEN IN ROME
Italian restaurants are easy. I go for calamari (not battered) or an antipasto appetiser, followed perhaps by chicken piccata, veal cutlets, grilled fish or grilled chicken. I then order some sautéed or steamed vegetables, such as courgettes, aubergine or perhaps capsicums sautéed in olive oil with lots of beautiful herbs. Avoid pasta dishes like the plague and remember that even a small piece of bread can contain more than 14g of carbohydrate.

TANDOORI WHATNOT
Not an easy task here since Indian dishes are a mixture of so many different kinds of food. This is one of the reasons it causes digestive disturbances for a lot of people. But it is do-able. I order Tandoori lamb, chicken or beef or a lamb curry without the rice. I also like chicken tikka and chicken tikka masala. I eat this with a cucumber salad perhaps, or some creamed spinach. Steer clear of all of the dishes made with rice, wheat or potatoes.

SIMPLE AND CLEAN
I love eating in Japanese restaurants, first because I find the food is so good in general and second, because it is one of the easiest places in the world to get simple low-carb foods. Order sashimi if you like it. But make sure you are eating at a *good* restaurant and that the raw fish is very fresh. Most of the fish the Japanese serve are rich in precious omega-3 fatty acids. If you have any doubts about the fish being served in a restaurant, do not under any circumstances eat it raw. There is always a risk of parasite contamination. Teppenyaki is an ideal dish. So is teriyaki chicken or beef and salad, seaweed broth, miso soup and tofu. Stay away from tempura of any kind since it is breaded and fried.

The body feels the things of our spirits that the mind never thought of.

Carl A. Hammerschlag

SHAKE IT AND GO

Whenever I'm travelling, in airlines, in the car or simply out for the day, I take a plastic shaker and a couple of little plastic bags containing a good dose of microfiltered whey protein plus some fibre. Then all I need to do is pour clean water into the shaker, add my fibre protein powder mix, shake it up and drink it. This is an excellent backup that I carry with me all the time so that I am not forced ever to eat food that I don't want. When stuck in a long meeting without food, I have even been known to go to the ladies room, mix up my drink and drink it. Then I don't have to worry whether the meeting goes on for hours and hours. Whatever else happens, I know at the very least that microfiltered whey protein will carry me through to the next decent meal.

FAST FOODS

The toughest restaurants, apart from fast-food chains, are those that are the so-called 'health food restaurants'. Their dishes are often choc full of high-carb-low-fat dishes riddled with flour, honey and raw sugar. If you get stuck in one of these it's generally best to go for a salad and see if they have some tofu you can eat with it. If you find yourself in a fast-food restaurant with no other choice, here are some suggestions:

❑ At McDonalds, try a McGrilled Chicken Classic Sandwich and get rid of the bread.

❑ At Wendy's, you might order chilli or a grilled chicken sandwich, again throwing away the bread.

❑ At Burger King, you might go for a BK Broiler without the mayonnaise.

❑ In all of these cases, it's best to ask for whatever you are ordering without mayonnaise, as commercial mayonnaise is full of trans-fatty acids – junk fats – which you don't want to eat.

Let's get something to eat. I'm thirsty.

William Powell

IT'S EASY

The truth is, once you get used to Age Power living, it becomes really easy to live this way. Only in the beginning do real adjustments need to take place. For we human beings are creatures of habit. Whatever habits we have been following for some time, whether they serve us in the highest possible way or not, they are always the ones we tend to fall back into. Learn to think ahead. When I worked with a group of people recently putting Age Power's Insulin Balance to the test, they found the only real challenge they had to face was learning to organise themselves. Film director, Danny Mulheron, was part of the group. He was used to arriving on set by 6 a.m. He decided he would get up an hour early to do some weight training before leaving home, so that he could arrive on the set on time, and then take aerobic walks late at night. He also organised his meals. Since most of the crew meals on shoots are so appalling that just about nobody would want to eat them, Danny cooked an extra protein meal the night before and carried that, together with a lot of lovely salad vegetables, to eat for lunch at work. To his amazement, he found within a week he had more energy, was less stressed and enjoyed life more than ever. Once you get organised, everything runs smoothly.

Only through being yourself can you give to the others in your world your greatest gifts. To do any less betrays both them and yourself.

Ken Carey

If you have to be some-place other than where you are, you'll never see the here and now.

Carl A. Hammerschlag

GREEN SUPREME

My doctor said I look like a million dollars – all green and wrinkled.

Red Skelton

Green foods regenerate and rejuvenate your body. As such, they are powerful anti-agers. The old adage 'eat your greens if you want to stay young and healthy' has become scientific fact. And the fun of it all is that, so far, advanced nutritional scientists know that green works wonders, although as yet we only partly understand why.

Green foods are superfoods. Not only do they help clean up your body and continue to detoxify, they also help protect it from future damage by offering a high level of synergistic nutrients, immune enhancers and specific phyto-chemicals – both identified and as yet unidentified – each of which works its own anti-ageing magic.

GREEN MAGIC

Dark green vegetables such as broccoli, Brussels sprouts, collards, kale, kohl rabi and mustard greens have hit the headlines, thanks to an overwhelming abundance of medical and scientific evidence that they help prevent cancer. What prevents cancer also prevents ageing.

Prestigious medical journals such as the *Federal Proceedings Report* and the *Journal of the National Cancer Institute* report that sulphoraphane and other plant factors in the brassicas inhibit the growth of cancer tumours, detoxify the body of poisonous and environmental chemicals, prevent colon cancer and increase your body's own supply of natural anti-ageing compounds. They also help lower LDL cholesterol. They improve elimination and they fight yeast infections such as Candida albicans. Adding a couple of florets of broccoli – better still the new broccoli sprouts – or a few leaves of kale to a salad, a soup or a glass of vegetable juice turns a food that is good for Age Power into something that is superb. But start slowly and gradually build up on your greens, especially if you have a sweet tooth or are addicted to sugar. In the beginning, the taste can seem pretty strong. Build up gradually and you will find that your wild craving for sugars and carbs has actually been transformed into a new craving for greens.

GET INTO GRASS

There is another group of green foods that has even more concentrated remarkable anti-ageing properties. I think of them as green lightening: cereal grasses such as green barley, alfalfa and wheat grass, as well as algae like spirulina, chlorella and finally, the seaweeds. These greens are even more powerful detoxifiers than the brassicas. They deep cleanse the body and help rid it of toxic waste including heavy metals like lead, cadmium and aluminium. They are also rich in minerals and trace elements to enhance metabolic processes long impaired as a result of living on a Western diet which is depleted of minerals and micronutrients.

GLORIOUS GREEN

So powerful is the life support offered by green superfoods, that the Japanese – who lead the world in nature-based health products – pay premium prices for them. Freshwater algae such as spirulina and chlorella as well as freeze-dried young green plants like alfalfa, wheat grass and barley are carefully prepared at low temperatures to produce powdered foods which can be stirred into a glass of water or a glass of vegetable juice. Prepared in this way they preserve most of the living properties of raw foods. The Japanese themselves call them wonder foods, for they are packed with minerals, amino acids (in a form that your system fairly soaks up the moment you swallow them) – and most important of all – enzymes, the very stuff of life itself.

Far from being destroyed in the stomach as was once believed, many enzymes are taken through the walls of the gut into the bloodstream where they help to create fresher skin, vitality and heightened resistance to stress and degeneration. While the physical by-products of stress – like most pollutants in our food and water – tend to be acid, green foods alkalinise

POWERFUL AND DELICATE

Chlorophyll is one of the most important elements in green food when it comes to what it can do for human health. To get the benefits from it you need to eat the foods raw, for chlorophyll is delicate and easily damaged by heat. This is one of the reasons why all the good green superfoods are processed at low heat in order to preserve the chlorophyll. For when it's heated the vital magnesium which it contains becomes disrupted and the chlorophyll loses its integrity. When taking any green supplements it is absolutely essential to make sure that it has not oxidised. For when chlorophyll breaks down slowly, it forms a deadly by-product called *phenophorbide* – a photosensitive chemical capable of producing serious illness. This is why in Japan there are strict regulations governing the freshness of green products and why when choosing any green product, from green barley and wheat grass to chlorella, aloe vera, johoba and spirulina or any mixture that contains any of these things, you want to make absolutely sure that you are getting top quality. (See Resources.)

your system. This restores balance and creates a feeling of being calm and in control during highly demanding times.

SEEDPOWER

A seed has more power for generating life and vitality than any other part of a plant. Little wonder, since seeds are primarily designed to grow new plants, not to provide us with food. Although the needs of a growing plant are not identical to our own needs, because seeds are a plant's future progeny, they contain a superb balance of protein, carbohydrate, fats, vitamins, minerals and plant factors necessary to launch a new plant. As such, they are the finest natural food that farming can provide us with.

ANTI-OX x 60

Recently, broccoli seeds have come on the market, sprouted for a few days. They are becoming available in supermarkets alongside the well-known alfalfa sprouts, snow pea sprouts, and mung beans. By now, everyone knows how good broccoli is for you but the seeds of broccoli are infinitely better. In fact, recent scientific research carried out in the United States indicates that they contain 60 times the levels of sulphoraphane – the most widely acclaimed phytonutrient in the war against cancer and ageing – than the broccoli itself.

EASY TO DIGEST

When you sprout a seed, enzymes which have been dormant spring into action, breaking down stored starch and turning it into simple natural sugars and splitting long chain proteins into smaller molecules that can be easily assimilated by your body when you eat them. In fact, sprouted seeds are in effect pre-digested and as such they have many times the nutritional efficiency of the seeds from which they are grown. They provide more nutrients gram for gram than any natural food known.

Seeds and grains are latent powerhouses of nutritional goodness and life energy, all of which can enhance an Age Power lifestyle. Their nutritional bounty helps fill the gaps created by years of living on depleted foods. You can buy them in packets and add spring water to germinate them. Let them grow for a few days in jars in your kitchen and you will harvest inexpensive fresh foods of phenomenal health-enhancing value. The vitamin content of seeds increases dramatically when they germinate. There is a huge rise in the levels of vitamins C, A, B-complex and especially B_1 and B_2, niacin, pantothenic acid and pyroxidine, biotin and folic acid and in chlorophyll. The vitamin B_2 in an oat grain, for instance, goes up 1300 percent almost as soon as the seed sprouts and by the time tiny leaves have formed, it has risen to 2000 percent.

Another attractive thing about seeds is their price. Basic seeds and grains are cheap gram for gram and these days many sprouted seeds are readily available in supermarkets and healthfood stores When you sprout seeds yourself with nothing but clean water, they become an easily accessible source of organically grown fresh vegetables, even for city dwellers. In an age when most fruit and vegetables are grown in artificially fertilised soils and treated with hormones, fungicides, insecticides, preservatives and all manner of other chemicals, the home-grown-in-a-jar sprouted seeds emerge as a pristine blessing – fresh, unpolluted and ready to eat in a minute by popping them into salads or just eating them as a snack.

FATHER OF ALL FOODS

The discovery that sprouted cereal grasses can enhance health tremendously is attributed to the Arabs, who used alfalfa to feed their horses, after discovering that it made the animals strong and fast. When they first tried this grass on men, they found there were so many benefits from eating that they named it al-fal-fa, which means 'father of all foods'.

BIG DADDY

Alfalfa contains eight enzymes which are known to promote beneficial chemical reactions improving the assimilation of the foods you eat. It is also rich in vitamins A, E, K and D as well as many of the plant nutrients such as flavonoids and the B-complex vitamins including pantothenic acid – particularly important for stress – B_{12} and B_6. Alfalfa, like the other seed grasses, also contains an abundance of alkaline minerals, especially calcium and iron, potassium and magnesium and the alfalfa seed is more than 40 percent complete protein. Again, like many of the other seed grasses, alfalfa boasts gentle plant hormones – oestrogen-like substances and compounds which can be enormously helpful in easing PMS and menopausal problems, simply because they are taken up by the hormone receptor sites in your body and help protect you from the dangerous effects of chemical oestrogen mimics in our environment and from drugs. In many ways, cereal grasses are the ideal fast foods.

Professor Takauki Shibamoto, chairman of the Environmental Toxicity Division, University of California at Davis, spent many years studying an anti-oxidant compound contained in the young green barley leaves called *2-0-GIV*. He discovered that this flavonoid inhibits lipid peroxidation at least as effectively as any other anti-oxidant including the vitamins

> There are currently in our environment well over fifty thousand toxic chemicals with which we come into contact regularly. These toxic chemicals can be mixed and matched to form billions of toxic assaults which trigger in us enzyme and hormonal reactions, glandular secretions, etc.
>
> *Roger Welsh*

and the carotenoids. Recent studies show that in addition to its anti-oxidant action, green barley extract taken as a supplement reduces inflammation, swelling and heat as well as pain. Its enzymes are capable of inactivating and breaking down carcinogens as well. So, like many of the other green grasses, it acts as a cancer fighter.

OLD AS HISTORY

The green tips of baby wheat plants and other grain plants were eaten as a delicacy in the Holy Land 2000 years ago. King Nebuchadnezzar of ancient Babylonia reportedly lived on nothing but young seed grasses for seven years in order to regain his health and mental clarity. Then in the nineteen twenties and thirties in the United States – before vitamin and mineral pills were in existence – bottled dehydrated cereal grass became a popular food supplement.

PERFECT MOMENTS

When rice, wheat, corn, oats, barley, rye or millet are planted, either in good healthy soil or grown in jars on your kitchen window, and are harvested at just the right moment – a few days after they begin to sprout – they are unbelievably rich in growth hormones as well as vitamins, minerals and plant factors. They are quite literally living foods – they carry a quality of energy that goes beyond anything we are able as yet to measure in chemical terms. The ungerminated seed is a little miracle of nature. It opens up and produces tiny leaves, photosynthesis produces simple sugars which are transformed into proteins, fatty acids, nucleic acid such as DNA and RNA, as well as complex carbohydrate through the action of enzymes and substrates produced from minerals in the water or soil. The peak of nutritional bounty in all cereal grasses – the moment when chlorophyll, protein and most of the vitamins and minerals reach their zenith – occurs just before *jointing*. This is the moment at which the young inter-nodal tissues in the grass leaf starts to elongate a form a stem. This is when cereal grasses are best harvested – usually between five and twelve days after planting. Afterwards, the chlorophyll, protein and vitamin content drops dramatically.

It was back in the late nineteen twenties that the power of cereal grasses came to the fore. The American chemist Charles Schnabel had been searching for a material that could be added to poultry feeds to improve egg production and lower chicken mortality. He wanted what he described as a 'blood building material'. By then scientists had identified chlorophyll – the green substance in plants – and noticed that it has a remarkable similarity in its chemical structure to haemoglobin, the oxygen carrying element in blood. Schnabel figured that 'green leaves should be the best source of blood'. So he began to feed all sorts of green things to chickens, from alfalfa to combinations of 20 green vegetables. He found them all wanting. Then he tried giving hens a green mixture which 'just happened to contain a large amount of immature wheat and oat sprouts'. Animals who got a mere 10 percent of this cereal grass feed responded amazingly. Winter egg production shot up from an average of 38 percent to 94 percent of summer levels, and the eggs that were produced had stronger shells and hatched healthier chickens.

FOOD FOR ALL

Intrigued by his success with chickens, Schnabel began to investigate every aspect of cereal grasses, from the soils that produced the most nutrition-ally-rich grasses, to the effect that eating dehydrated grasses had on the health of humans. He fed his own family of seven on them and was known to boast that none of them ever had a serious illness or decayed teeth. He even developed a vision on how to feed the hungry of the world on the extremely high quality protein from cereal grasses.

In the decades that followed, other scientists found that green cereal grass feeds – which contain natural plant steroid hormones – enhance fertility and improve lactation in many kinds of animals, including humans.

One morning I shot an elephant in my pyjamas. How he got into my pyjamas I'll never know.
Groucho Marx.

DRINK IT

There are three ways to go when it comes to making use of the anti-ageing properties of sprouted seed grasses. First, you can sprout the seeds themselves and use them in salads, snacks and stir fries. Second, you can buy extracts of seeds such as wheat and barley in powdered form. Third, you can drink the fresh juices themselves.

A SHOT OF LIFE

Wheat grass juice is one of my favourite foods and the best I have ever had was freshly extracted at the organic market held twice a week in Union Square in New York. You drink wheat juice by the shot glass and there are certain parallels between the experience of drinking it and the experience of drinking a shot of the best malt whisky. Not that the grass juices will make you drunk – far from it – but a glass of wheat grass juice has a similar ability to go right to your head the moment you drink it. So powerful is wheat grass juice that many people whose bodies are slightly toxic will actually be made ill by it, so it is a good idea if you are going to experiment with fresh cereal grass juice that you mix it with other vegetable juice in small quantities and gradually work up until your system detoxifies and you get used to its power.

These days most people prefer to get their sprouted grass seeds in the form of tablets or powders. These products often contain other healthful ingredients such as chlorella or herbal extracts. They vary tremendously in quality. Just because something is green and contains wheat grass does not mean that it is high quality so choose your supplements carefully.

THE AMAZING ALGAES

A near microscopic form of blue-green freshwater algae, spirulina is made up of translucent bubble-thin cells stacked end to end to form an incredibly beautiful deep green helix. Spirulina is one form of blue-green algae of which there are more than 1500 known species. The chemical make-up of each species is unique. All are rich in beta-carotene and other anti-oxidants, B-complex vitamins, iron and trace minerals, chlorophyll, enzymes and various other plant factors. Some species are also rich in gamma-linolenic acid (GLA), an omega-6 fatty acid that helps counter inflammation, lower cholesterol and may even help protect against heart disease.

THE BEST OF THE BEST

Because all green superfoods are full of life they degrade easily. This makes it essential to choose your green supplements carefully. The best are made from organic plants, processed at ultra low heat to preserve their enzymes and integrity and packed in glass to prevent the leaking of oxygen through plastics that causes oxidation. You can take supergreen foods as capsules, tablets or in powder form. Often you will find them mixed together. But the quality of the mixes varies tremendously from one manufacturer to another. The best green superfood I have ever found is a supplement called Pure Synergy™. It is a combination of 62 of nature's most potent and nourishing components including organic green juices, herbs, wild crafted algae and many other natural ingredients, all of them either wild or organically grown and carefully formulated in a synergistic way so that the energies of each balance the energies of the other. I begin each day with a drink of microfiltered whey protein, to which I add a little stevia and a teaspoon or two of Pure Synergy™ as well as some psyllium husks and organic flaxseeds for extra fibre. This makes a quick breakfast or a wonderful meal or snack on the run during the day. It is a perfect example of how high tech food production can work to our advantage when it is done with real integrity. (See Resources.)

Spirulina is also very rich in an unusual quality of protein which is alkaline rather than acid forming. It therefore can play an important part in detoxifying the body and also for helping you deal with high levels of stress. Rich in vitamins E, B_{12}, B_1, B_5 and B_6 as well as beta-carotene, spirulina also contains good quantities of the minerals zinc, copper, manganese and selenium as well as other anti-ageing phytonutrients including *phycocyanin*, a blue pigment structurally similar to beta-carotene which animal experiments have shown can enhance immune functions. The World Health Organisation, in attempting to deal with blindness due to vitamin A deficiency amongst malnourished children in India, found that when one gram of spirulina was added to their diet there was significant improvement. Recently, too, a

At 50, everyone has the face he deserves.

George Orwell

GREEN INHERITANCE

Some three and a half billion years ago these algae began to fix nitrogen and sugars and in the process, to release oxygen. If it had not been for the algae on the earth and the oxidation they produced, we would not have come into being. Nor would all the other animals who depend upon oxygen-based metabolism to survive. It is the algae that created the oxygen-rich atmosphere on which the rest of life was able to develop and the whole process took over one billion years to complete. Blue-green algae are microscopic organisms that are harvested from freshwater lakes, ponds and man-made tanks. In a very real way the algaes made human life possible. Using them as superfood supplements renews it.

report from the *Journal of the American Nutriceutical Association* indicated that a particular type of blue-green algae *Aphanizomenon flos-aquae* (AFA) has the ability to increase the surveillance activity of important immune cells. The researchers concluded that AFA may help prevent cancers by boosting immunity amongst mutant cells that can lead to the disease.

A SPOON A DAY

Adding between a teaspoon and a tablespoon of organic spirulina to a glass of water, juice or protein drink each day is a good way to reap the anti-ageing benefits it carries. As with all algae, however, it is important to use only the organically grown varieties for some wild algae products may be contaminated by environmental toxins, bacteria, animal wastes or other potentially harmful substances.

EMERALD TREASURE

Chlorella, another important green algae, is sometimes called the emerald food. Another great additive to protein drinks and juices, chlorella gets its name from its high chlorophyll content – the highest of any known plant. In addition, chlorella is rich in minerals, vitamin, fibre, nucleic acids, ammonia acids, enzymes and something called CGF – chlorella growth factor.

Chlorella contains the full spectrum of the carotenoids important for defending the cells against oxidation damage while other phyto-chemicals strengthen the immune system encouraging the production of interferon. Because chlorella enhances the growth of beneficial bacteria in the intestines, it also brings soothing and healing to the gastro-intestinal tract. It is used to advantage by people with Candida albicans, diverticulitis, Crohn's disease and ulcers. A number of animal studies confirm its healing effect on ulcers.

Chlorella also helps protect the liver from toxic injury and some practitioners claim it can even help prevent hangovers by promoting the removal of alcohol from the body. Most people take half a teaspoon to a teaspoon of chlorella a day, stirred into a glass of juice or other cold drink. Many vegans rely on chlorella as well as seaweeds and algae as a source of vitamin B_{12}, since in animal experiments, chlorella has been shown to elevate blood levels of this vitamin. Chlorella also contains more pantothenic acid than any other natural source plus many of the other important B vitamins, magnesium and other trace elements.

PROTEIN DETOX

Chlorella has long been cultivated in third world countries as an inexpensive substitute for animal proteins, for it is over 60 percent protein. But chlorella offers some other important properties as well. Its high concentration of chlorophyll makes it a powerful detoxifier of the body and allows it to play an important role in any purification programme. It helps eliminate many toxic metals including cadmium and even uranium.

EAT THE WEEDS

Sea vegetables, too, are a wonderful source of anti-ageing power. If you have never used sea vegetables for cooking, Age Power's Insulin Balance is a good excuse. They are not only delicious, bringing a wonderful spicy flavour to soups and salads, they are also the richest source of organic mineral salts in nature, especially iodine. Iodine is the mineral needed by the thyroid gland. As your thyroid gland is largely responsible for the body's metabolic rate – which tends to decrease with age – iodine is very important for energy.

TEA GREENS

Last, but by no means least, of the powerful anti-virus, anti-cancer anti-ageing green superfoods is green tea – the most popular of Asian drinks. For centuries green tea has been celebrated for its health benefits. It is literally riddled with anti-oxidants including polyphenols – bioflavonoids that act as super anti-oxidants to neutralise free radicals, lower cholesterol and blood pressure, block cancer proliferation, inhibit the growth of bacteria and viruses, improve digestion and help prevent against ulcers and strokes.

All of the more than 3000 varieties of tea grown come from the leaves of the same plant – *Camellia sinensis.* The three types of tea – black, oolong and green – vary only in the way that this plant is processed. The flavonoids green tea contains – mainly catechins with a ridiculously long name *epiglallocatechin-3-gallate* (EGCG) – are degraded soon after harvesting in most teas. However, in the case of green teas, the degradation process is

---

GREEN PROTECTION

Drinking green tea regularly may protect from cancer and ageing by preventing damage to DNA. Many studies indicate that drinking green tea regularly helps lower cholesterol and reduce the risk of heart disease and stroke. In animal studies, green tea has been shown to prevent the clumping of blood which contributes to arteriosclerosis and raises the risk of a heart attack. To reap the benefits of green tea, you need to drink it strong and this is a process most people have to ease themselves into, for full strength green tea has quite a bitter taste. Start weak and once you have become accustomed to the taste, increase the strength of the tea that you are drinking. There are no side effects known to drinking green tea except in very large quantities when the small amount of caffeine that it contains (usually 20 to 30 mg per cup compared to 150 mg. in a cup of coffee), may create an experience of nervousness or insomnia.

SEA GREENS

Seaweeds are also full of trace elements that are essential to the body, but in minute quantities. When boron, chromium, cobalt, calcium, iodine, manganese, magnesium, molibdenum, phosphorus, potassium, silicon, silver and sulphur (to mention only a few elements) are not present in the body, metabolism can experience big problems. Unlike the chalk which is added to bread to 'enrich' it with calcium and most of the mineral supplements you can buy in pill form in stores, the minerals in sea plants, like the minerals in all of the important green plants, are organic. This means that your body can easily make use of them to build energy.

Get to know the seaweeds and make use of them. Not only will they support a more youthful metabolism, you will find that your nails and hair and the rest of your body will be strengthened by a rich supply of minerals and trace elements that support the energy producing enzymes in the body. Seaweeds are readily available these days in healthfood stores and food shops. Make good use of them and they will take care of you well: Try

Arame	Kombu
Dulse	Laver Bread
Hiziki	Nori
Kelp	Wakami
Mixed sea salad	

prevented by steaming or panfrying the leaves, inactivating the enzyme that brings it about. Most researchers believe that it is this *EGCH catechin* that is primarily responsible for green tea's anti-ageing, disease preventing abilities.

When looking for green tea it is best to go for the finest traditional green teas or for gunpowder green tea, which you find in Asian speciality markets. An average cup of green tea contains 40 to 90 mg of EGCG. If you dislike the taste of this green powerhouse, you might like to go for supplements of green tea extract. In this case, read labels and limit your dose to somewhere between 350 and 500 mg of polyphenols a day. This is about what you would get in four to five cups of brewed green tea.

The widespread drinking of green tea is now believed to be one of the reasons why the rates of cancer in the Orient are so low compared with those in the West. If you feel you still need the odd boost from caffeine, try changing from your usual cup of tea or coffee to drinking green tea. Once you get used to the taste, you may well enjoy it. Certainly your body will. Now let's get into muscle.

KISS SARCOPENIA GOODBYE

There is no longer any doubt: exercise can save your life, while couch pot-atoism creates an existence that is nasty, sick and short.

Michael Colgan PhD

Age reversal is not just a total body process. It is a total *person* process which involves enhancing metabolic rate, increasing muscle mass and shrinking fat stores (nothing to do with how 'thin' or 'fat' you are by the way), as well as rediscovering your capacity for vitality and joy. The most powerful force for doing this is exercise. Yes, really. Better than any pill popping or expensive treatment, the right kind of exercise transforms your whole life.

Exercise can help you grow younger month by month, year by year. And just in case you think this is some kind of sales pitch for putting on your pink leg warmers and putting your back out, think again. As Evans and Rosenberg discovered in their endless investigations of the biomarkers, there are two kinds of exercise that help banish sarcopenia and reverse all those other biomarkers from blood pressure to Syndrome X: Aerobics or 'cardio' exercise and isotonics – strength through resistance exercise. They work synergistically to make your life better in just about every way.

Many flavonoids have anti-inflammatory properties. These properties can be particularly helpful for people who are overweight because obese people suffer from chronic low-grade inflammation, which increases their risk of heart disease. Of all the anti-oxidants, flavonoids have the most marked anti-inflammatory effects.

Jack Challam, Burt Berkson MD, PhD

POWER-UP

The goal of age power exercise is to reverse sarcopenia – the shrinking of muscle mass and the distortion of lean-body-mass-to-fat ratios. In the process you not only banish the gradual overall weakening of the body that may have developed over decades, you reverse virtually all the biomarkers in the process making you younger in medically measurable ways. It will firm your muscles, restore youthful contours and firmness and improve your self-image. It can:

- Reverse your biomarkers
- Prevent fat storage and reduce fat levels
- Keep your hormones at optimal levels
- Improve your heart's strength
- Make your skin look firmer and smoother and help it function in younger ways
- Protect you from arteriosclerosis
- Banish Syndrome X
- Lower your triglycerides
- Increase the level of high-density lipoproteins (HDL) – good guy cholesterol
- Strengthen your bones and prevent bone loss
- Increase lean muscle mass and your vitality
- Improve the oxygen-carrying capacity of your blood
- Lower high blood pressure
- Banish anxiety and depression
- Improve brain function
- Help you live longer

Muscle, to a far greater extent than most people realise, is responsible for the vitality of your whole physiological apparatus. It's why muscle mass and strength are our primary biomarkers – and why we believe that building muscle in the elderly is the key to their rejuvenation.

William Evans PhD and
Irwin Rosenberg MD

AEROBIC ENERGY

Aerobic exercise is always done at a speed and intensity which enables you to continue with it at a steady persevering pace so you are continuously processing oxygen with each movement. It does not require excessive speed or muscular strength. Never get out of breath while carrying out any aerobic activity. Smooth and steady are the keys to aerobic success – a driving force reversing both inner and outer biomarkers. Walk 30 minutes a day and reap the benefits (see Chapter 19).

AEROBIC CAPACITY

What's your VO2 Max? Biomarker Five – aerobic capacity – measures how much age-protecting oxygen your body can make use of each minute. As such it is the best indicator of overall fitness and functional capacity. Often referred to as VO2 Max, this can be measured in a gym or physiology lab using a treadmill test. It is a collective measurement of many physiological functions. Aerobic capacity indicates how well your lungs take in air, how much oxygen is coursing from your lungs into your bloodstream, how well your heart is pumping it to muscles and how well your capillaries are delivering it to your cells. Most people's VO2 Max declines as they move past 35. This decline is reversible. As you reverse it, your body grows younger, your mind clearer and your emotions more stable.

ISOTONIC POWER

The other form of exercise central to rejuvenating your body and reversing biomarkers is isotonic. Strength training or resistance exercise are designed to strengthen your muscles and your joints and to tip your lean-body-mass-to-fat ratio heavily towards more muscle. Isotonics will make your body leaner, stronger and more beautiful, no matter what your age or what condition you are in to begin with. It consists of strength-building practices such as weight training, as well as slow gentle stretching. Many sports activities like archery, even shuffleboard, fall into the isotonic category. But by far the most reliable and best form of isotonics consists of a regime using a couple of dumbbells and a set of leg weights, special rubber bands or gravity resistance movements like push-ups, lunges or squats. The Age Power Programme marries aerobics with isotonics and asks that you make this marriage an ordinary part of your day-to-day life, forever.

ISOTONICS REVERSE SYNDROME X

The most important physical activity of all for countering sarcopenia, isotonics banishes insulin resistance by building muscle, decreasing your body fat and increasing your body's energy-producing capacity within the mitochondria of your cells. The more often you move your muscles in resistance training, the more you build them. The more you build them, the more you increase your insulin sensitivity. Physically fit people secrete less insulin after eating carbohydrate foods than their couch potato cousins. Age Power's Exercise plus Insulin Balance eating is the most effective combination of rejuvenating power you will find anywhere.

CHECK IT OUT

There are a number of methods for measuring body composition. They are most often used by physiologists concerned with improving the performance of athletes. The procedure is sometimes done in sports clinics by hydrostatic weighing. With this method, the person sits on a chair in a tank of water to be weighed. The technique relies on Archimedes' principle that when a body is submerged, the buoyancy equals the weight of displaced water. Bone and muscle are denser than water, so a person who's got a higher LBM will weigh more in water, and a person with a higher percentage of body fat will weigh less. Some physiologists do the measurements using what is called an impedance unit, where a very small current is sent through pads placed on your wrist or ankle to determine LBM-to-fat ratios, or sound or light waves are sent through the body. These can give a ballpark reading, but only hydrostatic weighing is truly accurate. The most common way of measuring – although not by any means the most accurate – is done with skin callipers, where you pinch your skin at various parts of the body and then

> We feel that the older people's reduced muscle mass is almost wholly responsible for the gradual reduction of their basal metabolic rate.
>
> *William Evans PhD, and Irwin Rosenberg MD*

measure the thickness of the pinch. Some complex calculations later, you'll have determined your body mass ratio. Easiest of all is to reach down and pinch your own flesh with your fingers at the bottom of the ribs, on your thighs, upper arms, belly, bottom and hips. If your pinch is thicker than half an inch to one inch, your LBM-to-fat ratio is not as good as it could be.

YOU ARE YOUR LBM

Fat tissue is very different from muscle tissue. It does not need oxygen, does not create movement or activity and cannot repair itself. In fact, body fat is just about as close as you can get to dead flesh within a living system. Dr Vince Quas, American expert on body change and fat loss says it better than anyone else: 'Your lean body mass *is* you' he says. 'Your fat is *on* you.' Building more lean muscle through exercise is a fascinating metamorphosis. It does not change you in any intrinsic way, nor does it turn you into someone else's idea of the perfect body. It only makes you more what in essence you really are. It increases your sex drive and improves hormone levels for youthful skin. As your lean body mass slowly but inexorably begins to metamorphose, a body distorted over the years by stress, poor eating and lack of movement turns into a vital instrument for living your life more fully.

Because your body's fat tissues have a very low metabolic activity, they don't burn calories effectively, nor do they create high levels of energy and vitality. Only mitochondria in your muscle cells do this. The more muscle tissue you have the better your body burns calories, sheds fat and keeps it off. Also the more muscle you have, the more you are able to eat without gaining weight.

If you are over 35, if you are overweight and need to shed the excess, or if you are simply over fat (your lean body mass is not as good as it could be), unless you are already fit you need to know two things: How to increase your fat-burning and how to increase your muscle mass. But first you need to get a handle on just what your body composition is so you have something to measure your progress against.

Here is a simple method you can use as a quick rule of thumb.

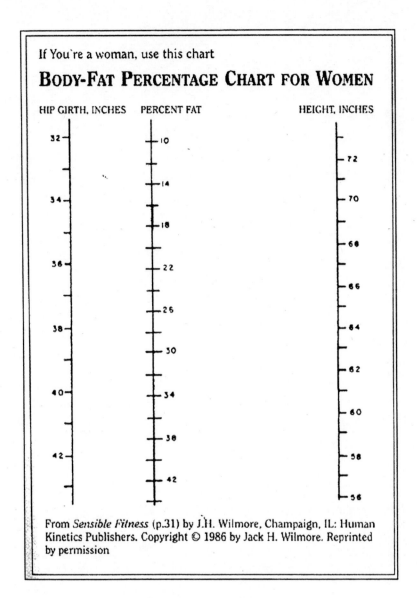

If You're a woman, use this chart

BODY-FAT PERCENTAGE CHART FOR WOMEN

HIP GIRTH, INCHES   PERCENT FAT   HEIGHT, INCHES

From *Sensible Fitness* (p.31) by J.H. Wilmore, Champaign, IL: Human Kinetics Publishers. Copyright © 1986 by Jack H. Wilmore. Reprinted by permission

Use a ruler to line up your hip measurement with your height.

For example: **If your hips measure 36.5 inches and you are 5 feet 2 inches tall, then your body fat is about 26 per cent.**

Your relative body-fat measurement is at the point where the ruler crosses the percentage fat line.

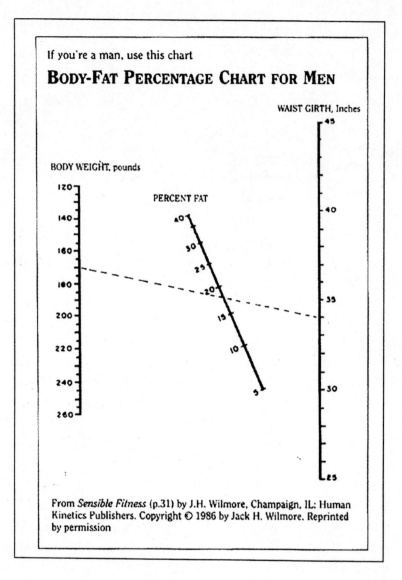

If you're a man, use this chart

Body-Fat Percentage Chart for Men

WAIST GIRTH, Inches

BODY WEIGHT, pounds

PERCENT FAT

From *Sensible Fitness* (p.31) by J.H. Wilmore, Champaign, IL: Human Kinetics Publishers. Copyright © 1986 by Jack H. Wilmore. Reprinted by permission

Use a ruler to line up your waist measurement with your body weight.

For example: **If you weigh 170 lbs and your waist is 34 inches then your body fat is about 18 percent.**

Your relative body-fat measurement is at the point where the ruler crosses the percentage fat line.

CHART YOUR PROGRESS

An ideal body fat for men over the age of 35 is somewhere between 15 and 22 percent, for women it hovers around 19 to 26 percent. But don't get obsessive about it all. The important thing is that you establish a starting point from which you can measure your progress. You are not trying to compete with top athletes, you are measuring yourself against yourself. The major issue is to get started in the right direction and gently, slowly yet inexorably, keep moving that way. This is what fundamental and permanent change is all about – real transformation stuff. Be sure to check out your overall fitness either with your doctor or in a gym before beginning any exercise programme and never push yourself hard. Not only is it unnecessary, it can actually be counter-productive when building lean body mass and burning excess fat. Let's look at isotonic exercise first.

SHAPE SHIFTING

Your LBM is always shifting. Being inactive makes it shrink. So does going on and off slimming diets. Crash dieting causes you to shed muscle tissue. Yet when lost weight is regained, it is regained as fat, forever decreasing the weight of your LBM. This is why the more you diet the flabbier you become. And because crash dieting shrinks LBM, it also lowers your metabolism. It becomes harder and harder to stay thin, and finally you need to starve yourself (and often ruin your health) to keep the scales right.

REAL TRANSFORMATION

I have always been fascinated by the idea of transformation. You know the kind of thing: Frogs into princes, Cinderella into belle of the ball. Most people believe that in real life transformation is not possible. They have never learned to work with muscle. Quite apart from all the mind-boggling new research into how the right kind of exercise can rejuvenate your body, I have discovered for myself that exercise is a great deal more than something you do to counteract ageing or protect yourself from heart disease. It can be used to fan the flames of creativity and help make you more true to yourself. Not only is such a transformation possible, it is virtually guaranteed – provided you are patient and provided you are willing to work hard.

Ten years ago, I decided to explore just what kind of transformation was possible by working intensively with isotonic exercise. I knew that skilled weight training (not the slap-about kind you see carried out in most gyms) is the fastest and most efficient way to do this. So I searched out someone who could work intensively with me as a trainer to shift the LBM-to-fat ratio in my own body. I found a Welsh champion weight lifter, Rhodri Thomas, who said he would take me on. When we began to work together I was scared to death that after the first two hours I would collapse in a heap. After all, I am no athlete.

IN AT THE DEEP END

We trained six days a week. Every day we would work with weights backed up by aerobic exercise such as running, swimming and cycling interspersed with other activities like squash and tennis – just for relaxation. I found to my amazement that I did not collapse. Instead I watched as all sorts of deep changes began to take place. Muscles I didn't know existed slowly and quietly began to surface through my flesh. I discovered that feelings, thoughts and past experiences are indeed held within the body. All sorts of old memories, emotions and fears seemed in some mysterious way to be locked in my muscles. When you work muscle intensively, such things sometimes come to the surface to be cleared away, much as the body is cleared of physical toxins during a detox programme. Frequently I found myself pushed to my absolute limits. Then the gym floor would be covered equally with my sweat and tears.

BECOME WHAT YOU ARE

Working with muscle in this way transforms the body externally by changing LBM-to-fat ratio and reshaping the body, which brings all sorts of wonderful rewards, including more energy, freedom from aches and pains, a lean, firm body and better hormonal balance. Even more wonderfully, it creates an internal transformation, developing from within a slow but steadily growing sense of self-confidence, clarity and independence. For many – myself included – this is a deep change virtually impossible to achieve any other way. It changed me on a psychological level too. It gave me confidence. Made me more authentic so that the inner and outer Leslie came closer and closer. It opened up a sense of all sorts of possibilities in my life that I would not have dreamed of before.

The results of the Human Genome Project have opened our eyes not to how people will die, but rather to what they need to do to live healthy, full lives based on genetic uniqueness.

Jeffrey Bland MD

So now when I think back to all those fairy tales about transformation, about frogs and princes, for the first time in my life I feel I am beginning to understand them and to understand what real transformation is about. It is not all glitzy, like in the movies. It is slow and inexorable. Yet it brings in its wake gifts beyond our wildest dreams. Now I wonder, would Cinderella have been prepared for union with her Prince Charming had she not for many years before strengthened her body and purified her spirit through hard work?

PURE ALCHEMY

The Chinese, who have probably delved into the whole process of rejuvenation more than any other culture, consider the whole process an alchemical one. They see it as a great art and science in which ultimately a person becomes more fully who they truly are, living out their physical, emotional, mental and spiritual potentials to the full. To put it another way, rejuvenation is a process in which 'base metal' undergoes a remarkable series of transformations first by being broken down into its *materia prima* (here is where detoxification comes in) and then transformed into 'gold'.

ISOTONIC MEDITATION

My experience was so very different than the clichéd image that people have of doing weights. I learned that it is a precise art and science. It is also incredibly stilling to the mind. When you are working with dumb-bells or barbells you are fully present with the experience. You work a specific muscle group, while the rest of your body is still – a state very much like meditation.

To promote fat loss, always do your isotonics on an empty stomach. This way you use up the glycogen in your body quickly, and then turn to fat burning for energy.

HOW TO BEGIN

Check out your overall fitness first. This you can do at a gym. Remember, it doesn't matter where you begin, for exercising at the right level for you will slowly, yet inexorably, build strength, beauty and power. Remember that when you are doing strength training with weights, they need to be heavy enough to challenge you without causing injury. Don't be worried if you feel a bit sore after your first few workouts. What you should not feel is serious pain.

Every time you lift and lower a weight, you form a repetition or 'rep'. Most reps take you six to seven seconds to complete – two or three seconds to lift the weights, one second to hold it, and three to four seconds to lower it. You always want to pick up a weight that you can lift at least eight times. The last rep should be the most difficult. As you work out and gain more strength, you will find you will need to increase the weight of some of your dumbbells. If you can perform more than 12 reps in a row with no difficulty, this is an indication that your strength has increased so much you need a slightly heavier weight.

A workout usually takes between 20 and 30 minutes to complete. The American College of Sports Medicine suggests 12 reps for each exercise, while people over 50 sometimes use somewhat lighter weights, light enough to allow 10 to 15 reps. The number of times you carry out each rep is called a set. For instance, eight leg extensions followed by a couple of minutes rest is considered one set. Begin any resistance training by doing a five to six minute warm-up, such as marching, dancing to music or some other form of aerobic activity. This warms up cold muscles and protects from injuries. After doing your strength training, you will want to do a stretch and cool down which lengthens the muscles and helps prevent the build-up of lactic acid, which can cause aches.

BREAK DOWN TO BUILD UP

Strength training works in a unique way. It is not while you are doing the exercises that you are building lean body mass – increasing muscle density. Working out with a set of weights actually breaks down muscle tissue, causing very small tears in it. It is between 24 and 48 hours later, in response to these minor tears, that the body reacts and builds new muscle tissue. This makes it important to give yourself plenty of time between each exercise session for new muscle to be built. If you choose to carry out four sessions of strength training or weight training each week, you will need to exercise a different muscle group each of the four days. Say, shoulders Monday, legs Tuesday, skip a day for recovery, then do chest and back on Thursday, and then arms on Friday, then skip two days and begin the programme all over again.

ACHES AND PAINS

When doing weight training or strength training it is pretty inevitable that you will experience some *delayed onset muscle soreness*. These are the common aches and pains all exercisers get at one time or another – regardless of how fit they are – on challenging their muscles. You body is telling you that the microscopic tears that take place in muscle cells and the minor swelling that accompanies them has happened. Within the next 48 hours or so your body will restore those tears and in the process create new muscle tissue for vitality and fat burning. This is how muscles adapt and this is an important part of the power for regeneration and rejuvenation that isotonic exercise brings.

Fat only burns in the mitochondria of muscle cells and the more muscle you have, the more fat you can burn. For this you need resistance training but not every day. Four sessions a week are ideal. Two days of training followed by a day of rest, another two days of training and two days of rest. On the three days when you are not doing your strength training with dumbbells or gym equipment, this is an excellent time to do some sort of ridge flexibility exercises such as yoga, Feldenkrais or Traeger, which can enhance your body's ability to deal with stress and help re-pattern your body neurologically. Many people find that these exercises are a tremendous boon to weight loss, not because biochemically they bring about significant fat burning, but rather because they help rebalance the autonomic nervous system so that you can handle stress much better and don't find yourself heading for the refrigerator every time something becomes difficult.

EQUIPMENT OPTIONS

Here are a number of different ways to approach strength training. They include:

FREE WEIGHTS

For general strength and fitness, these are the best. Even top weightlifters depend heavily on free weights to develop their strength and skill. They consist of hand weights and ankle weights and they are great for use at home. Buy a pair of weights in say, 3lb, 5lb and 8lb dumbbells (although when choosing dumbbells make sure you pick them up and try the exercises you are going to do with them first). The heaviest weight should leave your muscle fatigued at the end of six to eight repetitions, but not be so heavy that you cannot lift it.

WEIGHT MACHINES

This is the kind of equipment you will find in gyms. They're very popular, and it's easy to become dazzled by the technology. Some of the equipment is particularly useful when doing exercises such as leg extensions or leg curls. It's easier to do these on weight machines than in any other way. Mostly, however, free weights are better than weight machines. For weight machines tend to limit your range of motion and in doing so, negate the benefits gained by the balance itself that is established when you are actually moving free weights up and down.

RUBBER BANDS OR TUBING

These can be good for travel. The rubber bands are huge versions of the office type, in different colours. The tubes, again in different colours, have lightweight plastic or nylon bars attached to them. Using either, you can mimic the effect of using weights and carry out a range of exercises for both upper and lower body. I prefer the giant rubber bands to the rubber tubing and plastic bars, for I find that the rubber tubing can very easily cause injury if you happen to slip or let go of it while you are exercising. (See Resources.)

GRAVITY RESISTANCE

There are lots of exercises that use resistance to gravity to build strength without the need for any special equipment. Push-ups, lunges, squats and sit-ups use your own body weight against gravity to increase strength. Even top athletes who use weight machines and free weights often tend to do many of their exercises through simple resistance, especially the abdominal or 'abs' exercises.

WATER WORKS

Exercising in water, and using its natural resistance, is enormously valuable for anyone with arthritis or other muscular or skeletal difficulties. It is gentle on the joints and makes it possible for you to gain strength without putting strain where it shouldn't be put. Many gyms and pools offer water resistance workouts.

BANISH THE BLUES

Exercise tranquillises your body and improves your mood. In part this comes from a decrease in the muscle irritability and increase in deep muscle heat which it brings about. Partly, too, it is the result of the way exercise alters brain chemistry. Aerobic exercise has at least two important effects on the brain. First, it encourages the production of noradrenaline and norepinephrine, the neurotransmitter which makes you feel 'up'. Athletes have high levels of this hormone while endogenously depressed people usually show very low levels. Putting sedentary people into a regular exercise programme quite soon leads to an increase in noradrenaline and therefore to an improvement in mood, making them more optimistic and giving them feelings of having power over their life. Second, exercise greatly increases the body's production of beta-endorphins – natural opiates produced in the pituitary gland and in various structures of the brain which, through their action on the central nervous system, have a calming effect on the whole body as well as uplifting mind and mood. Study after study has shown that when chronically depressed people get into exercise programmes, even as simple as taking long brisk walks a few times a week, their depression lifts.

VIDEO HELP

I have looked at dozens of exercise videos and the only ones that I have seen which are excellent for beginner or intermediate people wanting to do weight training were made by Michael Colgan. Like all good programmes, they begin with a few minutes of movement to warm up the body and end with flexibility exercises for stretching and cooling down.

> Research shows that two weeks of complete bed rest can cause as much calcium loss from the bones as one whole year's worth of ageing.
>
> *William Evans and Irwin Rosenberg*

When I have used these tapes with people who are wanting specifically to regenerate and rejuvenate their bodies, the results have been phenomenal. And the people become so enthusiastic about them that they continue, because the tapes are easy to use and the exercises are so effective, month after month. Sadly the Colgan videos have been replaced in some countries by a set of similar videos by Nancy Papp using rubber bands. They too are good – great for travel too – but the Colgan videos which use dumbbells and leg weights are far better (see Resources).

WARM UP

It is important at the beginning of any exercise session that you spend a few minutes doing aerobic activity. Never pick up a weight when your muscles are cold. You can try running on the spot, slow, steady jumping jacks, using a rowing machine (my favourite) or bouncing on a rebounder. To begin with, your total exercise session may last only fifteen to twenty minutes, in which case you will want to devote five minutes at the begin-ning to the aerobic warm-up. Later on it can be longer. I generally row on the rowing machine for about ten minutes at a slow, steady pace to get my heart and lungs moving and warm up before beginning my weights. As the length of your exercise session grows week by week, until it is ideally forty-five minutes to an hour at a time, so will the time you spend on your aerobic activities at the beginning and end of the session and perhaps in the middle too.

STRETCH OUT

After this initial warm-up period, which should last long enough for you to feel fully warmed up, spend five to ten minutes stretching. Stretch slowly and smoothly towards the ceiling, towards your toes, to the side; never jerk when stretching. Breathe deeply. Stretching before a workout and after a warm-up allows major muscle groups along with associated tendons and ligaments to be gently eased, reducing the possibility of injury. Now you are ready for your muscle work.

THE COOL DOWN

It is important to spend a few minutes at the end of a weights session doing some kind of aerobic activity to cool down. How long depends on the length of your weights session. You can go through the same kind of activity you used at the beginning of your session but to ensure you stay warm, add an extra sweater. After a workout your body cools down fast and you don't want to become chilled.

STRETCH OUT AGAIN

Then do some more stretching for a couple of minutes. You will find that your body stretches more easily now, because your muscles are full of blood and energised. Go slowly and enjoy the feeling. It can be wonderful.

MORE HGH – MORE ENERGY

Another bonus rejuvenator that comes with practising isotonics is you increase the levels of human growth hormone (HGH).

YOUTH HORMONE

HGH is an anabolic, or tissue building, hormone. Produced in the pituitary, a tiny gland at the base of the skull, it is secreted on and off during the day. It boosts growth in children, aids in tissue repair, helps direct the metabolism to burn fat instead of storing it and to mobilise fat stores. In recent years there has been an enormous amount of research into the effects of introducing growth hormone by injection. Doctors use it with patients who have suffered severe burns or massive injuries to soft tissue and for people recovering from major surgery. They also give it to children who lack it to prevent dwarfism. By injecting small amounts of growth hormone under the skin, doctors promote healing and ensure growth. It's extremely expensive stuff.

People under 25 have lots of it, and are far more sensitive to the chemicals in the body which stimulate its release. As we get older, our production of HGH decreases dramatically, along with our sensitivity to the chemicals that trigger it. This is caused by a number of things, not only the passage of time. Living on the standard Western diet, which emphasises carbohydrates and junk fats, our blood glucose levels tend to increase which inhibits the normal flow of growth hormone released in the body. And we tend to get heavier – between the ages of 19 and 50, in fact, the average woman gains 15lb. This further inhibits release of growth hormone. That's the bad news. The good news is that the body has a tremendous capacity for regeneration and transformation. Age Power's Insulin Balance, coupled with resistance training – working out with weights – can help to increase your levels of growth hormone.

THESE THINGS INHIBIT THE RELEASE
OF GROWTH HORMONE

- ❑ High blood glucose levels
- ❑ High free fatty acid levels
- ❑ Obesity
- ❑ Pregnancy

FAT INTO MUSCLE

Recently, researchers have been exploring the use of HGH to prevent ageing. In one study reported in the *New England Journal of Medicine,* Dr Daniel Rudman of the Medical College of Wisconsin discovered that very small amounts of growth hormone, injected just under the skin of men aged 61 to 81, increased their lean body mass by 8.8 percent and decreased their body fat by 14.4 percent. Bone density was increased in the spine and the men's skin thickened by an amazing 7.1 percent. The men did not exercise or change their diet during the study. In Dr Rudman's opinion, so powerful were the transformative and rejuvenating changes that they were 'equivalent in magnitude to the changes incurred during 10-20 years of [reversing] ageing'. A number of studies show that injecting athletes with HGH even for only four to six weeks decreases their body fat dramatically and increases their lean body mass. In a very real sense, growth hormone is the elixir of youth. No wonder it is currently touted as the be-all and end-all for rejuvenation and is being offered at enormous expense at clinics in Mexico and Eastern Europe. By making use of the tools of Age Power, you can get yours for free.

TURN ON NATURALLY

By far the most powerful rejuvenating effects from increased levels of human growth hormone are brought about by the way you eat and live. Most of what stimulates the production of growth hormone are things over which we have control. These will help you do it:

- ❑ A carbohydrate restricted diet
- ❑ An adequate protein diet
- ❑ Deep sleep
- ❑ Isotonic exercise
- ❑ Decreasing blood glucose levels
- ❑ Increasing protein levels

Now let's look at how aerobics – the second branch of Age Power Exercise – can be used to reverse your biomarkers.

SHED FAT

Losing weight is the wrong goal. You should forget about your weight and concentrate on shedding fat and gaining muscle.

William Evans PhD and Irwin Rosenberg MD

The media is full of advice about how to use exercise to burn fat and shed excess weight – a major concern of three quarters of men and woman over 35. Most of it revolves around silly formulae which purport to calculate how many calories you burn while carrying out a specific activity. They are based on the idea that what exercise will do for you is simply burn off calories so that you can eat more and still stay slim. Such an approach is naïve and inaccurate.

Just as inaccurate is the idea – still pushed by too many so-called experts in the field of weight loss – that for fat shedding, you need to do your aerobics at 70 percent of your maximum heart rate (more about this in a moment). It does not work. Sadly the science of using exercise to dissolve away body fat while building lean body mass – the kind of exercise that will quite literally rejuvenate your body in medically measurable ways – is known to few.

For many years, following 'received opinion', I ran five miles a day, six days a week, only to find that, contrary to what the so-called experts in exercise physiology insisted would happen, I actually gained weight rather than losing it. For a long time I didn't understand why. It was my old friend Dr Michael Colgan, Director of the Colgan Institute of Nutritional Science in the USA, past advisor to the US Olympics Committee on Nutrition, who straightened me out.

In his early 60s, Colgan is one of the fittest men that I have ever known. He works with top athletes, designing nutritional training programmes that are at the leading edge. What Colgan can't do with a body is not worth doing. It was he who made me aware that what we have been told to do to reduce body fat is wrong.

FAT MATTERS

You will remember from Chapter 4, Meet the Biomarkers, that shedding fat is far more than a matter of narcissism. It is central to de-ageing your body. Adipose tissue – fat stores – is highly metabolically inactive. In excess it contributes nothing either in terms of energy for metabolism or overall vitality. Shedding fat the Age Power way builds muscle and shifts brain chemistry so you think more clearly, experience more confidence and gain greater emotional stability. In the process of fat shedding and building muscle you will increase your metabolic rate – the third biomarker – which tends in most people to decrease with age. You also shift the distribution of fat on your body as body fat percentage – the fourth biomarker – decreases. Meanwhile your basal metabolic rate and aerobic capacity improves – biomarker five. As aerobic capacity increases your heart grows stronger and your resistance to fatigue soars. Meanwhile, hormone levels return to more youthful levels and balance so that your whole body is rejuvenated.

LOW INTENSITY BURNS FAT

Pick up most books on weight loss and they will tell you to use aerobics to burn fat, exercising aerobically to a level that is 70 percent of your maximum heart rate. The reasoning goes something like this. At your training heart rate you should be moving just beneath the aerobic/anaerobic threshold. This means the highest level of movement that you can carry out where your body is burning mostly fat. Sounds great in theory, but don't you believe it.

> The amount of fat burned by exercise depends on the fuel mixture used by the body to do that exercise. Most programmes burn mainly sugar, leaving body fat virtually untouched.
>
> *Michael Colgan*

NOT HARD BUT LONG

To burn fat, aerobic exercise must *not* be high intensity. When you exercise too hard or become breathless while working out, the energy which feeds your movement is drawn not from your fat stores but from glycogen in your liver and your muscles. Exercise for fat shedding which works best is *moderate*, aerobic and of *long* duration, since only this kind of aerobics burns both glycogen *and* fat. After thirty minutes of brisk sustained walking your body makes an important shift so that only 50 percent of its energy comes from glycogen and the rest from your fat stores. Studies in exercise physiology show that the minimal aerobic threshold to shed fat demands continuous movement of at least 30 minutes duration, carried out at least three times a week. Less than that and you are really wasting your time. The important thing to remember about fat burning is to exercise not *hard* but *long*.

TRAINING HEART RATE

The training heart rate was originally created by exercise physiologists as a measure of cardiovascular fitness. And, for the last half century, researchers have established that exercising at the training heart rate does indeed enhance general fitness. It strengthens the lungs and the heart, improving the vital capacity of the body and increases VO2 Max. If you are already lean and fit, it will certainly make you fitter. But it won't make you leaner.

He's so old he gets winded playing checkers.

Ed Wynn

FORGET YOUR TRAINING RATE

There is another major problem with trying to calculate your ideal training rate – the point below which you need to train to be in an aerobic state (using lots of oxygen). If you go above it, you reach an anaerobic threshold and your body burns mostly protein and sugar. Your anaerobic/aerobic threshold depends far more on how fit you are than how old you are. Most people who need to shift fat from their bodies and enhance their lean-body-mass-to-fat ratio, tend to be highly unfit. If you are calculating your aerobic/anaerobic threshold using the standard method given above, the figure you will get will be far too high. This is why you see so many overweight women in aerobic classes and overweight men jogging around the park, panting like mad. Their bodies' ability to use fat for fuel becomes negligible at such a pace. Meanwhile, their muscles are being cannibalised for energy with every step they take. There is a better way.

GET INTO OXYGEN

Body fat is interesting stuff. It is very calorically dense. This means that it needs lots of oxygen, masses of it in fact, for it to be metabolised – broken down – so that it can be put into the bloodstream and used as energy. The moment you exercise at your training heart rate you are moving out of the level at which your body is supplied with masses of oxygen, so your body will tend to turn its attention *away* from fat burning towards whatever other tissue it can find to supply its energy. In effect, it will stop burning your stored *fat* and increase its burning of *protein* and *glucose,* for these tissues require less oxygen to be burnt.

Unlike your fat stores, muscle stores and circulating glucose in the system are easily burnt, even when the oxygen supply to the cells is poor. Exercise too vigorously, say running, rowing or sprinting, and your body never gets enough oxygen to burn fat efficiently. For as the intensity of your exercise increases, the amount of oxygen available decreases. When this happens, your body has to look for more and more sugar and protein to maintain the effort.

SLOW DOWN

The optimal intensity of exercise for fat shedding is far lower than your training heart rate. It is between 40 to 55 percent of your maximum heart rate. So long as you are trying to shed fat in your body, forget running, rowing and all that high tech aerobic equipment and those exhausting aerobics classes, unless you do them very slowly and gently. Get walking.

A daily walk of 30 minutes will burn far more fat than killing yourself at the gym. And little wonder. Our Paleolithic ancestors walked long distances on foot gathering food and carrying it back to their families. They only ran in short bursts when they needed to, to survive. The only aerobic activity amongst our ancient ancestors which was regular and continuous was walking.

TORTOISE OR HARE

At the Cooper Institute for Aerobics Research in Dallas, exercise physiologists divided 235 sedentary but otherwise healthy men and women between the ages of 30 and 60 into two groups. To one group they gave a vigorous regular exercise, between 20 and 60 minutes of it, biking or swimming, for example, up to five days a week. The other group spent a total of 30 minutes a day in low-to-moderate intensity activities such as climbing stairs, walking and doing household or garden chores such as leaf raking or vacuuming. Six months later, exercise physiologists measured the improvements in both groups. They discovered that there were no significant differences in the degree of improvements in heart and lung fitness, blood pressure and even body fat percentage. In effect, they showed that a moderate physical activity of walking and day-to-day chores on a regular basis is every bit as effective in making significant improvements in human biomarkers as more vigorous exercise.

In another study, exercise physiologists worked with 40 obese women between the ages of 21 and 60. Again, they divided them into two groups. One group carried out lifestyle activities including walking, climbing stairs and doing household chores. The others were put into structured exercise programmes where

> The second day of a diet is always easier than the first. By the second day you're off it.
>
> *Jackie Gleason*

they were vigorously exercising, much as those in the Dallas study were. All participants were also put onto a calorie restricted diet. After four months, when the measurements of the groups were taken, both showed significant improvements in lowered blood pressure, increased oxygen intake, reduced LDL (bad) cholesterol and fat loss. But what was particularly interesting, was that a year later when researchers did a follow-up on the group, those who had been taking only moderate physical activity such as walking and doing day-to-day chores had actually regained significantly less weight than those in the structured group. In no small part, this happens because the more you can incorporate low-to-moderate intensity exercise in your day-to-day life, the easier it becomes to continue to do it, forever.

GENTLY DOES IT TO CLEAR INSULIN RESISTANCE

Low intensity aerobics is also great for clearing insulin resistance, provided you do it regularly and for long enough periods. It burns fat, increases insulin sensitivity and helps balance blood sugar.

With the people I have worked with to help them create Age Power lifestyles, I ask that they begin to walk 20 minutes a day, every day. Within three weeks they increase their walks to 30 minutes a day – more if they like. They report what in the beginning seemed like a chore, a month later has become a sheer pleasure. Many find that once they get into their walking programme and shift their way of living, others in their family are drawn to the same thing. There is more than one marriage, I am told, which has been improved by partners going for a 30 minute walk together once a day. One friend of mine – a film director – found the only time he had to walk was late at night. His partner became intrigued with the whole idea of taking a walk with him before bed. It has since become a ritual that both of them look forward to. There is a great deal more to be gained from walking than simply the benefits of the physical activity. If you are lucky enough to be able to walk down tree-lined streets or even in a park, you benefit from the contact with living things, be they trees, grass, flowers, bird life or just the fresh open air.

WHEN AND HOW

How long you exercise matters for fat burning. Most people think that you start to burn fat as soon as you begin to move your body. This is not how it happens. Getting your body to burn fat instead of sugar depends on complex hormonal responses involving the way in which adrenal hormones and insulin trigger your fat cells to release triglycerides from them, and raise free fatty acids in your blood. This takes time. Just how much time depends on your metabolism, whether or not you have eaten before exercising and the level of intensity of the activity. Although the whole period of aerobic activity builds fitness and helps enhance your VO2 Max, when it comes to burning fat, you can discard the first 20 minutes of your walk knowing that you won't actually be burning fat until this period of time has passed, when these hormonal shifts have had an opportunity to happen.

Because of this time lag it is best, if possible, when exercising to shrink body fat, to do your walks (or whatever kind of low intensity aerobic exercise) after you have done isotonic resistance training or weight training. For the weight training itself brings about the response needed to trigger fat burning. Once you have done half an hour of weights, then head out for your walk, knowing that you will get the very best breakdown of free fatty acids and that fat burning will continue so long as you continue to walk. There is another bonus too: Fat burning will not end when the walk ends. This kind of exercise, in which you begin with resistance training and then go on to low intensity aerobic walking, increases your resting metabolic rate enough that it remains elevated for several hours. This means that you will burn more fat. In fact, much of the fat burning takes place after the exercise sessions are over. And this increase in metabolic rate happens not only to very overweight people, but even to those who have a few pounds of excess fat to shed. A raised metabolic rate triggered in this way not only means that you will burn a lot of extra calories that day, exercise physiologists have discovered that far more of those calories will be drawn from your fat stores.

> The benefit of moderate physical activity goes well beyond the heart. Lung capacity goes up, cancer rates go down. Regular exercise not only helps burn calories but adjusts the body's metabolic rate to offset the metabolic slowdown that occurs with dieting.
>
> *Robert Ornstein, PhD and David Sobel, MD, Healthy Pleasures*

BREATHE FREE

To get the most out of walking do it for at least half an hour, every day. Choose some place you want to walk to and wearing low-heeled shoes and loose comfortable clothes, set out with your arms swinging free from the shoulders. Breathe deeply and carry your body high. Every few minutes draw in a breath and then after a few seconds, without exhaling, draw in another and after a further interval of a few seconds, still another. After the third inhalation vigorously expel all your air. This helps inflate your chest to its full capacity. Most of us don't breathe fully or deeply, so we miss out on the full benefits of oxygen for brain and body. After a walk of say, two, three or four miles, if possible take off your clothes and rub down your skin with a flannel that has been dipped in cold water, or take a brief cold shower followed by a brisk rub with a Turkish towel. This will leave you refreshed and renewed and with energy to spare in the hours ahead.

SET YOUR BODY CLOCK

The best time to exercise for the highest level of fat burning is the early morning *before* you eat. Exercising in the early morning on an empty stomach raises your metabolic rate and keeps it high throughout the day. If you chose to do your exercise in the evening instead, some of this raised metabolic state simply goes unused. For when you go to bed, metabolism drops dramatically. Whatever low intensity aerobic exercise you choose, do it every day. For only if it is done with regularity does it bring about an increase in basal metabolic rate. Skip a day and your body quickly slips back into the lower level metabolic state you had before you began to do your daily walks.

I will tell you what I learned myself. For me a long, five or six mile walk helps. And one must go alone and every day.

Brenda Ueland

ACTION PLAN

Start today to exercise – walking is good. If you are not used to exercise begin with only 10 minutes a day and work up gradually adding another 10 minutes every few days.

- ❏ Find a friend and make a pact to exercise together.
- ❏ Make a note of how you feel on the days you do and don't exercise and compare them.
- ❏ Let yourself daydream about how your body will change in the next few months. The imagination is potent fuel to drive Age Power.

WALK NOW EAT LATER

Food can also interfere with fat burning. Many exercise programmes urge you to eat something before you begin. This is a bad idea. Aerobic exercise only does the very best for your body when it is carried out on an empty stomach. Water is great however. Drink as much of it as you can. To get the full benefits of fat burning, you have to exercise in the presence of relatively low blood sugar hormones. When you put food or energy drinks into your body this immediately releases sugar into your blood stream. Then your body will use that sugar rather than fat as its energy source. So the best time to do your exercise is immediately on waking when your body is free of food. If you are a coffee lover, provided you are not a habitual coffee drinker, this is a time when a cup of coffee can encourage fat loss. If you drink it – only one cup – a few minutes before beginning an exercise programme, the caffeine it contains actually triggers the adrenal hormones, which in turn release free fatty acids, encouraging your body to enter fat burning mode. If, however, you are someone who drinks coffee habitually, this trigger will not work, for your body will no longer respond to it.

THE TEN SECRETS OF FAT
LOSS THROUGH EXERCISE

1. Check with your doctor or an exercise physiologist before beginning. Never launch into vigorous exercise or weight training when you are not used to it. Take things easy to start with – you will be amazed at how quickly your body will gain strength and power.

2. Go for low intensity aerobic exercise, keeping within 40 to 55 percent of your training heart rate. This will ensure that your body burns maximum levels of stored fat.

3. Drink water.

4. Combine isotonics such as weight training with low intensity aerobic walking to build muscle mass, keep hormone levels high and enhance basal metabolic rate – creating a fat burning body.

5. Do your weight training four times a week before your cardio-vascular walk. This way your free fatty acids are mobilised so your body can use them for energy instead of protein or sugar.

6. Do your low intensity aerobic exercise ideally for 30 to 45 minutes a time, six or seven days a week.

7. Exercise first thing in the morning for maximum fat loss throughout the day.

8. Try drinking a cup of strong black unsweetened coffee half an hour before taking your walk to enhance the release of fat into the blood stream for burning. If you do, don't drink coffee at any other time.

9. Make it fun. Exercise should never be a chore. In the beginning it takes a little bit of dedication to get into, but very quickly you will find it can become a game. Play with it and enjoy it.

10. Organise your life. To get the best from exercise you have to set aside the time for it and this can take a little bit of organisation, especially at the beginning. You may need to shift your priorities a bit. Remember that everything you do for yourself such as setting aside the time to exercise regularly, ultimately will benefit all around you as you become stronger, more vital and leaner with each passing day. But be patient. Permanent change in the body takes time. Muscle is slow to build. Exercising in this way brings about steady, lasting, permanent change, for the better.

PART FIVE:
BRAIN BODY ALCHEMY

BRAINSTORM

The brain is a wonderful organ; it starts working the moment you get up in the morning and does not stop until you get into the office.

Unknown

Scientists once believed that the loss of our brain cells with age was inevitable, and once lost, there was no possibility of growing new ones. We now know this is not true. Your brain can grow new neurons regardless of your age, so long as your body is functioning well, is supplied with adequate minerals, vitamins, protein and essential fatty acids, and so long as you continue to challenge yourself.

The most remarkable organ in your body is also the most vulnerable. Made up of 10 billion – maybe more – closely packed cells called *neurons*, your brain is about the size of a large grapefruit. It weighs between three and three and a half pounds. Despite its small size, it is thousands of times more complex than the most advanced computer. Although it makes up a mere two percent of your whole body mass, your brain uses more than 25 percent of your body's basic fuels to do its job. And what a job it is: Your brain oversees every function in your body, co-ordinating signals and processes by means of thousands of nerves which make it possible for you to feel, taste, touch, wonder, dream, smell and interact with the world around you. So efficient is this magnificent organ at storing memories that you can instantaneously recall an event which took place 50 years ago, while the fragrance of a lipstick can take you back to the excitement of your first kiss.

SECRETS OF THE SENSES

We talk about the way our eyes see, our tongue tastes and our nose smells. In truth it is your brain doing all of these things. Sense organs are merely an interface between your environment and your inner life. Collecting information from the world around us, they pass it on to the brain which acts within milliseconds as a central processor, producing a response. Everything you want to do with your life, from learning new skills, changing a behaviour pattern, cooking dinner, making love or painting a picture, can only take place thanks to your brain's ability to process new information and to recall both short- and long-term memory. If this ability declines – as it does with many people as they get older – your whole life becomes less vital. Your capacity to learn diminishes and you begin to live like an automaton – by conditioned reflex. Most important of all, your sense of self and your ability to tap into states of expanded consciousness – peak experiences – is severely impaired. So is the unfolding of your unique soul energy as you live your life, making it difficult for you to create what you want to create. Before long you can no longer make clear, consistent and wise decisions. You can even come to the point where you do not *know* what you think and feel. If this gets bad enough a human being can become – as some people do – little more than a 'vegetable'.

DON'T LOSE IT

Loss of mental capacity is the greatest fear most people have about getting older. Not without reason. Half of the men and women over the age of 85 today have some degree of mental dysfunction. Age-related degeneration, left unchecked, makes heavy demands on your brain – so heavy that between the ages of 20 and 90, some lose 10 percent of their brain mass. As many as 100,000 nerve cells die each day. More than 40 percent of these cells may be lost from the neo-cortex – centre of rational thought. This does not need to happen. Anything you do to protect your body from accelerated ageing – Age Power's Insulin Balance, anti-oxidants, exercise, herbs, natural hormones – you also do for your brain. But even more so.

As you go the way of life, you will see a great chasm. Jump. It is not as wide as you think.

Joseph Campbell

THE POWER OF THREE

There are three main areas of the brain which need special care:

Central Nervous System: Together, the brain stem and the spinal column make up the central nervous system – the most primal brain. It looks after our primitive emotions and keeps our basic metabolic processes going, including breathing and blood pressure. Nothing in your body works right if it gets out of kilter.

Cerebellum: Centre of your lower brain, it deals with posture, balance and the co-ordination of movement in your body.

Forebrain: The biggest part of your brain, it is made up of the cerebrum, which accounts for 70 percent of the brain's weight. It looks after 'higher functions' like decision-making, calculating maths, speech, writing and creativity. The forebrain consists of two large hemispheres plus a number of other important structures clustered together in its centre. These include the pituitary gland and the limbic system. Within this area you find two very small but vitally important centres of control – the *hypothalamus* and the *hippocampus*. This cluster of structures looks after appetite, thirst, temperature regulation and control. The hypothalamus, under the direction of the hippocampus, sends out a number of releasing hormones to the pituitary to regulate the body's hormonal cascades. Your ability to reason is centred in the neo-cortex. Memory is primarily located within the hippocampus. The hippocampus is highly vulnerable to oxidation damage (see page 77). If this occurs it leads to loss of memory and degenerative brain conditions like Alzheimer's and Parkinson's.

A fully grown brain with its billions upon billions of neurons, each with many branches, has an estimated 100 trillion connections. It is important to understand how these connections work and how to keep them working if you are to prevent a decline in brain power as your get older. So bear with me.

INSIDE YOUR NERVOUS SYSTEM

Neurons look like strange sea creatures with hundreds of stringy filaments radiating out from their centre, called *dendrites,* as well as another stringy filament known as an *axon.* The dendrites carry nerve impulses towards a cell's body. The axon looks after transporting them away. Each axon branches into a number of terminals which reach up like tentacles towards the dendrites of nearby cells. The dendrites and axons between nerve cells never touch. Instead, in between them you find a microscopic gap known as a *synapse.* The transmission of impulses from one cell to another takes place across these synapses, thanks to the release of compounds known as *neurotransmitters,* which flow from an axon to the neighbouring dendrites. Brain chemicals make it possible for a nerve impulse to be carried instantaneously from one cell to another. So long as you have adequate neurotransmitters, the process takes place smoothly – as it does in healthy young people. But there are many things in our day to day lives which can interfere with it. Food additives in convenience foods, for instance, or chemicals in the environment can be the triggers for emotional instability, attention deficit problems and many other mental disorders. So can inadequate supplies of vitamins, minerals, amino acids and essential fatty acids needed for your body to manufacture essential neurotransmitters.

BEWARE MEMORY LOSS

As we get older, many of the neurotransmitters, including the two particularly involved in memory – *serotonin* and *acetylcholine* – formed out of essential nutrients from you diet, decrease. As they do, so does your brain power. This is called *age-related cognitive decline* (ARCD). Your moods can be affected. You can become depressed or anxious. Sleep can be disturbed so that in time, the whole quality of your life is undermined. Most of the consciousness-altering drugs designed to deal with anxiety, depression and other psychiatric disorders, do their work by *artificially* shifting the levels and balance of neurotransmitters. Such symptomatic treatments carry destructive side effects and can themselves lead to more rapid degeneration when used long term. There are *better* ways.

In the past 30 years, biochemists and practitioners of natural medicine have done much to explore how specific nutri-

> Old principals never die, they just lose their faculties.
>
> *Harry Allen*

> Several medical conditions can also play a role in the decline of cognitive functioning. The most common include hypertension, atherosclerosis and stroke. We must also recognise that, in older age groups, there are medicines prescribed for a variety of conditions that could have negative effects on brain health.
>
> *Ray Sahelian MD*

ents and natural substances can help a flagging brain re-establish optimum levels of the important neurotransmitters and restore its functioning – safely and *without* side-effects. We will look at some of these later. While it would be good to be able to take a pill and have everything fixed for us, this 'magic bullet' approach on its own, even one based on natural 'brain enhancers' – just won't work. Here are the facts: The most important thing of all when it comes to protecting your brain from degeneration and rejuvenating brain function is the *way you live*. Let's look at diet first – with an eye to glucose.

BRAIN FUEL

The primary brain fuel is glucose, carried on the bloodstream through the *blood brain barrier* – a membrane which separates your brain from your circulatory system. Because the brain is so vulnerable to chemical disruption, and because more than twenty-five percent of your blood supply is destined to feed the brain, the blood brain barrier is designed to keep most of the other components in your blood out of your brain – especially potentially damaging chemicals. If any breaks in the blood brain barrier occur so that molecules which don't belong there are allowed to leak through, this can set off an immunological response, disrupting brain function and creating all sorts of physical and mental disorders.

Glucose is the fuel needed by the mitochondria in brain cells for them to make enough energy for the brain to do its work. You must not have *too much*, or *too little*. If there is not enough glucose and if there are no ketones to replace it (ketones are an alternative brain fuel), then nerve cells eventually die. When they do, you can end up feeling fuzzy minded or even suffer mood disorders. On the other hand, if too much glucose passes the brain barrier, this can be equally destructive. It can cause nerve death.

Unlike cells in the rest of your body, brain cells do not depend on insulin to regulate and transport glucose into them. Inside your brain, how much glucose gets transported into its cells is determined by how much there happens to be in your blood. For optimal quantities to arrive in your brain, your blood sugar needs to remain relatively stable. Stability requires

> A sea of toxins surrounds you, from environmental chemicals in solvents, plastics and adhesives to poisons in make-up, moisturisers, nail polish, hair dyes and shampoos. Even food and soil are inundated with pesticides and herbicides; not to mention the contaminants and parasites lurking in water. Everything you touch, taste, breathe and eat is propelling the leading engine of the detoxification process, your liver, into overdrive.
>
> *Anne Louise Gittleman*

BEWARE EXCESS GLUCOSE

In excess, glucose can be one of the most damaging things in the world to brain functioning. One of the fastest ways to age your brain rapidly is to follow the standard low-fat-high-carbohydrate diet based on convenience foods riddled with junk fats. Yet as a result of pressures from food manufacturers and general ignorance about nutrition, governments are still trying to sell us the famous 'food pyramid' and to convince us this is a healthy way to live. Don't listen. What is great for the profits of multi-national corporations is not good for your brain.

good insulin sensitivity in your body as a whole, to keep blood sugar balanced. This can only come from a way of eating that is not high in refined foods like sugar and flour. When you eat them in excess – as most people do these days – too much glucose is released too quickly into your bloodstream, predisposing you to insulin resistance or Syndrome X, and to rapid degeneration in the brain as well as in the body as a whole.

BEWARE OF AGES

When too much glucose crosses the blood brain barrier and enters your brain, this can also trigger the formation of something known as *advanced glycosylation-endproducts* – AGEs. AGEs can cause major free radical damage, as well as a depletion in available oxygen and atherosclerosis. AGEs foster the development of plaques made up of a particularly destructive kind of protein called *beta ameloid*. You find it in large quantities in the brains of people with Alzheimer's disease.

STRESS MATTERS

Most of the brain's cortical-sensitive neurons are located within the hippocampus which conveys information to the rest of the body by triggering hormonal cascades. The hippocampus is also responsible for turning short-term memory into long-term memory. Damage or significant loss to hippocampal neurons which can happen when cortisol levels are too high, can also interfere with brain function.

One of the first improvements people notice when they follow Age Power's Insulin Balance, is how their thinking becomes clearer and their emotions far more stable, as their bodies stop experiencing huge peaks and troughs in blood sugar. So dramatic is this experience that many are stunned to find how much their lives change, even within a week or two, by making simple shifts in the way they are eating.

STRESS KILLS

Insulin ushers nutrients and energy into the cells and so reduces blood glucose levels, making less available to pass through the blood brain barrier. On the other hand, glucagon, the hormone which is the antagonist to insulin, restores blood glucose levels, provided it is doing its job efficiently. This is how good energy balance is established.

In people with unstable blood sugar and insulin resistance, however, the system breaks down. Their body tends to produce too much of the stress hormone *cortisol* – the body's primary back-up to glucagon – in an attempt to restore blood glucose balance. The problem is that, while cortisol does indeed raise levels of glucose in the blood, when it comes to the health of your brain, this stress hormone is one of the most destructive hormones the brain ever has to deal with.

There are significant qualitative as well as quantitative differences between age related (senescent) and disease related (pathological) processes ellipses ... Health and functional status in late life are increasingly seen as under our own control.

Dr John Rowe

Adrenaline is another blood-sugar elevating hormone which the brain uses in a pinch when there is not enough glucose available. In excess, adrenaline can also disrupt mood, creating a sense of anxiety or fear. This may be accompanied by panic attacks and heart irregularities, dry mouth or rapid heart beat. All these things can happen when excess adrenaline is secreted in an attempt to restore falling blood sugar levels. What this all adds up to is the fact that any kind of prolonged stress, be it mental, physical or emotional, is potentially destructive to the brain, causing stress hormones to rise and stay high for long periods. This may sound complicated but it all adds up to three simple rules if you want to protect your brain.

PROTECT YOUR BRAIN

❏   Maintain stable blood sugar levels and get rid of any insulin resistance present in your body. The primary force behind this is the Age Power's Insulin Balance way of living (see Chapter 15) including the right kind of regular exercise.

❏   Learn to make stress work for you rather than against you and use whatever nutritional support you need for good sleep and stress management.

❏   Make good use of appropriate leading-edge natural brain enhancers (see Chapter 21).

SHE'S GOTTA HAVE IT

The other thing which the brain absolutely cannot do without is oxygen. It hungers for it. A fifth of the oxygen you take into your body goes directly to your brain. When blood vessels attempting to transport it become blocked or stiff as a result of the build-up of plaque so that oxygen to the brain is reduced, you may get an inexorable loss of brain function. This can show itself in the form of depression, anxiety, an inability to concentrate or remember, fatigue, mood swings, confusion and an increased possibility that you will experience a stroke. The moment that the oxygen supply to the brain is reduced, free radical damage to the cells soars. So does the formation of AGEs.

EXERCISE HIGH

Regular exercise – walking briskly for 30 to 45 minutes a day – is an effective way to keep oxygen and nutrients flowing to the brain via clean blood vessels, which remain good carriers as the years go by. As well as preventing blockages to the blood flow and protecting the arteries, the exercise you do influences the production of a useful substance called *brain derived growth factor* (BDGF) which helps protect neurons. BDGF also exerts a positive effect on mood. When you are fit and exercise regularly, your brain produces a high level of blissful substances known as *endorphins* – the body's natural feel-good opiates. Exercise also stimulates the thyroid so that your whole metabolism functions better. While involved in physical activity, you lose anxiety and tend to focus on what you are doing in the moment rather than mulling over – as we all tend to do – the worries and concerns of your life. Like regular meditation, this enhances brain health and helps protect from age degeneration.

STRETCH YOURSELF

It is not just moving your body that matters either. You need to exercise your mind continually as well. That old adage 'use it or lose it' is absolutely true. The brain loss that occurs to most people as they get older is by no means inevitable. It depends on all of the things we have just been looking at, as well as on how much you continue to stretch yourself to learn new skills and face new challenges year after year. Numerous studies show that people with higher levels of education are far less likely to develop Alzheimer's disease than the general population, probably because they remain more active mentally, both in work and leisure time.

TUNE IN – TURN ON

Like a thoroughbred, your brain needs to be put through its paces. It requires constant challenges in order to stay in peak form. When we are young, such challenges present themselves automatically. As we get older and more 'comfortable' with life, we often have to go out of our way to find them. Stop and think of all the things that you have long wanted to do but have never done. Do you want to take up a musical instrument? Learn a new language? Learn to sky dive or to scuba dive? Take up Tai Chi or Salsa dancing? Learn philosophy? Whatever it is you fancy, do it for the sake of your brain. The more of your brain you use, the less of it you will lose.

In many instances, people claim that they smoke, drink alcohol or take drugs because it calms them. In reality, these substances complicate matters. The relaxation or chemical high these drugs induce is short-lived and ultimately adds more stress to the system . . . individuals suffering from stress-related disorders, anxiety, depression or other psychological conditions must absolutely stop drinking coffee and other sources of caffeine, alcohol, smoking and other destructive habits. Instead choose health.

Michael T. Murray, ND

FAT HEAD

To function in top form, your brain needs fats but they must be the right kinds of fats. This is not surprising since more than 60 percent of its complex structure is derived from fats of one kind or another – including the much maligned but absolutely essential cholesterol.

Fats make up more than three quarters of the protective insulating tissue known as the myelin sheath which covers all of the nerve fibres in your body. If ever these myelin sheaths begin to break down, neurons can be laid bare. You can end up with any number of neurological and psychological disturbances from mood disorders to epilepsy and multiple sclerosis. Like other cells in the body, neurons are covered by membranes made mostly from essential fatty acids in a phospholipid form. It is this phospholipid membrane which guards the integrity as well as ensuring semi-permeability of brain cell membranes. What determines the quality of phospholipids which your cell membranes are made from is the kind of fats that you eat. Fill up on convenience foods full of saturated fats and trans-fatty acids – junk fats – and the structure and function of your nerve cells become altered. Cell membranes become less fluid. Essential nutrients and oxygen can't enter brain cells to nourish them adequately.

ESSENTIAL OMEGA 3S

Most people are on far too many convenience foods riddled with trans-fatty acids and sugar – both of which are destructive to the brain. The average Western diet is highly deficient in the omega-3 fats (found in good quantities in fatty fish and flaxseed oils) so that the phospholipid-based cell membranes, which a body produces from eating this way, are not up to scratch when it comes to enabling the neurons to perform vital functions. Brain cells cannot hold water properly. Nor do they have adequate access to vital nutrients and electrolytes. Neither are they efficient at eliminating wastes. The standard diet of manufactured foods creates a deficiency of omega-3 fatty acids as well as an imbalance between the omega-3 and the omega-6 essential fatty acid groups so your body suffers and your brain becomes a major target for degeneration.

> An innovative study of 'self complexity' finds that men and women who are complex and diverse, whose selves reach out in different directions, suffer fewer signs of life stresses. They report less depression and fewer foul moods, colds, coughs, stomach pains, headaches and muscle aches than their less complex counterparts.
>
> *Robert Ornstein, PhD and David Sobel, MD*

GO FISH

The balance between the two groups of essential fats – omega-3 and omega-6 – has to be right. Most of us get far too much omega-6 and too little omega-3. In a study published in the American Journal of Epidemiology, researchers reported that people whose intake was very high in linoleic acid – an omega-6 fat – often experience impaired cognition. In practical terms, this means that people who eat a lot of margarine and vegetable oils such as safflower, sunflower, corn, peanut and soya oil did not think as clearly as those who took in a much higher amount of omega-3 fatty acids – those who eat a lot of fish. The fish eaters had much better mental functions. Supplements of omega-3 oils – especially DHA – can radically improve the way you think or feel. Many researchers now believe that attention deficit disorder and hyperactivity in children together with learning disabilities and behaviour problems, has a great deal to do with the fact that the convenience foods kids are now raised on severely disrupt mental functions and growth. This phenomenon begins in the womb when a pregnant woman is already eating junk fats. Highly processed golden oils and the margarines made from them

BRAIN FOOD

How To Get More Omega-3 Essential Fatty Acids In Your Diet

❏ Eat more cold-water fish such as salmon, trout, tuna, sardines, herrings and anchovies.

❏ Add omega-3 rich flaxseed oil to salad dressings and drizzle it over cooked vegetables or porridge.

❏ Add chopped walnuts or ground flaxseeds to salads and other dishes.

❏ Go for organic and free-range chickens and meats where animals have grazed on omega-3-rich grass and insects (rather than those fattened up on omega-6-rich grains).

❏ Eat game such as venison, pheasant and wild duck; they have a fatty-acid profile more closely resembling the fatty-acid profiles of the wild meats our ancestors ate.

❏ Eat more green vegetables – the darker the better. Good sources of omega-3 fatty acids include romaine lettuce, mesclun mixed greens, rocket, kale, collards, mustard greens, swiss chard and lamb's lettuce.

❏ If you don't like fatty fish or any of the other food ideas listed here, consider taking a good quality omega-3 fish oil supplement. (Be sure to store it in the fridge).

form the basis of much of the fat in our foods today. Coupled with the high level of saturated fats in the average diet, they interfere with brain cell receptors, making it impossible for the brain's signalling chemistry to transmit messages effectively across synapses between one cell and another. The myelin sheath along nerve fibres can break down, further disrupting brain functioning. Eating junk fats, which now make up the lion's share of fat in the Western diet, is like taking poison into your brain. Stay away from foods which contain them.

This is the foundation of lasting brain function. Now let's look at some of the bells and whistles – recently discovered brain enhancing nutrients and substances which can help a healthy well-functioning brain rise to new levels of vitality and power. But unless you get these basics right, leading-edge brain supplements are not going to make up the gap.

BOTTOM LINE

How well your brain functions as the years pass depends almost entirely on how well you look after your body as a whole. Follow the Age Power's Insulin Balance – based on natural unprocessed foods, including good quantities of low-glycaemic and low-density carbohydrates like broccoli and the green vegetables, together with plenty of omega-3 fats from cold water fish like wild salmon, mackerel, sardines and herring. It also means avoiding sugar, high-glycaemic and high-density carbohydrates such as refined flour and all the convenience foods containing it. Make these adjustments to your life while increasing the amount of exercise you get day in and day out. Continue to challenge your brain by learning something new. Not only will these changes help protect you from loss of brain function and all of the degenerative conditions associated with it, you should be able to look forward to better brain function with each decade that passes.

LEADING-EDGE BRAIN

Patient: Doctor, I think I'm suffering from lack of memory.
Doctor: How long have you had this problem?
Patient: What problem is that?

Mark Brown

We thrive on beauty and wonder to keep our brain working well so our experience of life can grow richer, more intricate and more complex as the years pass. Fine tune your brain and nervous system with state-of-the-art natural substances. They can intensify your experience of excitement, deep relaxation, sensuality and memory. They may even enhance your creativity and your capacity for joy.

Each time you experience anything, learn anything or encounter anything, your brain forges new connections. To hold onto new facts, experiences and memories, neurons actually grow new dendrites. These dendrites reach out towards other neurons creating links that have never existed before. This is a major reason why it is so important, as you grow older, not to become complacent with your life, get into a rut or allow it to narrow by doing the same things all the time in the same way. Your brain and life-long personal development needs a rich environment filled with smells and textures, sights and sounds, as well as new ideas and the best possible biochemical medium to thrive.

THE AMAZING NEUROTRANSMITTERS

So far, scientists have identified more than fifty *neurotransmitters* – also called *neuromodulators* – which affect the brain. Many are found only within the brain and central nervous system. While there is no need to concern yourself with all fifty, it is useful to be aware of those which appear to be the most important. Some dazzling advances in brain enhancement have come out of the knowledge we now have about how to increase these compounds naturally. By doing so, you can improve brain functions and life as a whole. For instance choline, some of the B complex vitamins and minerals such as potassium are necessary in truly adequate quantities (not the easiest thing to get as you grow older) for nerves to fire properly. There is also a rapidly developing awareness of how to use natural compounds, such as acetyl L-carnitine and phosphatidylserine as well as herbs from Ginkgo to Kava Kava, to help deal with depression, insomnia and other nervous system-related symptoms. Let's look at the most important neurotransmitters and what roles they play in keeping your brain young, your emotions balanced and your body vital. Then we will examine the natural substances you can use to enhance them.

SEROTONIN
PEACE AND MEMORY

Serotonin is one of two neurotransmitters that look after learning and memory. It has many other health-enhancing properties as well. This is an inhibitory neurotransmitter – fundamentally calming to the brain and to the rest of the body. Serotonin plays a vital role in regulating appetite and sleep, both of which go awry when insufficient serotonin is available. Low serotonin can produce insomnia and appetite disorders including hunger which is never sated. When you have adequate serotonin you feel satisfied as well as relaxed and comfortable. Serotonin improves memory. In animal studies, when serotonin levels are increased, the ability to store memories and to learn is enhanced. Drinking alcohol decreases your brain's ability to concentrate and to remember. Studies show that when people have been given drugs or natural substances which produce greater concentrations of serotonin at the synapse, alcohol-related memory deficit does not occur.

Your body makes serotonin by converting the amino acid tryptophan into another metabolite 5-hydroxy tryptophan (5-HTP) and then changing 5-HTP into serotonin itself. Some of your serotonin then gets converted into melatonin – the hormone used to regulate your body clock. Serotonin behaves as a vaso-constrictor. It is also found in your digestive system and in blood platelets where it helps control blood clotting. Much migraine has been linked to a serotonin deficiency. Many popular migraine drugs are serotonin *agonists*. This means they heighten serotonin levels in the brain.

> Age is . . . (something that) doesn't matter unless you're a cheese.
>
> *Billie Burke*

> He's so full of alcohol, if you put a lighted wick in his mouth he'd burn for three days.
>
> *Groucho Marx*

Increasing serotonin is a goal of many of the anti-depressant drugs such as Prozac, too. They try to correct or mitigate imbalances in the *amines* – also known as *monoamines* – which include serotonin, dopamine, adrenaline and noradrenaline. Many anti-depressant drugs act by increasing specific amino amines in the brain. While they may be successful in temporarily alleviating depression, all of these drugs cause serious side-effects including increased insomnia, anxiety, allergic reactions and nervousness. There are better, easier, and more natural ways of increasing serotonin. They include taking supplements of 5-HTP on an empty stomach or using an extract of St. John's Wort (see page 439).

Caution: Do not use 5HTP and or St. John's Wort if you are currently on tranquillisers. Ask for help to gradually get off the drugs before using them.

MOOD MAKER – SEROTONIN

How serotonin levels affect mood and behaviour

Adequate Serotonin	Low Serotonin
Good concentration	Poor attention span
Easy going attitude	Hot-headed responses
Responsive behaviour	Reactive behaviour
No carbohydrate cravings	Cravings (particularly carbs and sweets)
Good sleep patterns	Insomnia
Dream recall	Poor dream recall
Rational thinking	Impulsive behaviour
Loving responses	Anger
Good natured personality	Bad temper

ACETYLCHOLINE
FOR CONCENTRATION

The other biggie when it comes to protecting memory is acetylcholine. Depletion of this neurotransmitter is a major contributor to Alzheimer's disease. A deficiency of acetylcholine shows up in the post mortem brains of people who have had it. Biopsies taken from living Alzheimer's patients indicate that they have a lowered ability to make acetylcholine. Older people who maintain clear memory show little, if any, deficit of this important neurotransmitter. Acetylcholine is one of the most abundant neurotransmitters in your body and one of the most important. It acts as a messenger between muscles and nerve cells. It improves memory functions and enhances concentration. Using drugs or nutrients to increase the brain's acetylcholine levels can bring about significant improvements in memory, not only with older people who have experienced memory loss, but in people of any age with poor memory.

You cannot take supplements of acetylcholine to raise acetylcholine levels in the brain. For it is broken down by your digestive system and therefore cannot cross the blood brain barrier to be used by the brain. Nevertheless, many independent studies show that taking some of the natural dietary supplements of choline, pantothenic acid, vitamin B_1, B_6, vitamin C and the minerals calcium and zinc does help increase acetylcholine in the brain. These are the substances your body uses to manufacture this vital neurotransmitter. Combined with Age Power's Insulin Balance they can help raise acetylcholine levels and improve memory. Many people claim that taking lecithin, which contains choline, works to enhance acetylcholine levels. Most of the experiments designed to verify this belief have not been successful however. Experimental studies which have been successful in raising aceytlcholine have employed somewhere between three to 20 grams of phosphatidyl-choline (see page 322) a day to do the job. Best of all is to use phosphatidyl-choline together with foods high in choline such as lecithin, wheat germ and soya.

As with any programme designed to improve brain function it is never enough only to tackle the issues at a biochemical level alone. Enhanced acetylcholine levels, memory and cognition can also improve significantly and long term if you also challenge your brain by continuing to learn in new ways.

Several studies have found caffeine intake to be extremely high in individuals with psychiatric disorders, and the degree of fatigue they experienced was often related to how much caffeine was ingested.

Michael T. Murray

MEMORY MAGIC

Supplying your body with the natural metabolites, vitamins and herbs it can use for memory enhancement can sometimes work wonders. The cocktail below, based around acetyl L-carnitine is designed to supply the nuts and bolts to help preserve cell receptors and to promote optimal learning and attention. Take acetyl L-carnitine first thing in the morning on an empty stomach. The other ingredients can be taken with meals:

Acetyl L-carnitine	1500mg
Phosphatidylserine	400mg
Zinc	20mg
Chelated Magnesium	300mg
EPA/DHA omega-3s	750mg
Extract of Ginkgo	200mg
Extract of Bilberry	100mg
Tincture of Gotu kola	20drops

DOPAMINE
FOR BALANCE

This neurotransmitter is essential to good motor co-ordination, motivation, insulin regulation, immune function, short-term memory, clear cognition, physical energy and balanced emotions. Dopamine is also involved in sexual drive and in helping to balance the autonomic nervous system. Dopamine sends messages to your pituitary gland to release growth hormone. Growth hormone helps keep your body young and fat free, builds muscles and helps repair damage to tissues. To manufacture enough dopamine, in addition to an excellent diet supplying all the essential nutrients, your body needs good quantities of the amino acids phenylalanine and tyrosine. It also needs optimal quantities of vitamin B_6, vitamin B_{12} and folic acid which serve as co-factors to the enzymes that make the manufacture of dopamine possible. Supplying adequate quantities (by diet and nutritional supplement – see page 314) of these nutrients can hugely improve all of the functions dopamine looks after in your body. A decline in dopamine activity in the brain is linked to the learning and coordination problems associated with Parkinson's disease.

NORADRENALINE
FOR VITALITY

Your body makes this neurotransmitter from dopamine, with the help of vitamins B_3, B_6 and C plus a little of the mineral copper. It is one of the 'feel good' brain chemicals found in good quantities in the blood of highly active people like athletes. People with long-term depression have very low levels of noradrenaline. Your body uses noradrenaline, also known as *norepinephrine,* to regulate many activities from sexual response and appetite to how well you burn energy. Like acetylcholine and dopamine, noradrenaline also plays an important part in learning, memory and regulating your moods. Regular exercise increases noradrenaline – a major reason it makes people feel so good.

THE GABA SYSTEM
TO KEEP YOUR COOL

Glutamine, gamma aminobutyric acid and glutamate amino acids, together are known as the GABA system. Discovered in 1950, they are the 'calmers' – the most important inhibitory neurotransmitters in the brain. They work to balance and control levels of the stimulatory neurotransmitters such as noradrenaline. These three are also important if you are to experience deep relaxation and to sleep well. Many tranquillising drugs like Valium manipulate levels of the GABA system to calm you. Some studies indicate that supplements of L-glutamine can improve levels of the GABA system in your brain, in the process helping to eliminate food cravings as well as alcohol cravings. L-glutamine has also shown good results in the treatment of Alzheimer's patients. Taking GABA itself is *not* a good way of increasing GABA since it does not easily cross the blood brain barrier. Chemists are still searching for a way of overcoming this.

NEUROTRANSMITTERS –
WHAT THEY DO

❑ **Serotonin** – alters mood, controls appetite, brings calm, improves memory
❑ **Aceytlcholine** – enhances learning, improves concentration
❑ **Dopamine** – affects insulin regulation, short-term memory, clear thinking, physical energy, emotional balance, sex drive
❑ **Noradrenaline** – affects arousal, alertness and mood
❑ **GABA** – brings calm and relaxation

CLEAN UP AND THRIVE

The single most important thing you can do to create a healthy balance in your neurotransmitters and improve the overall functioning of your brain is to detoxify your body. Because the brain or the nervous system is so high in the levels of the special kinds of fats known as phospholipids, it is highly vulnerable to free radical damage. To guard these phospholipids, the body needs to remain as free as possible from toxicity. It also needs high levels of anti-oxidants – vitamins and minerals as well as phytonutrients. Animal studies show that when sufficient anti-oxidants are not available in the diet, the brain is rapidly damaged by the formation of a pigment known as *lipofuscin* in brain cells. How much lipofuscin accumulates in your brain determines to a large extent how rapidly your brain is ageing. This is why anti-oxidants play such an important role in protecting the brain and ensuring that it functions optimally as the years pass. Your first line of defence is to make sure that toxicity, from poor diet, environmental pollution, drugs, alcohol, prolonged stress and lack of exercise, is not allowed to build up in the body and cause oxidation damage. When it does, your brain takes the brunt of the damage. As this happens you can become prone to changes in mood, memory and cognition associated with ageing. If your liver is working properly and you have adequate supplies of enzymes that support detoxification, then you are miles ahead of most people when it comes to protecting your brain from degeneration.

> Participants in a forty-one year study at Johns Hopkins University who didn't express tension and emotion at age twenty-three were twice as likely to die by age fifty-five than those who freely expressed anxieties.
>
> *Anne Louise Gittleman*

THE TROUBLE WITH ALCOHOL

Scientists have long known that brain damage and dementia result from the toxic effects of alcohol. Now, thanks to researcher Charles Leiber at the Mt. Sinai School of Medicine in New York City, we are beginning to understand why. Leiber and his colleagues have discovered it is not alcohol itself that is the problem. It is the fact that, when alcohol is metabolised by the liver in the body's attempt to detoxify itself, this process produces free radicals. If these cannot be adequately cleared they can bring about damage to delicate tissues of the heart, brain and kidneys – in no small part because they destroy phospholipids in the nervous system.

STRESS EQUATIONS

How well your liver detoxifies alcohol is a highly individual thing. Not only does it depend on your genetically inherited ability to detoxify, it is also determined by how many other toxic substances such as caffeine, drugs, heavy metals, environmental chemicals and excess hormones it is also trying to cope with. Studies show that patients with chronic liver problems have significantly diminished mental functioning and much less success at work. Your long-term stress levels matter too. Not only is stress damaging to the brain because of the excessive cortisol it creates which destroys some brain cells and damages others, being under heavy stress also tends to make people consume more alcohol and medication and to work longer hours because they are less able to function efficiently. This creates a cycle of yet more stress, further build-up of toxicity and further putting delicate brain cells at risk.

As far back as the nineteen eighties, reports in scientific literature suggested that people who are exposed to industrial chemicals have a higher incidence of Parkinson's disease and Alzheimer's disease than those who are not. In the late-eighties, men in their late 20s or early 30s were already starting to demonstrate the symptoms of Parkinson's disease, apparently as a result of exposure to the toxic chemical MTPT, one of hundreds – perhaps thousands – of toxins that can affect the nervous system and increase damage to your neurons. These are toxic chemicals from the environment such as herbicides, pesticides and xenohormones, as well as destructive chemicals in plastics and drugs. For those with a diminished ability to clear these *excotoxins* through the action of the liver, brain damage eventually becomes inevitable unless the liver is strengthened and the body detoxified. It is likely that people with a high risk of neurological disorders are those who have a history of long-term exposure to excotoxins coupled with poor detoxification capacity. So you want to be careful of the chemicals that you use in your environment.

THE CLEAN OUT

❑ Clear out chemicals in your home and use non-toxic cleaners and natural, biodegradable products instead.

❑ Steer clear of unnecessary drugs including hormones, including those involved in birth control or hormone replacement therapy.

❑ Limit your alcohol and caffeine intake.

❑ Supply your brain, as well as your body as a whole, with adequate quantities of the nutrients essential to brain functioning including those minerals specifically needed to spur the activity of the liver's detoxifying enzymes: manganese, copper, zinc, selenium and molybdenum.

❑ Learn the secrets of ongoing detoxification and practise them.

❑ Consider supporting your liver with milk thistle to strengthen it.

B IS FOR BRAIN

To initiate any neuro-protective programme for the brain you need good nutrition plus a broad base multi-vitamin and mineral supplement, whose nutrients are within both the safe and the effective ranges for anyone who has marginal nutritional deficiencies. This includes most of us these days. Certain vitamins are particularly important for your brain, including the entire B vitamin complex from thiamine (vitamin B_1) right through to cobalamine (vitamin B_{12}). You need adequate B vitamins to make neurotransmitters. If you are low in any one of them, you are likely to be low in others. Even mild deficiencies in some of the B vitamins can cause significant difficulties – from anxiety and depression to loss of memory, confusion and sleep disorders.

One of the problems with B complex vitamins is that they are often difficult to absorb with food, particularly as we get older. Many people over sixty do not eat enough or eat well enough to supply the B vitamins they need. One way to enhance your B vitamin uptake is to eat organic lamb's liver a couple of times a week. Not only is it an excellent source of almost all the B complex, it boasts other stress protective ingredients, some of which have not even been identified yet. For some reason, eating liver has gone out of fashion in the last 20 years – probably because so much liver available these days comes from unhealthy animals. The last thing you would want to eat is the liver from any unhealthy animal. So go organic whenever you can.

Two B vitamins are particularly important for the brain – vitamin B_{12} and folic acid. Close behind them follows vitamin B_6 (pyroxidine), essential in making haemoglobin – the oxygen-carrying red pigment in your blood. Vitamin B_5 (pantothenic acid) is essential for your body to make Coenzyme A for ATP – your main fuel – as well as neurotransmitter chemicals which transfer information in your brain from one nerve to the next.

BIG B_{12}

Studies show that most people over the age of 50 are deficient in cobalamine (B_{12}). B_{12} is not easy to absorb from foods anyway. As we get older, the amount of hydrochloric acid and pepsin in the stomach tends to diminish. So does a special substance called intrinsic factor. All three are necessary for you to absorb B_{12} from your food, but with age, most people on a Western diet of convenience foods make progressively less and less of them. By the age of 60 or 65, unless you are one of the lucky ones and have lived primarily on a natural diet, you may well be unable to absorb all the B_{12} you need from your food. There are two ways you can tackle the problem if you think you are not getting enough B_{12}: You can try taking good quality digestive enzymes (readily available in your local health food store); or you can speak to your doctor about B_{12} injections, as B_{12} taken in this form does not require good digestion for absorption.

SECRETS OF B$_{12}$

One of the symptoms of B$_{12}$ deficiency is classic *senility* – something fairly easy to detect with blood tests since it shows itself as an obvious form of anaemia. Mild B$_{12}$ deficiency is harder to detect. According to one recent study, 40 percent of the population over 67 have sub-optimal levels of this vitamin and 12 percent have outright deficiencies. Because B$_{12}$ is also hard to absorb when taken orally, most doctors trained in nutrition prefer to use periodic injections of B$_{12}$. The usual dose is 1cc containing one milligram of the vitamin given each month. To get a similar amount of the vitamin into your system orally, the general consensus is that you need to take over 1000mcg as a supplement – and remember, no matter how much you take orally you will not absorb it without adequate intrinsic factor and good digestion.

FORGOTTEN POWER

Folic acid deficiency is the most common vitamin deficiency in the world for many different reasons. First, with the exception of liver, animal foods are very low in folic acid while green leafed plants are a good source. Our Paleolithc ancestors got 200 to 400 times the level of folic acid we get today because they ate so many green leafy herbs and vegetables. Nowadays, few people eat them often enough. Second, all sorts of drugs – from the oestrogens and the barbiturates to alcohol – interfere with the metabolism of folic acid. This vitamin is delicate and easily destroyed by light or heat. Also known as folate or folacin, it functions together with vitamin B$_{12}$ in many of your body's most important processes such as DNA synthesis and the division of cells. Folate is absolutely essential to the healthy development of the nervous system of a foetus and young child. Where folic acid deficiencies occur in pregnancy, they are linked to many different birth defects including spina bifida and neural tube disorders. You also often find folic acid deficiency in people with osteoporosis, arteriosclerosis and depression. A folic acid deficiency can even produce abnormal pap smears in women. I believe that just about everyone would benefit from taking a supplement of at least 800mcg of folic acid a day. Most doctors still rely on blood tests for anaemia to determine whether a person is deficient in folic acid. This is by no means the most efficient way of determining your folate status. Measuring the level of homocysteine in the blood is much more reliable for determining both folate and B_{12} status.

YOUR BRAIN AND IMMUNITY

Many chemical messengers from the immune system affect your brain too. Especially *cytokines* – interferons, interleukins and tumour necrosis factor. Brain neurotransmitters affect your immune system too. For instance, your white blood cells are covered with serotonin receptors. This is why when you are ill your brain goes out of kilter too.

LOW HOMOCYSTEINE MEANS GOOD HEALTH

Homocysteine is an intermediate compound involved in converting the sulphur based amino acid *methionine* to *cysteine*. When you are deficient in folic acid, vitamin B_6 or B_{12}, you will experience an increase in the level of homocysteine – a compound increasingly linked to a great number of degenerative conditions including arteriosclerosis, the build-up of plaque in your arteries. Homocysteine damages arteries, directly interfering with the integrity of the blood vessel walls. High levels of homocysteine also interfere with the healthy formation of new collagen, the main protein in your skin and bones. So important are homocysteine levels in your body, they are now considered an independent risk factor in the development of every kind of vascular disease, stroke and heart attack as well as in osteoporosis. Keep them low. When it comes to the brain, high levels of homocysteine can make you prone to Alzheimer's disease. People with this condition show low levels of B_{12} and folic acid plus elevated blood levels of homocysteine. In one study of two groups of people aged 55 and over – one of which had Alzheimer's disease and the other which did not – researchers discovered that those with the highest levels of homocysteine were four and a half times more at risk of having Alzheimer's disease than those with the lowest. Measuring homocysteine levels should be standard practice, but as yet, few doctors do this.

> Regardless of the 'disease' the reward for most people who adopt a more positive mental attitude, eat a healthy diet, exercise regularly and utilise natural, health promoting measures is a healthier life filed with very high levels of energy, joy, vitality and a tremendous passion for living.
>
> *Michael T. Murray*

Homocysteine is relatively easy to lower with supplements of vitamin B_{12}, folic acid and vitamin B_6. B_6 is easy, simply take 50mg of B_6 supplement a day. Sadly, however, it can be difficult to get a high enough dose of folic acid as a nutritional supplement. Official recommendations for folic acid levels hover at somewhere between 400 and 800mcg. This is far lower than experts in functional and nutrition based medicine deem necessary to lower homocysteine and guard the health of your brain and body overall. Informed doctors and nutritional biochemists insist that even healthy people over 35 should supplement their diet with somewhere between 4 and 8mg a day (a milligram is 100 micrograms). If there is any history of stroke, heart disease, osteoporosis or early senility in your family, they insist you are likely to need significantly more.

Vitamin B_{12}, folic acid and a form of methionine known as S-adenosyl-methionine (SAMe) work together as 'methyl donors'. This means that they *give* methyl molecules – important in the production of DNA and brain neurotransmitters as well as in the detoxification of the body (see pages 107–8). Folic acid supplementation enhances methylation reactions in the brain and brings about an increase in the neurotransmitter serotonin. This is probably why both folic acid and the other methyl donors also exert an anti-depressive effect on people using them as supplements.

Any folic acid supplementation should always include vitamin B_{12} (from 400 to 1000mg daily, or by injection if digestion is poor) otherwise supplementing with folic acid can cover up an underlying vitamin B_{12} deficiency. Folic acid has to be used very carefully in epileptics since, in some people, it may increase seizures. It works particularly well with vitamin B_{12}, B_6 and choline (the recommended dose of choline is 150-500mg a day). SAMe has recently become one of the hottest new anti-ageing supplements (see page 92). It works well, especially well, with these important B complex vitamins to enhance brain functioning.

Homocysteine may represent a metabolic link in the cause of arteriosclerosis vascular diseases and old-age dementias. Excessive homocysteine is an independent risk factor for coronary artery disease, peripheral vascular disease and cerebrovascular disease. Homocysteine is a reliable marker of vitamin B_{12} deficiency, a common condition in the elderly, which is known to induce neurological deficits including cognitive impairment. A high prevalence of folate deficiency has been reported in geriatric patients suffering from depression and dementia.

Dr Lucilla Parnetti

GOOD SOURCES FOR B VITAMINS

Try to include some of these foods in your diet every day.

- ❑ Alfalfa
- ❑ Asparagus
- ❑ Brewer's yeast
- ❑ Brown rice
- ❑ Brussels sprouts
- ❑ Buckwheat
- ❑ Egg yolk
- ❑ Fresh peas
- ❑ Kidney beans
- ❑ Lentils
- ❑ Lima beans
- ❑ Nuts
- ❑ Oats
- ❑ Seeds
- ❑ Soya products
- ❑ Wheatgerm

It is a good idea to take a top quality B 100 Complex supplement once or twice a day also.

GET INTO ANTI-OXIDANTS

Anti-oxidants look after your brain, since most of the damage done to the brain occurs as a result of free radical oxidation. The anti-oxidants most people are familiar with are vitamin C and vitamin E. Both are important to the brain because they are found in particularly high levels within the nervous system. Evidence increases each year that the higher your intake of anti-oxidants over a period of years, the better your mental functions will be later in life. A good intake of anti-oxidants will significantly lower your risk of Parkinson's disease, Alzheimer's disease and other degenerative brain conditions. How much vitamin C? Most experts agree somewhere between 500 and 1500mg per day is essential while 400 to 800 international units of vitamin E is considered a good generally recommended dose. Other important anti-oxidants for brain care include selenium, beta-carotene and the other carotinoids, flavonoids, sulphur-containing amino acids such as methionine and cysteine, and

Co-enzyme Q10. When it comes to anti-oxidants, whatever you do to look after your whole body will do great things for your brain as well.

SPACE AGE BRAIN SUPPORT

In recent years a great many natural substances – either metabolites that occur in the human body or occur naturally in our foods or herbs – have become popular brain-helpers because they offer protection from brain-related age degeneration and all of the emotional and mental dramas that accompany it. There are many known brain boosters which are now considered to be safe and user friendly. Most are available over the counter. Some, such as DHEA and melatonin, can be purchased freely in one country but not in another. Others such as Ginkgo biloba extract, acetyl L-carnitine, blueberry or bilberry extracts are widely available just about everywhere. Each has specific actions. If these actions coincide with a particular need you have they are well worth looking at as possible supplements. But remember what comes first is diet and lifestyle. No brain-enhancer, no matter how effective, can work its wonders in a neglected, malnourished, toxic body. Here is my favourite list:

ALPHA-LIPOIC ACID

Often called a master nutrient, alpha-lipoic acid is so unique and important for health that small amounts of it are made by your body. It helps burn glucose and convert it into energy to power your brain as well as every organ in the body and it provides noticeable cognitive effects. It also offers high-level anti-oxidant protection against free radical damage. It even enhances the actions of other anti-oxidants such as vitamins, minerals and phytonutrients which you should be getting in your diet. It helps preserve the functions of vitamins C and E. So powerful an effect can alpha-lipoic acid have on improving the function of the brain, that in the early nineties the German government approved it as a treatment for diabetic polyneuropathy – a serious nerve disorder. It also helps prevent Syndrome X and glucose problems. It increases your brain's ability to produce energy while protecting it from nerve damage. It reduces

> Within you lie all the chemicals required for every emotion you can possibly experience. The key is not to take drugs to try and duplicate these feelings, but rather to learn how to create the feelings inside of you so that you can conjure them up whenever you want. Your mind is a powerful tool. You can use your mind to create powerful positive emotions that give you a natural high to help you better cope with stress.
>
> *Michael T. Murray*

the formation of AGEs, neutralises free radicals, lowers glucose levels and reduces insulin resistance. The recommended dose to help prevent Syndrome X and as a general anti-oxidant supplement is from 50 to 100mg daily. To help *reverse* glucose intolerance and Syndrome X, 100 to 200mg daily.

ACETYL L-CARNITINE

Another important anti-oxidant is acetyl L-carnitine, which has more than 50 controlled studies under its belt and which demonstrate its remark-able ability to boost overall anti-oxidant actions. Used as a supplement, it has been shown to increase intelligence, prevent loss of brain function and enhance memory. In no small part this is because acetyl L-carnitine helps restore normal acetylcholine metabolism, improving memory and cognition. Acetyl L-carnitine is used to treat depression and memory loss in the aged, to counter Alzheimer's disease and to improve mental processes in people of any age. The generally recommended dose is 500 to 2000mg per day.

Caution: Acetyl L-carnitine is well tolerated. However, a high dose can induce restlessness, agitation and very occasionally nausea in a very few people.

GINKGO BILOBA

A standardised extract of Ginkgo biloba containing 24 percent *ginkgoflavo-glycosides* has shown itself again and again to be an effective anti-ageing supplement offering particular enhancement to the brain. It can be useful to improve short-term memory and to counter depression. Ginkgo is the world's oldest living tree species. Its heritage goes back more than two hundred million years. Throughout recorded history, ginkgo has been associated with longevity thanks to its ability as a plant to resist disease, pollution and insect attack. It has long been considered a powerful promoter of longevity. Ginkgo is useful both for its anti-oxidant proper-ties and – thanks to its ability to enhance blood flow and oxygen supply to the brain – known to improve many symptoms of brain ageing, including memory loss, headaches, dizziness, ringing in the ears, depression and dementia. When using ginkgo, look for a standardised extract of 24 percent ginkgoflavoglycosides, as this is what has been most studied and is confirmed to be effective. Ginkgo enhances the synthesis of ATP, bringing more energy to the brain and the body as a whole. Most studies with gingko use daily doses of 120 to 160mg (50:1 concentration 24 percent flavonoids). For anti-ageing maintenance 40 to 50 mg three times a day is generally considered a good dose. Practitioners of natural medicine often double these quantities when they are seeking therapeutic effects from this marvellous plant. You need a few weeks for positive results to be fully appreciated.

PHOSPHATIDYLSERINE

The major phospholipid in the brain, phosphatidylserine can work wonders wherever there is a deficiency of the omega-3 fats or the methyl donors (vitamin B_{12}, folic acid and SAMe) which prevents the brain from making adequate quantities of phosphatidylserine by itself. Supplements of this important phospholipid have been used effectively to clear depression and to improve mental functions in the elderly, thanks to phosphatidylserine's ability to orchestrate many important tasks. These include stimulating the release of brain neurotransmitters, regulating the availability of glucose and activating the transport of nutrients into the cells. For your brain to learn efficiently it needs adequate levels of phosphatidylserine. Levels tend to decline with age. Generally recommended supplementation of vegetable-based phosphatidylserine is between 80 and 100mg three times daily.

DMAE

A naturally occurring nutrient found in fatty fish such as sardines and anchovies, dimethyl-amino-ethanol, or DMAE, also occurs in small quantities in the human brain. It is available as a nutritional supplement, useful thanks to its ability to accelerate the brain synthesis of acetylcholine, important in preventing loss of memory and maximising mental ability. DMAE increases learning ability and intelligence. It extends the lifespan of laboratory animals. It improves memory and elevates mood. For many, small does of DMAE taken daily seems to increase physical and mental energy so they experience less fatigue and more sound sleep. DMAE is no quick fix remedy, it usually takes three to four weeks for DMAE to take effect. As a supplement, it is recommended that you start with a dose of 50 to 100mg three times a day, then if you feel you need more gradually increase the dose to 500 to 1000mg a day. In many, even the low doses are enough to do the trick. DMAE is probably the best version of choline you can get, but don't forget to eat plenty of egg yolks as well since they are unquestionably the best dietary source of phosphatidylserine.

Caution: DMAE is another brain enhancer not to be used by anyone suffering from epilepsy unless closely monitored by a doctor. Nor is it suitable for manic depressives. Taking too much of it can result in insomnia and muscular tension in some people.

DHA

Known as *docosahexaenoic acid*, DHA is essential for the brain to function properly at all ages, from womb to 120. It is an omega-3 fat which we take in from our foods, usually together with another important omega-3 fatty acid, EPA. Both are found in cold water fish such as sardines, mackerel, herring, wild salmon and cod. DHA is a must as a supplement unless you eat masses of fatty fish. It helps regulate nerve transmission, maintain essential oxygen in the brain cells, regulates smooth muscle and autonomic reflexes, protects from inflammation and regulates fluid pressure in the eyes and blood vessels. It also enhances the production of protective 'good' prostaglandins as well as hormones important for countering degeneration. The recommended daily dose as a supplement hovers between 400 and 600mg of DHA, best taken with EPA two to four times a day. A good rule of thumb is to take 300mg of EPA for every 200mg of DHA.

PHOSPHATIDYL-CHOLINE

Like vitamin B_{12}, SAMe and folic acid, choline is a methyl donor essential for proper liver function and detoxification. When taken in the form of phosphatidyl-choline as a supplement, it helps enhance the levels of acetylcholine, improving memory as well as a host of other brain functions. Phosphatidyl-choline can be particularly helpful for Alzheimer's patients. It is also used to treat liver disorders, elevated cholesterol and bi-polar depression. The best phosphatidyl-choline supplements contain 90 percent phosphatidyl-choline. When buying them, you generally get what you pay for. The standard recommended dose is 350mg three times a day, with meals. In the treatment of Alzheimer's disease and bi-polar depression, doctors have used 5000 to 10000mg to bring about considerable improvement.

Caution: High doses must always be used under the supervision of a doctor trained in nutritional medicine as, in a very few cases, they may actually worsen depression, reduce appetite and create nausea and gastrointestinal disturbances.

SMART DRUGS NOT SO SMART

Smart drugs are fascinating. Substances such as deprenyl, hydergine, vinpocetine, piracetam and other prescription drugs are now used to manipulate brain chemistry. In some countries, a few of them are legal. In most countries they are only available by prescription. My attitude to smart drugs in simple: First, since you can do so many effective things to improve brain functioning and counter degeneration without them, they seldom seem necessary. Second, they are not natural to the body, they are foreign chemicals. As such, your body does not have the metabolic ability to detoxify itself of them and therefore they can cause side-effects. Third, I believe if you are going to use them at all that you need to do so under the care of a physician who has much experience of their use for maximising brain health. There are too many potential side-effects.

10 STEPS TO A LEADING-EDGE BRAIN

1. **Go For Age Power Insulin Balance:** Forget high-carb-low-fat diets forever. Make sure you have plenty of good quality protein from fish, organic chicken and organic meat, eggs and soya as well as lots of phytonutrients from low-glycaemic, low-density carbohydrate vegetables such as broccoli, spinach, bok choy, fresh herbs and low-glycaemic fruits like berries and melons (see Chapter 14).

2. **Get Moving:** Physical exercise increases the circulation to your brain. Mental exercise helps create new synapse connections, protect you from the loss of brain cells and can even help you grow new ones.

3. **Manage Stress:** The number one enemy to brain health is stress, because of the effect of cortisol and other stress related compounds which actively destroy brain cells. Take up meditation. Use consciousness-enhancing quantum mind technology (see Chapter 26), give yourself plenty of time for relaxation. Above all, choose how you live your life in line with what you really want yourself, rather than living by someone else's rules.

4. **Steer Clear of Poisons:** Use organic food, avoid herbicides, pesticides, drugs and other compounds that can poison your body and stress your liver. Clear your home and workspace of chemical cleaners, air-fresheners and other products There are strong links between a build-up of these elements in the brain and the development of such diseases as Alzheimer's and Parkinson's.

5. **Get a Hair Analysis Every Five Years:** A simple hair analysis carried out in a medical laboratory can check for levels of heavy metals such as cadmium, aluminium and lead which build up to damage brain tissue. If you find that they are present, put yourself through a controlled detoxification programme.

6. **Keep Alcohol to a Minimum**: In any amount, alcohol damages brain tissue. If you are going to drink at all, make it infrequent and drink only the very best. Forget the plonk. Top quality wine is better than beer or distilled alcohol such as whisky.

7. **Look After Your Liver**: Support the health of your liver with periodic detoxification (see pages 107–8) supported by liver protective plants such as milk thistle and other supplements such as phosphatidylcholine. Damage to the liver invariably brings damage to the brain.

8. **Limit Coffee**: Steer clear of artificial stimulants such as coffee or any other compounds which over-stimulate the brain, including any kind of stimulating drugs. Like stress, they can cause potential damage to brain tissue taken over a long period of time.

9. **Steer Clear of Drugs**: Both prescription drugs, over-the-counter drugs and illegal drugs have side-effects that negatively undermine the health of the liver and the brain when taken over the long term. Stay away from them. Don't take drugs of any kind unless they are absolutely necessary for life. Experiment. See what one or more of the Space Age Brain Supporters can do for you.

DE-AGEING THE MATRIX

We have a genius for overlooking openings to extraordinary life.

Michael Murphy

The ineffable power of youth – too often lost with the passing of years, is regained through making changes in how you live, then needs to be carefully nurtured throughout the whole of your life. There is no better way to do this than Live Cell Therapy – 'the treatment of Kings'.

Cell therapy has long been considered the most controversial of all natural treatments for revitalising the body. The injection of fresh animal embryo cells into living organisms (even the injection of lyophilised preparations of animal cells) has long been outlawed in Britain and the United States where, for half a century, it has been the focus of hostility, both from powerful multi-national pharmaceutical companies and from the orthodox medical community who remain ignorant of its benefits.

It is no accident that Live Cell Therapy, known as LCT, has been called the therapy of Kings. This is a treatment in which carefully selected living embryonic cells are injected into a patient to rejuvenate the body. Popes and Emperors, the wealthy, the powerful and the gifted from the world of art and entertainment, all secretly avail themselves of this remarkable treatment. Those who take it regularly, every two or three years, claim that LCT not only slows degeneration and enhances immunity, it reverses premature ageing. Because of its powerful rejuvenating and regenerating properties, it is tempting to assume that LCT is a fountain of youth – a cure-all – which will restore youthful functioning to any body. This is not the case. Like all genuinely holistic treatments on which an Age Power approach is based, Live Cell Therapy needs to be used as part of an integrated multi-dimensional biological approach to high level health which includes regular detoxification, a diet high in fresh low-glycaemic fruits and vegetables, regular exercise and keeping alcohol to a minimum while eliminating drugs not essential to life.

> To me old age is always fifteen years older than I am.
>
> *Bernard Baruch*

ROYAL ROAD TO VITALITY

When your body is young, it has the ability easily to evolve, regenerate and adjust itself to stressors of all kinds. It can create and use energy efficiently. And, provided it is supplied with good nutrition, clean water and air, as well as a lifestyle which supports the highest level of your genetic expression – it will continue to thrive year after year. Cells in a youthful body resonate optimally on an energetic level within an electromagnetic semi-conductive matrix of connective tissue. All your cells, which are the physical building blocks of life itself, developed from one unified cell when you were but an embryo, thanks to the myriad processes of cell division. They continue throughout the whole of our lives to renew and replace themselves, provided the biological terrain in which they are held has good energy and balance. What happens as we grow older is that the ability of our cells to regenerate slows down. LCT addresses these issues with supreme skill.

When we are exposed to poor nutrition, processed sugar and alcohol, stress, heavy metals and artificial hormones in the environment, or bacteria, viruses and parasites, these things interfere with our ability to renew ourselves. They can disturb the perfect structure, form and function of DNA and undermine health. Our bodies develop toxicity. Our tissues become too acid. We experience a high level of oxidation damage from excessive free radicals and undergo destructive hormonal changes. This leads to gradual malfunction on a cellular, organ, hormonal and immune level. The tissue matrix itself is the most important fundamental biological level at which degeneration takes place, and it is at this level that the most profound regeneration and rejuvenation can be instigated. There is no better way to do this than Live Cell Therapy – the most controversial as well as the most potent natural treatment in the world for revitalising body and mind.

REVERSE THE RAVAGES

Live Cell Therapy is a form of non-toxic holistic medicine which aims to reverse the ravages of degeneration by the intra-muscular injection of healthy embryonic animal cells – usually the cells from a foetal lamb. It improves overall health, enhances immunity, increases vitality and counters both the physical and emotional effects of ageing. It has been shown to restore sexual potency, enhance healing, reverse Parkinson's disease as well as other age-related brain degenerative conditions in some people. The list of conditions and diseases that its proponents report cell therapy to have alleviated is so long it would be hard to cover them all. Here are a few:

- ❏ Adult Onset diabetes
- ❏ Hormonal imbalances including those associated with menopause
- ❏ Chronic brain diseases in children
- ❏ Depressive neuro-vegetative disorders and depressive moods
- ❏ Chronic liver disease
- ❏ Epilepsy
- ❏ Herpes
- ❏ Hardening of the arteries
- ❏ Skin problems
- ❏ Circulatory problems
- ❏ Chronic fatigue

Yet in one sense to speak specifically about the conditions which cell therapy can 'treat' is to misunderstand its very nature. Because properly selected and administered embryonic animal cells can restore more youthful function, structure and form at such a fundamental level as the tissue matrix itself. This treatment can help regenerate the whole being. It is important to look at LCT in this 'total person' way in order to understand the many gifts it has to offer.

YOUNG AND SAFE

Live Cell Therapy relies on a carefully chosen 'cocktail' of fresh embry-onic animal cells taken from specially prepared organ-specific tissues – the brain, the liver, the thyroid, the adrenals and so forth – being injected into the body. What makes such 'implants' valuable is the fact that cells from the unborn are *immunologically naïve*. Because they are in a primi-tive state of development, the human body does not yet recognise them as *antigens* – distinctive proteins identified as 'foreign' and then rejected by your body. This is why, unlike organs transplanted by surgery such as the kidneys or the heart, LCT injections rarely cause immune or allergic reactions. Therefore they pose no danger of being rejected.

The non-antigenic quality of embryo cells plays an important role in the development of the life of every mammal. For instance, each of us has a different blood group from our mother and a completely different tissue type. Yet, thanks to immunological naivety and to the protection offered by the placenta and the umbilical cord, a baby can live at peace in the body of its mother for nine months without being hurt by her immune reactions or harming her. So when embryo cells are injected into the human body, it accepts them.

SMEAR TACTICS

In the mid-sixties, a US Federal Court ordered the destruction of some small shipments of lyophilised cell products sent to New York by comp-anies in Germany and Switzerland. By 1984 the FDA had banned all importation of cellular powders and extracts intended for injection. In 1996, the FDA issued warnings against pills containing cellular extracts manufactured by a Mexican company who had been attempting to distribute them in the United States. Since the fifties, numerous warnings have been issued by 'official bodies'. LCT has been the focus of smear campaigns which have claimed that cases of serious illness from Guilliam-Barré syndrome, to blistering skin disease, have occurred as a result of it.

> By studying DNA, molec-ular biologists have verified that all living organisms are genetically related.
>
> *David Suzuki and Amanda McConnell*

> Middle age is when your age starts to show around your middle.
>
> *Bob Hope*

In the seventies an American Medical Association report in a consumer magazine alleged that two men, given injections of foetal sheep cells, died from gangrene. If you try to investigate the source of such assertions you discover ignorance, unfounded aggression and fear of natural methods from the industrial-medical complex, as well as an enormous volume of misinformation. Why?

WEBS OF PREJUDICE

Conventional drug-based medicine and the assumptions which lie behind it are based on a completely different approach to the treatment of the body than natural medicine. Orthodox medicine treats the symptoms of ageing or disease by giving artificially produced, often toxic drugs, based on the belief that disease is an externally caused phenomena, and the notion that any abnormality needs a 'magic-bullet' approach to banish it. Because the average doctor works with drugs, he must constantly evaluate the 'risk to benefit' relationship of whatever drug or combination of drugs he is using to alter the perceived symptom or disease state. Live Cell Therapy, like other natural holistic approaches, is designed to supply whatever enhances the body's energetic and biochemical terrain, allowing its own natural potentials for self-healing and vitality to emerge. By supplying non-human low antigenic foetal cellular components including DNA, RNA enzymes and other important components of the tissue matrix, LCT injections call on the ability of foetal cells to renew our biological functions. While drugs work *symptomatically*, not *causally*, and only for as long as we continue to take them, biological treatments, such as Live Cell Therapy, bring long-term results because they are capable of regenerating the life functions of an organ long term.

Most orthodox doctors remain without knowledge of LCT, its history and its methodology. They tend to speak of Live Cell Therapy as an 'unscientific treatment' for they remain ignorant of the several thousands of scientific publications that have carried papers written about it. They remain unaware that by now several millions of people have safely received this treatment in Europe, in centres carefully monitored by the Swiss, Russian and German governments.

One of the great ironies of the criticism levelled at Live Cell Therapy is that the orthodox medical profession in the English-speaking world often claims that LCT is no more than an expensive hoax used to pamper the spoilt and gullible. Yet in European clinics in recent years, within the halls of the same medical orthodoxy, variations on Live Cell Therapy, such as *stem cell therapy* and *foetal cell transplants* are on their way to becoming big businesses and demand huge government grants.

SECRETS OF STEM CELLS

In stem cell therapy immature cells from human embryos, stem cells – those which have not yet differentiated into specific types of cells – are being used experimentally to repair bone, cartilage, tendon and other injured or aged tissues, as well as to treat many other conditions from Parkinson's and Alzheimer's disease to humanity's most devastating degenerative illnesses. The problem is, to obtain these little 'magic nuts and bolts' of human tissues, they have to destroy the embryos. Here's how it works: A human egg is fertilised or cloned to form an embryo. Then the embryo is allowed to divide again and again. Within a few days, the embryo takes the shape of a spear, called a *blastocyst*. Within a week or two, embryonic *stem cells* begin to be visible. At this point, these cells are capable of turning into any tissue in the body. The stem cells are then removed from the embryo and grown in a Petrie dish. As they divide, they create a whole line of stem cells. By feeding them various nutrients and other factors in the laboratory, scientists attempt to turn stem cells into any of the body's more than 200 tissues, for instance to make islets of Langerhans cells for the regeneration of the pancreas. This, researchers hope, may provide a cure for diabetes. Other scientists are attempting to turn stem cells into nerve cells, which they hope may be useful in the treatment of Alzheimer's and Parkinson's disease. Still others are using them in the hope of repairing spinal cord injuries, or turning them into muscle cells which they think could repair or replace a damaged heart.

BRAVE NEW WORLDS

Each of the ways used to get human embryos presents its own ethical challenges. The most acceptable way to the majority of people is to use embryos left over from fertility treatments. Fertility technicians routinely fuse more than one egg with sperm so that if implanting a fertilised egg doesn't work first time round, they can have another go at creating a pregnancy. The second source is through aborted foetuses. John Gearhart, the Johns Hopkins biologist who is one of two men credited with first culturing stem cells, takes his cells from foetuses donated by women at a nearby abortion clinic. The third option is cloning. A few companies in the United States such as Advanced Cell Technology of Worcester, Massachusetts, acknowledge that they have not only been trying to create cloned human embryos, a few have now succeeded. These rudimentary cloned human beings are euphemistically referred to as 'entities'. At places such as the Jones Institute in Virginia in the United States, where the first test-tube baby was conceived, sperms and eggs are mixed with the express purpose of creating embryos as stem cells donors. All of these methods are accompanied by high-sounding polemics about how necessary all this is to find cures for suffering human beings. In the meantime, the surrounding questionable ethics in such practices burgeon.

STEM CELLS VS LCT

Those doctors and scientists who are knowledgeable both about the leading-edge research into human stem cell and foetal cell therapy, as well as Live Cell Therapy which uses animal embryos instead – most often lamb cells – generally agree that, quite apart from moral considerations, the dangers of harvesting human embryonic cells for any of these treatments, far outweigh those attributed to the use of properly administered animal foetal cells. Among numerous cautions that are being issued about the use of human stem cells are warnings they may transmit AIDS. What surprises me about all this is that within the rapidly burgeoning human stem cell and human foetal cell transplant scientific community, there is virtually no recognition of an important truth – one which European doctors working with LCT have known for almost a century: Thanks to the biological closeness of all mammal tissue and the immunilogically naïve characteristics of all embryo tissue, cells from *any* mammalian embryo – human, rabbit, sheep – will do equally well in bringing about regeneration of structure, function and form when administered to the human body. Will the two camps ever get together? One can only hope. However, because the basic paradigms from which they operate are so diametrically opposed to each other, and because stem cell treatments are becoming big business, I suspect it is not likely.

You do not have to face the truth if you hire a belief system to do it in your place.

Ken Carey

CHALK AND CHEESE

Allopathic medicine works superbly in treating an emergency or an acute problem – anything from trauma and broken bones to acute inflammation or infection and by stemming rapid tissue failure. Live Cell Therapy, by contrast, is much more appropriate for alleviating long-term diminished functioning. Like many natural anti-ageing therapies, LCT is far more appropriate than most orthodox medical procedures in the treatment of chronic degenerative diseases, immune incompetence, premature ageing, chronic allergies and endocrine dysfunctions. Neither approach can guarantee any miraculous cures or absolute successes, but when applied with wisdom and confidence, each has something valuable to offer.

LIKE HEALS LIKE

Live Cell Therapy is a natural extension of one of the oldest natural treatments in the world. It is part of a whole tradition of natural medicine – a way of thinking about health and healing that works. As far back as 1600BC, Egyptian hieroglyphics recommended the use of animal organs to improve human vitality. In 360BC Aristotle spoke of the value of live healing preparations taken from animal or human origins. In the Middle Ages, the Swiss philosopher and physician Paraselsus, who first pointed out that the cell is the unit of organisation for all life, observed that 'like heals like'. He said 'the heart heals the heart, the kidney heals the kidney'. This is exactly what happens in cell therapy treatment. Cells from an animal foetal liver are used to enhance the functioning of an ailing human liver. Cells from an unborn animal spleen are given as a treatment for a troubled human spleen.

> The human organism is not a helpless, defenceless victim attacked at every turn by agents of disease, whether germs or stressors. We resist breakdown and disease through a remarkable internal health maintenance system regulated by the brain.
>
> *Robert Ornstein, PhD and David Sobel, MD*

EMBRYONIC POWER

In 1912, at the Rockefeller Institute in New York, a brilliant French physiologist and Nobel Laureate, Alexis Carrel, initiated a world famous anti-ageing study using fibroblast cells – connective tissue cells – from a chicken embryo. These are widely distributed throughout an organism. His experiment was instrumental both in forming scientific opinion about the ageing process for more than half a century and also in initiating modern cell therapy. Carrel grew his cell structure in a glass vessel, nourishing it with a crude *embryo* extract. To the amazement of the scientific community his living cells outlived even Carrel himself. They went on multiplying for more than thirty years – keeping alive fragments of a chicken heart a quarter of a century after the chicken itself had died. Some scientists believe that Carrel had shown that living cells are apparently immortal. Others insisted that these cells were kept alive only as a result of being fed the embryonic serum. Their hypothesis triggered a vast number of research projects in search of the 'natural youth serum' – the elixir of life.

NEW AGE BEGINS

The man considered the father of modern cell therapy is Swiss surgeon Paul Niehans. Niehans became interested in endocrinology while he was head of staff at a renowned hospital in Switzerland. At that time, some of his colleagues were experimenting with animal gland implants into their patients whose organs had malfunctioned. But many of these attempts failed. Niehans discovered that he could imbed fine slivers of organic tissue into a patient's muscle pockets and get the results they were after. Gradually he developed an even better method: Injecting cell suspensions of specific animal organs, glands and tissues into the buttocks of his patients using large hypodermic needles.

The first injection Niehans gave was in 1931 to a woman suffering from severe convulsions. She had been transferred to his care following an unsuccessful operation on her thyroid gland. The Swiss surgeon ground up the para-thyroid gland of a newborn ox into very tiny pieces, put them into suspension using a saline solution and injected them

> Oh, to be seventy again!
> *James Oliver Wendell Jr,*
> *at the age of 86, on*
> *seeing a pretty girl*

into his patient's body. He assumed that the beneficial effects, if any, would be short lived, just like an effective hormone, and that he would have to repeat the injection. 'But to my great surprise the injection of fresh cells not only failed to provoke an immune response, but the effect lasted longer than any synthetic hormone, any implant, or any surgical graft,' Niehans reported. His patient was still free of cramps in 1956. Niehans had recognised, long before any understanding of immune reactions was present in the scientific community, that foetal cells are more easily tolerated by a patient and also have a far more powerful therapeutic effect than any other kind of living tissues. From then on he began to work not only with glands – which was customary in endocrinology, his speciality – but other types of tissues too: Heart, liver, brain etc. Niehans was also the first to use different types of cells from unborn donor animals together.

CHARISMATIC AND OPINIONATED

An eccentric outspoken and opinioned man, Niehans fought hard – and some say not always honestly – with anyone opposing him. Niehans and his practices became a locus of controversy. This fact, coupled with the *unorthodox* – that is the non-drug nature – of the treatment he developed – gave both the doctor and Live Cell Therapy itself a controversial image. Yet Niehans applied his discoveries to over 50,000 people with major success. They included the great celebrities of the time from Charles de Gaulle, Joan Crawford, Somerset Maugham and Charlie Chaplin to Dwight and Mimi Eisenhower, Winston Churchill and the Duke and Duchess of Windsor, as well as Noel Coward, Joseph Kennedy and Picasso. Niehans continued his research and his work well into the Sixties. He was even summoned to the Vatican by Pope Pious XII to inject fresh cells into the critically ailing man. The Holy Father continued to take Live Cell Therapy for another four years, insisting that the Swiss doctor had saved his life. He even went so far as to admit Professor Niehans to a membership in the Papal Academy of Sciences.

Unfortunately for the English-speaking world most of Niehan's work was only published in Germany. It was not until 1967 that an English version of his original book, *Cell Research and Cellular Therapy*, became available from a Swiss publisher. In the forty-odd years since his death, more than five million cell therapy treatments have been given in West Germany alone.

PROOF OF THE PUDDING

Cell therapy is often challenged on the grounds that there is no evidence it has any beneficial effect on the body. Yet, since the early fifties, literally thousands of experiments and clinical reports have been published about it – half of them from University-based scientists in European medical communities. Most are not available in English and therefore remain outside the access of the British and American scientific community. These reports not only support the contention that cell therapy can be a highly effective treatment for a wide variety of illnesses and degenerative conditions, they also indicate that European scientists have a considerable understanding of how cell injections bring their remarkable benefits to the human body. This is something which doctors involved in human-based foetal cell transplants and stem cell therapy admit they are still at a loss to explain – probably because they are still imprisoned by the materialistic medical paradigm, inherited from Newtonian physics, that largely ignores the energetic nature of living systems.

Cell therapy consists of several injections made all at once. The injections are made up of cells and tissues from animal embryos, which have been carefully chosen to meet the individual needs of the patient. These are determined by the doctor giving the treatment from the results of blood and urine tests, as well as electrocardiograms and other standard medical assessments, as well as the case history of the patient.

LIFE ENERGY COCKTAIL

The LCT doctor chooses cells from many different foetal tissues. They range from cartilage, connective tissue, lung and bronchial to eye, para-thyroid, pituitary, spleen, ovaries or testes, muscle and thymus. There are nearly 40 different possibilities in all. Once a patient's *cell cocktail* has been prepared from freshly sacrificed foetal lamb tissue, it is immediately injected into the muscle. The patient is required to spend a day or two in bed so that the biological actions initiated by the fresh cells can do their work. Almost immediately on receipt of vital embryonic cells, the body begins to respond. Cell therapists, as far back as Niehans himself, have always believed that cells from each specific tissue migrate to the site of that particular tissue in the human body injected with them and settle there. It is a belief still highly criticised by the orthodox medical community who pooh pooh the idea as nonsensical.

BLIND IRONY

One of the ironies which surrounds the ignorance among the medical orthodoxy about using foetal cells from one species to treat another is that they don't seem aware that Live Cell Therapy has been working successfully for decades without human embryos. The results of recent research projects show that organ-specific foetal cells from one animal can be used to heal another, and that metabolic chemicals from organ-specific cells of the donor animal do indeed make their way to the targeted organ just as LCT practitioners have always said they do. Researchers at such prestigious institutions as New York Medical College, Cornell University and Henry Ford Hospital in the US discovered that:

❑ Old rats performed better on a test of memory and learning after scientists injected brain cells from aborted human foetuses. The injected cells were able to travel to the damaged area in the brain and produce substances there to enhance healing.

❑ Bone marrow cells grown from human embryonic tissue, marked with a green fluorescent protein so scientists could trace where they went, were injected into mice with artificially induced heart attacks and within nine days settled into the rodent hearts and restored heart functions.

❑ Human stem cells isolated from bone marrow were injected into rats with artificially caused heart attacks. They rebuilt the damaged heart enabling the rats to build new capillaries and tissues and to restore functions.

Why, one wonders, are not the same scientists carrying out similar experiments using animals cells to restore human functions?

HOMING CELLS

In the 1970s at the University of Heidelberg, Doctors H. Lettré and F. Schmidt showed that this does indeed occur. Using radioactive markers they traced the material from animal foetal cells injected into humans and discovered that they do indeed end up in the target organ: thymus to thymus, spleen to spleen. Their research was landmark. Yet it is still largely ignored. It did however do much to prove that embryonic animal cellular material is indeed transported by the human host to counterpart organs and tissues, just as LCT doctors have always claimed.

The mechanism by which this cellular homing and recognition takes place appears to be dependant on the host's *microphages* and *macrophages* (white blood cells) carrying growth factor fractions from the donor. This mechanism is unlikely ever to be explained in biochemical terms alone. It probably has to do with the unique energy frequencies – often known as *tensegriti* – emitted by the DNA coils and membrane fibre optics in living cells, which was described as far back as the 1920s by scientists Tesla and Lakhovsky. It seems that in all living organisms, like seeks a resonance with like. Cells probably tend to congregate, due not so much to chemical or mechanical binding sites, but rather to vibrational signals.

HOLOGRAPHIC BODY

All vibrations react and interact with other vibrations throughout the universe. For the universe appears to be organised in a holographic way and all beings are part of that hologram. Looked at from such a leading-edge point of view, it is likely that, when injected, embryonic live cells do not traverse the body in a random way looking for binding sites. They are much more likely to home in on each other much as an aeroplane does to a radio beacon. What appears to happen in the living body injected with embryonic cells is that human microphages – white blood cells – migrate to the site of the injection. There they link up with particles from the implanted cells and break them down into smaller particles. The whole process of breakdown takes as little as twenty-four hours. By that time the embryo cells have been absorbed by these microphages which are in turn engulfed by enlarged white blood cells – the macrophages. By now the patient's macrophages hold the foetal DNA which resonates at the same frequency as the host's own target cells.

Live Cell Therapy adds powerful resonant themes to enhance ageing or sickly tissue and to help re-establish a harmonious vibrational order within the symphony of the body. Live Cell Therapy appears to be following the most basic laws of biophysics, although few are, as yet, aware of it. The biologic materials from the break-down embryo cells are rapidly distributed throughout the body in an exponentially declining curve. The main energetic activity appears to take place about forty-eight hours after the first injection. Laboratory investigations indicate that the degree of absorption of substances from a particular organ or tissue in the body is directly related to the need of that organ or tissue for regeneration.

> To return to the root is to find the meaning, but to pursue appearances is to miss the source.
>
> *Zen Patriarch, Sengtsan,*
> *sixth-century poor*
> *hermit monk*

BETTER AND BETTER

Over half of patients given the treatment report they feel
better within the first two weeks. Live cells stimulate repair
processes in different organs at different speeds, depending
upon how rapidly specific organs or tissues renew themselves.
Despite the rapid assimilation of embryo cell material, it can
be months before the person receiving cell therapy experiences full benefits. This is because cell therapy, unlike drug
treatments or the artificial stimulation which comes with using
specific hormones, works *biologically* – at the speed of nature.

When improvement comes – in seven out of 10 people – it is often dramatic.
The conditions for which cell therapy has a good reputation include many
disorders for which stem cell and foetal cell transplants are currently being
tried: Down's syndrome, brain damage in early childhood, constitutional
sicknesses and diseases of the immune system such as anti-body deficiency syndromes as well as blood ailments including sickle cell anaemia.
LCT also works remarkably well in the treatment of skin diseases, neurological disorders including the early stages of Parkinson's disease, and for
infertility, endocrine imbalances and circulatory disorders. Where clinical
reports in cell therapy are most abundant and most glowing are its ability
to counter age-dependent weakness: restoring loss of sexual function, revitalising the body, banishing aches and pains and bringing a higher level
of vitality to the whole organism.

On a biochemical level, German Professor Franz Schmidt, renowned
throughout the world for his treatment of children with cell therapy, points
out that foetal tissue contains a high concentration of biochemical
substances such as peptides, enzymes and their substrates, designed to
bring about high growth rate of foetal structures. These substances, he
believes, when injected into the body, can be absorbed by it and made
use of in whatever way it needs to enhance its own living processes. In
effect they heighten cell aliveness and when you heighten aliveness in
such a way, you ultimately improve the condition of the whole organism.

DEEPEST IRONY

In the 1908s as Western orthodoxy began to *legitimise* foetal cell therapy,
in other words to find some inroad that would make it acceptable within
the orthodox medical paradigm, Doctor Michael Osband reported in the

New England Journal of Medicine that in 1981, 10 out of 17 children treated for an immuno-suppressive condition called histiocytosis, experienced complete remission after being treated with daily intra-muscular injections of thymus extract taken from five-day-old calves. This was the first reported use of a crude form of animal Live Cell Therapy under controlled conditions carried out within the United States.

In 1983 the American Paralysis Association Convention was presented evidence that cells from aborted human foetuses, when injected into animals, proved useful in the repair of spinal cord accidents and degenerative diseases. Later on in the eighties Doctor Kevin Lafferty at the University of Colorado Medical Centre reported 'good results' in 16 out of 17 diabetic patients who were treated with 'implanted cells' from foetal pancreases. At the time of the Chernobyl disaster, foetal cell transplants hit the headlines when Robert Gale from the University of California went to the Soviet Union to implant liver cells from aborted human foetuses into some of the victims. It was Gale's hope that these cells would multiply and supplant the bone marrow by restoring the victim's ability to produce blood cells destroyed through radiation exposure. Sadly, his patients died from their burns before the results of therapy could be assessed.

THE BEST IS YET TO COME

We will probably never know the complete answer to how foetal cells from either the same or another species work their wonders when injected into a body. What does seem apparent is that genetic information is transferred both energetically and chemically to the host cells, yet not incorporated into the genes of the host's cells so it cannot be transmitted to an offspring. Some believe it is the incompatibility of sequence addresses at either end of an animal gene, which allows utilisation in the human cell, but prevents familial genetic effects.

To know consists in
opening out a way
Whence the imprisoned
splendour may escape.
Robert Browning

On a biochemical level, one of the factors from embryo tissues which appears to be particularly important in bringing about enhancement of energy, is the presence of specific growth factors which are found in high concentrations in embryos. When embryo tissue is introduced to the body, these growth factors stimulate the body's repair mechanisms, both at a cellular level and throughout the immune system, resulting in a total revitalisation of the organism.

PATIENT REPORTS

According to Dr Claus Martin, director of the Institute for Live Cell Therapy in Rottach-Egern, Germany – the most experienced practitioner in LCT in the world today – 'Live Cell Therapy is so far our only available form of molecular bio-engineering therapy. That is why it is probably the best way to stay young longer and healthier'. In one study, Martin and his associates compared the complaints and the state of patients' health before and six months after treatment, looking at more than 370 participants. The results showed more than eighty percent of patients valued the therapy both as a method for alleviating their complaints and improving health.

PERSONAL ODYSSEY

A highly trained surgeon from an orthodox background, Martin came to look at cell therapy only as a result of a family health problem for which he could find no solution. His oldest son, Patrick, had developed Perthe's disease – a kind of degeneration of the hipbone in which the centre of bone growth breaks up and the bone doesn't develop. This results in the child living in constant pain. In Patrick's case it was so bad that he could no longer walk. Martin consulted all the top specialists in the world. They insisted that his son needed a complex operation in which the hipbone is cut and turned around. This would mean the child remained in a cast for two months. And afterwards, according to other parents who allowed the operation on their children, there was likelihood that he would suffer great pain and remain crippled for the rest of his life. Martin had heard about Schmidt's work with children using cell therapy in Aschaffenberg. He contacted Schmidt to find that he had treated 10 children with Perthe's disease with good results. So he decided to give it a try. He administered the embryo tissue himself and, to his amazement, in two months Patrick began to walk again. Within a year x-rays showed that the hip joints were completely normal.

> The real voyage of discovery consists not in seeking new landscapes, but in having new eyes.
>
> *Marcel Proust*

That was many years ago. Patrick is now a tall, handsome, athletic, perfectly normal adult. Martin took this experience as an indication that he should pursue cell therapy as a career. This he has done, and has established what is widely accepted as the best clinic in the world for LCT.

LIVE CELLS BEST

Cell therapy comes in three different forms: fresh cells taken from live embryos and injected almost immediately, deep frozen cells, and lyophilised or freeze-dried cells purchased from pharmaceutical houses. The potency of the treatment in terms of its healing and regenerative capacities depends both on which form is given and on the medical wisdom of the person giving it. Live cells from lamb embryos are best, with deep frozen next and lyophilised last.

Martin's carefully selected clients – and I have interviewed many between the ages of 30 and 95 – undergo a standard battery of medical tests in order to determine which cocktail of tissues is to be administered to them. The protocols at the clinic are of the highest order, yet the atmosphere is relaxed and friendly. The reports of success from those who continue to return either annually or biennially for ongoing anti-ageing support are excellent. It is an interesting experience to spend time with men and women who continue to avail themselves of this remarkable natural treatment on a regular basis. You meet people in their 80s and 90s who have the vitality of those of 25 with sharp brains, a wonderful sense of humour and a dynamism that puts most of us to shame.

NO CURE-ALL

It is important to look upon cell therapy as part of an integrated multi-dimensional approach to anti-ageing. There is no question that people who receive the greatest benefits from Live Cell Therapy treatment are those who, in between treatments, take good care of their own bodies, supporting their health and well-being with excellent diet, anti-oxidant nutrients and who steer clear of destructive excess. Few of the people I interviewed – even people past the age of 70 – are on any form of long-term drug therapy. When I asked one gentleman why this was the case, he laughed out loud and said 'Who needs it?'

There are very few clinics that carry out Live Cell Therapy. Most of what is *called* Live Cell Therapy in fact uses lyophilised cells which by no means offers the range of therapeutic and life-enhancing benefits that do fresh live cells.

Recently, as a result of reports of allergic reactions to injections of lyophilised and frozen cells by untrained practitioners, authorities in West Germany forced a halt to the selling of commercially manufactured cell therapy preparations. Around their actions there has been much controversy and speculation. There have even been suggestions that pressures from pharmaceutical companies are behind such changes, since, in reality, reports of allergic reactions, even to manufactured preparations for cell therapy, are very few and far between. In any case, as of now, this splendid biological therapy of kings is only available at a handful of clinics throughout the world, and then only in its original – and best as it happens – form: Fresh cells from live-embryos. To me it is sad to think that a biological treatment of such value continues to be available only to those fortunate enough to know about it and well off enough to afford it.

Thanks to new research into stem cells and foetal cell transplant, there is a growing interest in biological alternatives to drug treatments. As a result of growing moral concerns over using human foetal material in any kind of treatment, in the next few years a renaissance may well take place. The treatment of kings just might, for the first time in its history, be properly honoured by the scientific community for its power. Hopefully this is a first step. For in a world in which degenerative diseases – for which we have no effective treatments in the orthodox repertoire of drug therapies – have reached epidemic proportions, we cannot afford to ignore the clinical experience of physicians skilled in the use of Live Cell Therapy for restoring harmony and balance to the person as a whole. Past the age of 40, if there is one therapy that I hold to be valuable above all else, it is this.

LIFE BREAKS THE RULES

'God is dead' – Nietzsche, 1886
'Nietzsche is dead' – God, 1900

Bumper Sticker

Now we come to the exciting stuff – energy. This is where life breaks all the rules. Biological science is just beginning to penetrate the mysteries of life energies. Until now, energy has remained the province of mystics, sages and leading-edge physicists. But when it comes to rejuvenating your body, energy is where it's at.

You may find some of this very unfamiliar. We are at the leading edge of science here, entering unknown territory. Successful rejuvenation depends on activating energies which support the life force from within. That's what all the tools and techniques of Age Power – from brisk walks and low-glycaemic carbs and extra Coenzyme-A to special forms of body work and meditation – can help you do. It is this life force which governs growth, nourishes us, sustains us, deep cleanses our bodies, regenerates our cells, heals us and makes us feel happy just to be alive. This ineffable life force is found in abundance in each of us as it is in all living things from bananas to hedgehogs. Different cultures call it by different names. The Indians speak of it as *Prana*. In Polynesia it is known as *Mana*. The Chinese call it *Qi*. These words describe various forms of subtle energy, which until the advent of quantum physics, remained unknown to Western science. Yet throughout history all forms of traditional medicine from Paracelsus to Chinese and Ayurvedic herbalism have worked with it. It is important to get the hang of how energy of all kinds can be used to enhance your own experience of living with age power.

BIOPHOTONS AND QUANTUM MAGIC

The eminent scientist Albert Szent-Györgyi, who won a Nobel prize for his work on oxidation and for isolating vitamin C, asked himself a question more than fifty years ago. He has spent almost every working moment of his life since in an attempt to answer it. He is often quoted as having posed the question at a dinner party: 'What is the difference between a living rat and a dead one?' According to the laws of classical chemistry and physics, there should be no fundamental difference. Szent-Györgyi's own reply is simple yet revolutionary – 'Some kind of electricity.'

Early in the twentieth century quantum physics established that wave particles in living systems behave as biophoton energies. These energies regulate and control enzyme activities, cell reproduction and the creation of vitality in living systems. Experiments, such as those reported in the March 1995 issue of *Scientific American* by Brumer and Shapiro, have helped establish the importance of particle/wave reactions in organisms. Like light bulbs, all atoms and molecules give out radiant bioenergies, both good and bad, when it comes to their effect on the human body. Science is beginning to understand how the interference wave forms from negative sources – generated either by internally manufactured toxins or by external exposure to environmental pollutants – can disrupt the body's harmonious biophoton energies and undermine homeostasis on which our health and protection from premature ageing depend.

There is currently much investigation taking place to determine how we can use various kinds of bioenergies constructively to support health and slow degeneration. Some of this is considered 'hard science' from electromagnetic techniques now used to rejuvenate bone and tissues to electronic diagnostic devices for diagnosing disease. Some of it is still considered 'alternative' by mainstream science – the use of visualisation for instance, spiritual healing as well as energy-based martial arts like Aikido or even Tai Chi. Within the next few decades we are going to hear a lot more about these biophoton energies and their effects on our health. For now, we can still make practical use of what knowledge has already emerged about how to influence the body on an energetic level for healing and regeneration.

ENERGY OF CONSCIOUSNESS

From the point of view of quantum physics, as human beings we are not only immersed in an energy field, our bodies, our minds, our selves *are* energy fields. These fields are constantly contracting and expanding as our thoughts, diet and lifestyle change. The aim of any form of natural treatment, from dietary change or detoxification to hydrotherapy, exercise and meditation, is to enhance positive bio-energies in an organism and to create greater order in your body, biochemically, psychologically and spiritually.

Man can learn nothing except by going from the known to the unknown.
Claude Bernard

PART TRUTHS

The biochemical view of ageing which we have mostly been looking at is based on the assumption that life can be entirely explained by an understanding of the laws of chemistry and physiology. It looks at the way that inorganic chemicals act and interact in a biological system to perpetuate the living state. Indeed, this is the whole point and purpose of biochemistry and molecular biology – the major scientific models involved in most of what is known about ageing. The only problem is that the living human body breaks all the rules.

To get full benefit from what is now known about life processes and age-retardation we must make good use of the biochemical model of ageing, but we also need to go beyond it. How? First by asking a few provocative – and largely unanswerable – questions like, 'What is the nature of life energy anyway?' And, 'How can we preserve it?' Second we need to take a look at theoretical models at the leading edge of science which can be applied to the ageing process. They include models built on the New Physics and on *information theory* as applied to biology. These new scientific paradigms not only bring a broader understanding of the ageing process, they also point the way to a more comprehensive and effective approach to Age Power. It involves both our response to radiation and electromagnetic influences in our environment, and the role that how we think and feel plays in in how rapidly or slowly we age.

By the end of the third decade of the twentieth century, virtually every major postulate of the earlier scientific conception had been controverted: the atom as solid, indestructible and separate building block of nature, space and time as independent absolutes, the strict mechanistic causality of all phenomena, the possibility of the objective observation of nature. Such fundamental transformation in the scientific world picture was staggering, and for no one was this more true than the physicists themselves.

Richard Tarnas

BREAK THE RULES

In physics, the first and second laws of thermodynamics focus on the nature of energy in the universe. These laws are an attempt to understand events in the universe by studying the kind of energy changes which accompany them. The *second law of thermodynamics* is particularly important in relation to ageing. It is called the law of *entropy*. It states simply that, left to their own devices, things in the universe become disordered: Iron rusts, buildings crumble, dead flowers decay, humans lose homeostasis, degenerate and eventually die. This is described in scientific language by saying that everything tends toward *maximum* entropy. Entropy describes a state of maximum disorder – chaos if you prefer – in which all useful energy has been decreased.

ORDER FROM CHAOS

What is so remarkable about a living human being – and what has been a great puzzle to some of the world's finest scientific minds – is this: Despite the second law of thermodynamics, we, like other living organisms, are able to remain highly ordered. In fact, so long as we remain alive our bodies are maintained in a condition of fantastic improbability despite the endless destructive processes continually going on in and around us. More than that, there is every indication that a healthy body – a healthy mind as well – regardless of age, is continually involved in creating yet more order. This we do both individually, thanks to the repair functions of our cells and enzymic systems, as well as from an evolutionary point of view since, with time, living species differentiate into ever more complex and highly structured organisms.

NEGENTROPIC WONDERS

Unlike the rocks and nails in the inorganic world, living organisms are capable of both becoming and of remaining superbly ordered through their capacity for recreating homeostasis and wholeness. This is how we maintain our bodies at a high degree of health. This 'ordering ability' makes no sense within the paradigms of Newtonian physics: There should be little difference in the chemical and physical processes taking place in a living body and those of a corpse – since both follow the same scientific laws. Yet there is every difference in the world. In life, events are able to maintain the system in quite exceptional harmony (in scientific terms a high degree of negative entropy or *negentropy*) despite the fact that events leading to maximum entropy in the universe as a whole should destroy it.

The stupendous juggling act that is cell life depends on a continuous supply of energy: without it the cell literally falls apart. Without energy the molecules, meant to be outside the cell, cannot be prevented from coming in, and those meant to be inside cannot be stopped from leaking out.

Guy Brown

LIFE'S PARADOX

In the words of Nobel laureate Albert Szent-Györgyi: 'Life is a paradox... the most basic rule of inanimate nature is that it tends toward equilibrium which is at the maximum of entropy and the minimum of free energy. The main characteristic of life is that it tends to decrease its entropy. It also tends to increase its free energy. Maximum entropy means complete randomness, disorder. Life is made possible by order, structure, a pattern which is the opposite of entropy. This pattern is our chief possession, it was developed over billions of years. The main aim of our existence is its conservation and transmission. Life is a revolt against the statistical rules of physics. Death means that the revolt subsided and statistical laws resumed their sway.'

From an energetic point of view, ageing is the process which transports your body from a youthful, highly ordered, homeostatic state towards maximum entropy – illness, degeneration and death. To protect your body from this destructive process we need to give it all the help we can to support our natural capacity for order on an energetic level. An effective anti-ageing programme needs to take negentrophic energy into account.

SUCK ORDER

Physicist and Nobel laureate Erwin Schrodinger took a close look at the scientific contradictions implicit in the living state and concluded that so long as the human body is alive, it avoids decaying into an inert state of equilibrium – death – through metabolism. In other words by eating, drinking and assimilating information, it *sucks order* from the environment. As far back as 1944 Schrodinger wrote: Every process, event, happening – call it what you will; in a word, everything that is going on in Nature means an increase of the entropy of the part of the world where it is going on. Thus a living organism continually increases its entropy – or as you may say, produces positive entropy – and thus tends to approach the dangerous state of maximum entropy, which is death. It can only keep aloof from it, i.e. alive, by continually drawing from its environment negative entropy . . . What an organism feeds upon is negative entropy . . . which is in itself a measure of order. *Thus the device by which an organism maintains itself stationary at a fairly high level of orderliness really consists in continually sucking orderliness from its environment.'*

Energetically, a human being is described as an *open system*. It continually exchanges energy with its environment – through the foods we eat, digest, assimilate and excrete, as well as the company we keep, ongoing radiation and electromagnetic fields we are exposed to, the way we exercise – even the thoughts we think. As such we are constantly processing *information* which comes to us and flows from us. We need a constant supply of the right kind of information from the outside world to keep our bodies functioning optimally, and we need to be able to dissipate any disorder and chaos – entropy – that has built up within our bodies and our lives.

Although most biochemists and all physicists know about Schrodinger's concept of living organisms feeding on negative entropy and it is covered in standard textbooks on biophysics and biochemistry, it is still largely ignored by most age researchers. Eminent scientific thinkers like Ludwig von Bertalanffy, author of *Robots, Men and Minds*, British scientist and philosopher Michael Polanyi and the Soviet biochemist I. I. Brekhman from the Far East Scientific Centre of the Academy of Sciences of the USSR, Vladivostok, are among a growing number who take it very seriously indeed.

THE OSTRICH SYNDROME

Life processes which cannot be explained within a particular scientific discipline have a long history either of being ignored or misinterpreted. It is often easier to bury your head in the sand. Yet these unanswered questions are central to an understanding of the ageing process. For when control processes go awry, disorder invades the organism and degeneration ensues. They are also biology's most intriguing problems and therefore make many biochemists very uncomfortable indeed, simply because they are unanswerable in biochemical terms. Where can we find the answers? Or at the very least, where should we be looking?

INFORMATION BREEDS ORDER

Brekhman refers to energy exchange in relation to his main interests: Food and natural medicines such as ginseng and Siberian ginseng, with a long history of use, which scientific research has shown to have non-specific abilities to strengthen an organism's vitality. Brekhman and his team have shown that the heating and processing of foods which we carry out can decrease the quality of structural information that they bring to an organism and thus their health-supporting and age-retarding properties. Fresh foods carry a higher degree of the structural information which your body can beneficially use, than do cooked or processed foods.

They discovered that foods high in 'structural information' enable animals to carry out physical tasks for significantly longer periods than processed foods low in structural information even when the foods compared are equal in calories and therefore, by orthodox biochemical standards, supplying an organism with the same amount of energy. They have even developed a means of measuring the structural information a particular food or herb carries in what they call 'significant units of action'. To retard the process of ageing and degeneration, then, both the quantity and quality of this information must be as close to the ideal needs of our organism as possible. In Schrodinger's words it needs to supply a high degree of orderliness.

These new paradigms have important implications when it comes to the nutritional control of the rate at which our body ages. They make it clear that slowing down the ageing process demands more than swallowing megadoses of vitamins, minerals and ordinary nutraceuticals to support to your body's anti-oxidant and immune systems. They imply that it is necessary to approach the whole question of food not only from the point of view of energy (calories) and materials (specific proteins, vitamins, minerals, fatty acids, etc) alone. And they are stimulating researchers to explore how nutrition for age-retardation is dependent on the complexity of the way all of this energy and material is woven together by nature.

> Many of the reasons for problems at the chemical level have to do with lifestyle choices that the whole person makes and lives out. Even the choice between a positive or negative attitude about life sets up a set of chemical alterations in the brain that affect the whole body . . . Restoration of the body's health (wholeness) begins with an understanding that supplying the body with 'good things' is foundational to becoming this whole person.
>
> *James F Balch MD*

NEW ENERGY PARADIGMS

In the 1960s the Polish priest and biophysicist Wlodzimierz Sedlac wrote prolifically describing biological structure in energetic ways. His work set an energy revolution in motion which, I believe, will eventually topple the chemical and mechanical paradigms which too rigidly still define human health. He described cells as *diode resonators*. Mitochondria work as *intracellular interferometers* and *inductance emission coils*. Cell membranes can be considered *photon resonators*. In Germany, the brilliant physicist Fritz Popp showed that when stimulated by a laser emission from the mitochondria, DNA emits far more UV light. In fact our cells give off powerful light energy. When they are dividing or dying they also emit UV light radiation. It is the *coherence* between UV light and electromagnetic organisation which appears to give each cell its ability to vibrate at specific frequencies. Cells behave much like radiotransmitters, enabling them to communicate within the superconducting semi-solid plasma of the body's liquid crystal matrix – the *mesenchyme*.

Doctors and scientists working with natural treatments have claimed for over 150 years that the mesenchyme is the seedbed of health and youth. Look after the state of the mesenchyme – your body's biological terrain – and the rest of the body will look after itself. Mathematics, biophysics and wave mechanics are beginning to describe biological systems as kinetic, electrical, magnetic, gravitational and mass energies – all of which fit into the cohesive field theory of universal energy at the leading-edge of modern physics. They also help us to understand some of what enhances negentropy and its ability to preserve health and what can undermine it from an energetic point of view.

GOOD VIBRATIONS

The right kind of food is not by any means the only kind of carrier of energetic as well as chemical information which is necessary to support the needs of the body for Age Power. We also need stimulation to the nervous system from changing environmental conditions, from pure water we can drink and clean air we can breathe. Even the effects of body movement are energetic in their implications. All of these things act as stimuli to an organism. In terms of ageing, their effects can either be either good or bad.

We need to make use of everything possible to ensure they are good. This is something which advocates of natural medicine have been doing for generations in two main ways. First by applying stimuli to enhance bodily responses and increase vitality. It is on this principle that most of the natural methods of healing – from water therapy to aerobic exercise – are based. Second by examining the quality of information which is coming to a person in terms of the environment in which you live. If it is the right kind of information, if the air you breathe is rich in negative ion particles, for instance, known to produce a sense of harmonious well-being in most people, then it is something which belongs in any holistic programme for Age Power. If it is not – if, instead, it is full of industrial pollutants and depleted in negative ions – then the opposite is true and we need to take whatever action we can either to change it or to protect ourselves from the negative effects of the kind of information our body is being forced to process.

CLEARING PSYCHIC ENTROPY

The order needed both to sustain a negentropic state and to maintain inner order living, as we do in a world of increasing chaos, is not only chemical and bioenergetic in nature. We also need to expand our consciousness with the passing of the years and to feed ourselves on a spiritual level so that two things happen:

- We shed steadily and inexorably whatever false notions, destructive habits and self-imposed limitations that each of us accrue growing up and wrestling with the challenges of day-to-day life.
- We need, as each year passes, to become more aware of the whispers of our soul which bring us in touch with what we love most and what both will bring us the greatest satisfaction in living as well as bring to our families, our work and the world around us the greatest gifts we have to offer.

> The more I work with the body . . . the more I appreciate and sympathise with a given 'disease' . . . the body no longer appears as a sick or irrational demon, but as a process with its own logic and wisdom.
>
> *Arnold Mindell*

This is where meditation can help, or autogenic training or some other method by which the psyche can be encouraged to dissipate its own confusion and entropy, and to drink order from the world around us.

THE ORDER OF CONSCIOUSNESS

Mechanistic science has completely ignored – left out altogether – one critical factor in its description of reality: the power of consciousness. By consciousness I mean both our everyday sense of awareness as well as the vast uncharted realms of the quantum mind which psychologists call the unconscious. In quantum realms you find the seat of our creative powers, our intuition, our dreams, our spiritual experiences and our sense of ultimate meaning and values.

Although consciousness is not something you can hold in your hand or draw a picture of, it has enormous power to affect material reality. This is not just an empty statement. Literally hundreds of researchers throughout the world have carried out well-designed multidisciplinary, multicultural research as part of what might be called the Human Consciousness Project. Their intention is to map the whole spectrum of the various states of human awareness, including those generally categorised as unconscious. In many ways their work parallels the research of the Human Genome Project where scientists are now intensively studying the whole sequence of human DNA in the endeavour to map all our gene sequences. The efforts of scientists and doctors involved in consciousness research have converged to form a surprisingly coherent picture of the various states of consciousness available to men and women and the remarkably different experiences that can come out of each one. They are also discovering that the quantum realms – source of creativity, mythology and spiritual experience – can be mapped just as we have mapped ordinary reality. This is some of the mind blowing stuff which is at the core of your journey into age power.

BREAKING THE MOULD

Yet despite all this most of us continue to follow the values of our society; we keep learning in school, buying the things we are told to buy and trying to make sense of a world while somewhere deep inside we feel that we are imprisoned. We experience very little sense of freedom. When things get really bad it can even seem we are living in a wasteland, a mechanical world without meaning or purpose. In short we have become separated from our own authentic power. Sometimes we get so far from it we come to doubt its very existence. And as far as the experience of freedom is concerned,

> In transpersonal states, we have the potential to experience ourselves as anything that is part of creation, as well as the creative principle itself. The same is true for other people who can experience themselves as anything and anybody else, including ourselves. In this sense, each human being is not only a small constituent part of the universe, but also the entire field of creation.
>
> *Stanislav Grof*

it is in such times that we become easy prey to the purveyors of facsimile. We keep buying the goods they tell us to buy, we keep playing the games they tell us to play only to discover they lead nowhere.

SUCKING SPIRITUAL ORDER

Our longing for freedom – really a passion for just being who we really are – asks that we reconnect with our instincts, for instinct is the voice of the multi-sensory quantum realms. In short, it asks that we come home to ourselves. You can do this without drugs, without gurus, without becoming a disciple or having to belong to any privileged group. You can do it regardless of your age, your physical condition or your religious beliefs. Freedom becomes part of your day-to-day experience as soon as you are ready to:

- Become an explorer of the multi-dimensional universe in which you live.
- Learn to recognise, honour and respect the beauty of the individual soul and give it authentic expression in your life.
- Allow your worldview to expand until it gets large enough to encompass the whole of reality
- Let go of the restrictions imposed on you from childhood, religion and education.
- Seek out your individual place within the order of the universe.
- Develop a deep and abiding friendship with the inhabitants of the multi-dimensional universe in which we make our homes – from the moles and the stars, the grass and the trees, the rocks and the quasars, to the helping spirits who guide, bless and inform us, the muses who inspire us, the angels who shine for us and the maggots who eat away decaying matter so that new life may come forth from old.
- Learn to build powerful bridges between the rich inner world of consciousness and your day-to-day existence.
- Commit yourself to bringing your own unique creations into being.

In its essence Age Power is a spiritual process as much as it is a physical one. It is designed to bring you home to that sense of bliss and wholeness which we all know should be in our lives but which we often experience only fleetingly. It is a process that depends on simple-to-use skills giving direct access to the wisdom that lies within *you* by awakening your awareness to who you really are and then living out your authentic power more and more with each passing year. As this happens the kind of

> The best and most beautiful things in the world cannot be seen or even touched. They must be felt with the heart.
>
> *Helen Keller*

order, which develops quite automatically from within, creates a sense of both excitement and joy about your life that no amount of brain enhancing chemicals can match. Age power is about moving into real freedom – the freedom to be who you are and to do with energy and joy what you want most to do.

GET INTO BLISS

In a very real sense your body is the universe, the world tree at the axis mundi rooted deep within the earth. It grows as you grow towards the heavens. A sanctuary, a fortress, a bird in flight towards heaven, the powers of your body are the powers of the universe. Celebrate them.

Leslie Kenton in Journey to Freedom

All thought, all feeling, every response to beauty and to horror is mediated through your body. Your body is the medium for experiencing everything in your life. As any healthy two-year-old knows, when your body is fully alive you are fully alive. One of the most ageing influences in our lives – something that destroys aliveness and our capacity for bliss – is the force of habit. The very best bodywork can help you rediscover it.

How often do you rejoice in your body? Feel at ease in your skin and in harmony with your world? If the answer is seldom, you are not alone. Most of us put up with our body. We think of it as some kind of cumbersome baggage we carry with us as we go about. There is exercise for the body and there is care for the body. Each is as important as the other. It is time to rediscover a childlike sense of aliveness. Your body not only feeds on food and exercise. It feeds on bliss too.

We all know, to our great frustration, that our patterns and our behaviour do not change merely because we want them to or because we hear a new idea somewhere. Ingrained habits can only change when their underlying re-inforcements change – accumulative experiences, emotional states, values, beliefs, expectations, moods and attitudes.

Dean Juhan

DE-GROOVE YOUR LIFE

Habitual ways of thinking, moving and feeling are rather like 'grooves' into which we conveniently let ourselves fall for protection from life's surprises. Such grooves can be useful. They bring us structure and a sense of security day to day. After all, none of us can live our whole life standing atop a cliff while the winds of change toss us about unceasingly.

Yet life grooves can be stultifying too – especially when we are not fully aware of the habits of thinking, moving and feeling we let ourselves fall into. Our grooves limit us by exchanging the sense of free, open, positive expectations about life which we had when we were young for strange self-protective prisons from which we gaze through the bars at what might have been. Too often habits block our power and authenticity. They needed to be 'detoxified'. Over time, in physical ways, these habits build muscular tensions and distort our physical structure producing bad posture, even causing chronic pain.

The way in which we have been taught to think of our body together with chronic holding patterns stand in the way of our shedding habitual ways of thinking as well as distorting our natural beauty. They make us look old and decrease our capacity for bliss. We also need to think of the body in new ways – as a wondrous medium for experiencing pleasure and joy, creativity and connections with the world around us – and to stop seeing it as an object to be criticised, disciplined and degraded because it does not meet some standard imposed upon us from the outside. This is often not an easy task. For instance don't get into this frame of mind after reading the previous two chapters.

We need to stop treating our bodies as objects. Your body is a living energetic system, one could even say the energy field of the soul, capable of infinite bliss, joy and pleasure. The very best bodywork can help you discover these things.

BEYOND EXERCISE

Physical exercise can be demanding. It commits you to doing something active which, in the doing of it, sometimes feels more of a chore than a joy. Bodywork is different – sheer pleasure is something we human beings need, the way we need food and air and love. In the past few years a greater variety of fine bodywork has become available – from Trager and Feldenkrais to traditional Tui Na massage from China and Nuad Bo'Raen from Thailand. Choose your bliss and follow it regularly. Not only can it alter the way you look and feel, it can help you cleanse your being of imprisoning ideas and holding patterns and release more of your energy and personal power.

> Outside of a dog, a book is man's best friend. Inside of a dog, it's too dark to read.
>
> *Groucho Marx*

> In some cases, visionary experiences occur during bodywork to form the first stages of actually acquiring a body. Many people are not aware of their physical bodies.
>
> *Arnold Mindell*

There are three different body therapies I am particularly fond of: Alexander Technique, Feldenkrais Method and Trager. Others, such as Rolfing, Watsu, Tui Na and classic Shiatsu are equally helpful – each in its own way.

TO ROLFE OR NOT TO ROLFE

Rolfing, otherwise known as Structural Integration, is a form of deep body work, the purpose of which is to restructure your musculoskeletal system completely by addressing in a physical way the patterns of tension which you hold in your facia – the body's connective tissue. 'Getting rolfed' means going through 10 one hour to two hour sessions during which the rolfer uses deep pressure from fingers and elbows to open up specific parts of your body that are chronically tense. Although it can be temporarily painful, rolfing is a superb way of releasing suppressed material in the body and in doing so, changing not only habitual holding patterns of bad posture and chronic pain, but also repressed fears and false assumptions. In the hands of a good practitioner, rolfing is nothing less than life transforming; but it is not a technique for the faint hearted. To find a practitioner get in touch with the Rolfe Institute of Structural Integration or look online at www.rolf.org.

ALEXANDER'S WAY

A body therapy which emphasises the proper alignment of the spine, head and neck, Alexander Technique was developed by Fredrick Matthias Alexander, a Shakespearian actor. It grew out of Alexander's belief that poor posture was what was interfering with his recurring loss of voice. The Alexander Technique is easy to learn. The practitioner shows you how, through simple movement, to restore you body's natural poise and muscle tension. Alexander Technique is particularly good for anyone with common back or neck problems or sciatica. It is also useful for tinnitus – the ringing in the ears often associated with long-term stress.

'. . . rocking, stretching, swinging, compressing, shimmering . . . with the sole purpose of feeling [the body's] patterns . . . ease, fluidity, spaciousness, connectedness, wholeness, liveliness, freedom, lightness – all the qualities of vibrant health . . .

Susan K. Holper

As we get older and balance becomes less good, the Alexander Technique is helpful for restoring balance. It is also used to improve function in people with Parkinson's disease, as well as to help clear depression, sprain injuries, migraines, panic attacks and other stress related disorders. So good is this technique for integrating the body that it is now taught in most drama and music schools. The best way to learn it is a one-on-one session which generally lasts from half an hour to an hour. The practitioner asks you to lie on a padded table while he or she gently moves your legs, arms and head, enabling you to let go of tension. He then observes how you walk, sit and stand, and through a combination of gentle touch and verbal instructions helps you re-educate how you perform simple movements like getting up out of the chair, sitting down, climbing stairs and all the other things we do day-in-day-out. One of the interesting experiences that people report after Alexander bodywork is that they feel taller and in a very real way Alexander does lengthen the spine. For more information check on the web at www.alexandertech.org.

SHIATSU

The traditional healing art from Japan, Shiatsu now comes in so many forms it is hard to list them all. Most can be both energising and relaxing and are excellent for the release of muscle pain, particularly around the area of the neck and shoulders. Shiatsu can be helpful to people who are lacking in energy, as well as those with chronic ailments from low back pain and nervous disorders, PMS and sexual dysfunction to digestive disturbances, asthma and sinus troubles. The aim of Shiatsu is to balance your body's energy flow so it is useful on a regular basis for maintaining general health. A session lasts half an hour to an hour and a half. It is generally given clothed. You lie on a padded surface on the floor while the practitioner works on your body using fingers, elbows and sometimes even feet, stretching and pressing, holding a point for a few seconds, then letting go. It's important to let your practitioner know what kind of pressure you like best. It varies tremendously from one person to another.

WATER BLISS

Watsu is the father of water-based bodywork. The name comes from 'WATer ShaitSU'. It was developed in the 1980s by Harold Dull while working with his Shiatsu students. Since then Watsu has evolved into one of the most profound bodyworks in the world. While other forms of bodywork are based on touch, Watsu – which involves being cradled in a warm pool while having your body gently stretched and glided through a series of flowing movements – necessitates bringing you to a new level of connection and trust with life. It's little wonder that Watsu has become so popular as a means of stress reduction. It is much more, however. It's used to rehabilitate people with disorders ranging from joint and muscle injuries to cerebral palsy and stroke. The warm weightlessness of Watsu helps calm your mind and puts you in deep touch with your body. As this happens, not only are tension and patterns of false thought released, you can be left with a fundamental sense of the essence of your being. It can help answer the questions: Who are you? Why are you in this body? On this planet? How do you fit into the grand scheme of things? To find a practitioner check out the website of Worldwide Aquatic Bodywork Association at www.waba.edu.

RUSSIAN JOYS

Developed by Russian physicist and accomplished athlete Dr Moshe Feldenkrais, the Feldenkrais Method uses gentle, blissful movement to retrain, and ultimately restructure, the nervous system. It actually helps your body create new neural and muscular pathways around areas of blockage or damage while integrating body and psyche. I know this sounds a big agenda, but it really does work. There are two ways of doing Feldenkrais: First you can have a Feldenkrais practitioner work on your body to help breakdown habitual movements which restrict you and re-educate your brain and nervous system to new patterns of movement. The second way is to be taught the movements yourself so that you can work on your own. In my opinion it is by far the best way.

Born in Russia in 1919, Moshe Feldenkrais worked for the British Admiralty during World War II, and then emigrated to Palestine, where, plagued by a knee problem brought on by a sports injury, he found a way of helping himself heal. He was highly resistant to the idea of orthopaedic surgery, which is what all of his physicians urged him to do. Feldenkrais began to explore how the body moves naturally. With his training as a scientist he also studied neuro-physiology and neuro-psychology. Before long he had not only written a classic examination of mind/body, he was also able to throw his crutches away. His knee had healed completely. Feldenkrais insisted that motor function and thought patterns are inseparable. Our emotions, such as sorrow, grief, joy and enthusiasm are encoded within our

> The key to developing a beautiful physical appearance is to start from the inside out by clearing away physical and emotional toxins.
>
> *Anne Louise Gittleman*

flesh and expressed through our body's intentions. He then went on to develop simple blissful ways of helping people develop an awareness of how the body moves and feels to experience life fully. The Feldenkrais Method aims to help you to come closer and closer to what he called *functional integration* – wholeness in the largest sense. When it comes to rejuvenating body and psyche his techniques are nothing short of revolutionary.

CREATIVE HELP

Feldenkrais' work is much praised by some of the world's top artists and scientists for whom it has proved nothing short of life changing – from the late Yehudi Menuhin and director Peter Brooke, to neuro-physiologist and brain expert Dr Carl Pribram. Until his death Dr Feldenkrais continued to perform what were amusingly called 'routine miracles' transforming the lives of the sick and the apparently well, by helping them expand their ability to move. Feldenkrais can greatly benefit people whose movements have been restricted by damage to the body, fibromyalgia, stroke or any other disabling conditions.

Feldenkrais is excellent for repetitive strain injury, muscle damage and sciatica. It is also a wonderful way to help athletes, musicians and actors enhance their performance. It helps older people expand their range of flexibility and motions, improve their body image and expand their consciousness.

A session of Feldenkrais can be private, lasting from 45 to 60 minutes, in which the practitioner gives you gentle hands-on guidance in performing movements related to whatever condition you have consulted him or her about. Classes in Feldenkrais movement – my favorite way of approaching this particular form of bodywork – consists of a teacher giving verbal instructions and guiding you in common movements, such as leaning, bending and even breathing. While working on the floor the instructor helps each participant to discover the ways he or she can move most easily and blissfully. The emphasis of Feldenkrais is very much on experiences, pleasure and ease. This is one of the things that attracts me most to it. In my opinion there is far too little bliss in our lives.

RESTORE ENERGETIC HOMEOSTASIS

Functional integration through Feldenkrais is really the physiological and psychological counterpart of biomedical and energetic homeostasis – an organism's attempt to maintain equilibrium – in the body. It introduces you to a centered, grounded way of living, where physical

> The old skin has to be shed before the new one can come.
>
> Joseph Campbell

and psychic movements are open, vital and creative. Over time the Feldenkrais techniques gradually and easily melt away emotional restrictions and the mechanical limitations of our thinking to which we are all prone as we grow older. Feldenkrais himself used to say, 'In a perfectly mature body which has grown without great emotional disturbances, movement tends gradually to conform to the mechanical requirements of the surrounding world. The nervous system has evolved under the influence of these laws and has fitted to them. However, in our society, we do, by the promise of great reward or intense punishment, so distort the even balance of the system that many acts become excluded or restricted. The result is that we have to provide special conditions for providing adult maturations of many rested functions. The majority of people have to be taught not only the special movements of the repertoire, but also to reform patterns of movements and attitudes that should never have been excluded or neglected.' A good web reference for Feldenkrais is www.feldenkrais.com.

THAI BODY SECRETS

Tui Na – pronounced 'twee-nah' – is a powerful and dynamic approach to working with the body which brings together stretching and pressure applied to acupuncture points, channels and muscle groups. It is a form of two thousand-year-old Oriental bodywork therapy which uses the flow of qi through the meridians of the body as its therapeutic orientation. Tui Na seeks to establish a more harmonious flow of energy, allowing the body quite naturally to heal itself. Tui Na works beautifully in the treatment of musculoskeletal disorders, chronic stress problems related to digestion, breathing and reproduction. It is not a bodywork useful for someone who simply wants mild sedating relaxation. Tui Na makes use of an enormous number of hands-on techniques from gentle stroking to deep tissue work which can cause pain in its effort to balance the flow of qi in the body. A session lasts 30 to 60 minutes and is usually carried out on a loosely clothed body. For further information check out www.acupuncture.com\tuina\.

MYSTERIOUS PLAY

In many ways Trager is the most mysterious and the most magnificent of all the three major transformative forms of bodywork. It is the discovery of Milton Trager, MD, who came upon the principles on which it is based by accident at the age of 18. An American, born in Chicago in 1908, Milton Trager had a congenital spinal deformity, which contributed to a weak and sickly childhood. As so often happens with someone who needs to overcome adversity, it was looking for answers and solutions to his own challenges that led Trager eventually to achieve the graceful body of a dancer, gymnast and athlete. He was also a boxer.

The Trager approach relies on gentle rocking and fine movements of the body, which induce deep pleasant relaxation. Trager discovered that a very light hands on touch can alleviate all sorts of ailments in people. A Trager practitioner helps you feel what it is like to move freely and effortlessly. As this happens something much deeper occurs: You begin to experience a newer, higher level of balance, physically and emotionally. Homeostasis in the body becomes a much easier matter to maintain and you find deep-seated physical and mental challenges that may be causing your pain, emotional disorders or lack of confidence, or may in some other way be disrupting normal function, gradually clear. This leaves you a freer more vital human being.

Like Feldenkrais, there are two aspects to the Trager approach. In the first aspect the practitioner works on you while you passively receive the benefits, this is called tablework. The active aspect of the Trager approach is called Mentastics. Mentastics relies on natural, gentle movements, which you can do yourself to release deep-seated mental and physical patterns, facilitate wider mobility and mental clarity and increase energy. The Trager approach is a wonderful way of reducing stress, but it goes far further. It helps to make new connections between nervous system and muscle. As such, it is a wonderful way of rehabilitating motion for any one who has suffered from traumatic injury or stroke or who has any neuro-muscular disorder, such as muscular dystrophy, Parkinson's disease, multiple sclerosis or post-polio syndrome. Trager also improves breathing and is good for people with lung problems or any kind of

As I play with the body, I come upon patterns not in harmony – tough strands of muscle fibre trying to do some long-forgotten task, or a limpness of tissue that could be livelier. I invite a better possibility from my unconscious store, invoking softness, vitality and beauty. I am asking, not insisting, and my hands become softer, more responsive. I let go of each eagerness that arises in me. I keep paying attention to what I am feeling, staying in the moment, allowing, always allowing.

Susan K. Holfer

chronic pain. The Trager approach whether through tablework or Mentastics, enriches your ability to feel and expands your awareness of who you really are and how you can interact gracefully with the world around you.

A typical session of tablework lasts from an hour to an hour and a half, during which you are either fully clothed or in underwear. The Trager practitioner gently stretches and rocks various areas of your body and then is likely to instruct you how to do Mentastics.

> I am convinced that for every physical non-yielding condition, there is a psychic counter-part in the unconscious mind corresponding exactly to the degree of the physical manifestation. These patterns often develop in response to adverse circumstances such as accidents, surgery, illness, poor posture, emotional trauma, stresses of daily living, or poor movement habits. The purpose of my work is to break up these sensory and mental patterns which inhibit free movement and cause pain and disruption of normal function.
>
> *Milton Trager*

Moshe Feldenkrais and Milton Trager were good friends. In fact it was Trager, teaching his technique at Eslen Institute in Big Sur, California for many years, who brought Feldenkrais to Eslen. The two masters of bodywork used to work on each others bodies. It is almost impossible to describe how deep the effect of Trager can go. I have myself experienced profound transformation on the very deepest levels of creativity, physical well-being and view of reality, having done several sessions with a Trager practitioner named Jananda Bird in the UK. For further information on Trager take a look at the website www.trager.com.

Degrooving your life begins with the body and then moves on to the mind. Each of us is born free. Moving into age power brings us deeper connections with the power of authentic freedom from inside out.

> Happiness springs from how much of the time a person spends feeling good, not from the momentary peaks of ecstasy. Simple pleasures – hours spent walking on a sunny day, gardening, running with the dog, chopping wood or working on a new craft – are more allied with happiness than are strong, momentary feelings.
>
> *Robert Ornstein, PhD and David Sobel, MD*

BORN FREE

Age Power is a process by which we break Rousseau's chains – progressively and inexorably. The most exciting passage you ever make, Age Power liberates you from relentless forces of doubt, self-criticism, and fear, inherited growing up in an ethos which splits minds from bodies and teaches us not to trust the voice within.

As we grow older, far too many of us climb to the top of the ladder only to find it's leaning against the wrong wall. What's worse, in the process, we discover we have often lost touch with our dreams. So instead of awakening each morning with the child's sense of wonderment at what the day ahead will bring, we wake up with a sense of impossibility or with a sense of deep regret over a life that seems to have passed us by.

ENTER THE BLUES

It is little wonder. Growing older brings each of us face to face with loss, grief, sadness and disappointment. When you're 25, your whole life lies ahead of you. At 35, you get the first inkling that not all you dreamed of doing and being is likely to materialise. By the time you are 50, you often begin to look back more than you look forward, to wonder what it's all about and why so much of life has been painful. After all, you've been the good employee, mother, lover, artist, husband. You've put as much of yourself as you could into your work and connections with people. Yet something is missing. Maybe you find the rules you played by and the rules by which you have defined yourself are not enough. There's a great empty gap somewhere. Children have gone or are going. A job is lost. A marriage collapses. Maybe you experience a problem with your health which drugs, prescribed by a well-meaning doctor, can't shift. Perhaps you have been waiting for something to happen, for someone to come and rescue you from a life-less-than-perfect. Then you wake up one day to find that nobody is there. Even if you have a wonderful marriage and you love your job, sooner or later each of us

> Most of us don't become what we can because we can't see it's what we already are.
>
> *Carl A Hammerschlag*

comes face to face with a sense of isolation and loneliness that seems endemic in being human. Where do we go from here?

SOULSCAPE

Welcome. You have entered the region of the soul – a wide, deep, unchartered terrain which most of us spend our lives trying to avoid. Transformation – the kind of change that leads you progressively towards becoming more and more of who you truly are – is never comfortable. Neither does growth take place smoothly. Age Power is no Walt Disney movie. It asks that we take up the challenge of connecting at the very deepest levels with our own authenticity. In the process we inevitably go through an emotional and spiritual detoxification that can make the bad headache you get when you quit drinking coffee look like a picnic.

SEEDPOWER

Each human being is unique. Like the seed of a plant which has encoded within its genetic material the potential for everything it can become as a full blown flower, each of us comes into the world carrying a package of as yet unrealised potential for health, energy, creativity and joy. It is this physical, psychological and spiritual potential which creates our uniqueness. Age Power is about living that potential to its fullest, and coming into a sense of authentic freedom – the freedom to be just who you are without pretence or apologies. I believe there is no greater freedom in the world.

> Once again, life louses up the script.
>
> *Humphrey Bogart*

> Pain is inevitable. Suffering is optional.
>
> *Kathleen C Theisen*

> Loneliness is the way by which destiny endeavours to lead man to himself.
>
> *Hermann Hesse*

THE ZEN OF SOUL

When the Zen painter uses a brush to represent a leaf on a bamboo shaft, he creates a totally singular stroke – like no other leaf that ever existed. Yet within its uniqueness is encompassed universal beauty and life energy of the highest order. So it is with each of us. Within the individual genetic package which was you when you came into this life, was nestled your very own brand of seedpower – an essential soul energy that encompasses greater physical, creative and spiritual potential than you could ever hope to realise in 10 lifetimes. The more fully seedpower is allowed to unfold, the richer your experience of life becomes. So focussed is the energy of spirit within a tiny seed that it opens and reaches toward the light, regardless of what's in its way. Once I pulled up a weed growing in my garden to discover within its root a child's marble that had been crushed out of all recognition by the life force of the growing plant.

POWER FROM WITHIN

A wonderful thing about any little seed is that it doesn't take much for it to develop into the plant it's designed to be. Some good rich organic soil, a little rain and a dose of sunlight. The power and the intelligence that makes growth possible lies not *outside* of it but within the seed itself. People – you and me and the woman you saw when you left your home this morning – are just like plants. All we need is a good healthy environment which allows our unfolding to take place.

HITCHES AND GLITCHES

The problem is that few of us get it. For as we are unfolding – as we are passing through the superbly orchestrated phases of our physical and spiritual development – more often than not our environment does not provide the rich soil, clean water and sunlight we need for full unfolding. More often than not it truncates our development. Then, like a little plant trying to grow in depleted soil with too little water and not enough light, our psychological and spiritual growth becomes stunted. Like a seedling trying to push through the earth with a stone on top of it, we develop 'distortions'.

FISH AND DUCKS

All sorts of things can cause distortions: illnesses, accidents, emotional or physical abuse. Even being raised in a wonderful family if you happen to be a 'fish' when the rest of your family are 'ducks'. Distortions can be physical in nature – a sunken chest or an excess of fat to create a cushion against the harsh world. They can also be emotional, leaving us with a sense that there is something *wrong* with us, that we cannot rely on our own judgment, that we are unworthy, or incompetent, or guilty, even though we may have no idea why or how. And they can be spiritual.

PSYCHIC TERRAIN

When we grow up in a terrain in which our own brand of seedpower can't flourish – when we feel ourselves to be isolated and living in the boxed up world of only five senses, when we think we need to follow other people's rules in order to find out how to love – then we can end up experiencing discouragement or despair. It can seem as though we have nowhere to go, nothing to do and no purpose in remaining alive. Such feelings are common in the wide population as they age. They develop through all sorts of causes. The most common fall into three categories: Our parental training, our religious training and our restricted world-view. It begins when we are kids. We grow up trying to conform to our parent's expectations. We have to. We need their love and care to survive. We learn that we can have love by being 'good'.

Seldom does being 'good' have much to do with being who you are. It's usually about being quiet when someone is talking. It's about using the right fork or not sucking your thumb or not telling the truth in case what you say offends the neighbours. Such imperatives become encoded within our body and our psyche as though they were major rules by which we should live our lives. We fear if we cannot do this we will not get the love and care we need. That's how we learn to play roles. One of the great things about growing older is that we have the ability to let go of these roles when we choose to do so. Organised religion does its share of imprisoning, too. Some religions have

> Sometimes I lie awake at night, and I ask 'Where have I gone wrong?' Then a voice says to me, 'This is going to take more than one night.'
>
> *Charlie Brown*

endless lists of 'dos' and 'don'ts'. Others traffic in fear, based on the notion that our God is the only God.

AUTHENTICITY

As we grow older, the outer forms of religion tend to be replaced by a growing awareness of the luminous quality of life and an awesome sense that in some way we are part of it. If we are lucky, as we grow older, we also come to realise that freedom, authenticity and creative power depend little on the external circumstances in which we find ourselves. Nor need they be limited by age or condition.

REAL THING

One of the most moving accounts I have ever read of this experience came from a political dissonant imprisoned in a concentration camp in the early forties. It told how he came to experience the true nature of freedom, creativity and wholeness while living in the most inhumane conditions of physical incarceration imaginable. He reclaimed his freedom in the only way any of us ever will – by coming to live from ever deeper layers of himself. Eventually his soul and his outer personality became authentic echoes of each other. As this happens to each one of us, the distortions we have carried – the false beliefs, destructive parental training or negative habit patterns formed throughout our lives – fall away. As they do, a genuine rejuvenation occurs – emotionally, physically and spiritually. This liberates life energy and shifts the whole way we look upon reality by allowing us simply to be who we are without pretensions or self-limiting assumptions to unconsciously block our experience of being fully alive. It leaves us able – if not sooner, then later – to make full use of our potentials. Far too much vitality lies stillborn beneath patterns of addictive behaviour, fear and heavy psychological baggage – the kind of

> Do you know what's wrong with you?
> No. What?
> Nothing.
>
> *Audrey Hepburn and Cary Grant in* Charade

> Matter is transparent and malleable in relation to the spirit.
>
> *Pierre Teilhard de Chardin*

> The galaxies exist in you, not printed as mere images within your skull, but in your every cell, your every atom.
>
> *George Leonard*

stuff we all carry around with us to thwart our energy and make being who we are hard work.

THE CALL

Beneath whatever physical, emotional or mental rubbish we accumulate, freedom breathes softly waiting for our call. Embracing it is essential for our fulfilment. This asks that we let go of careless ways of eating and living that degrade our health and distort our thinking. It asks too that we ease our grip on fear and frustrations developed over the years and learn to reassert our trust in our essential self. The wonderful thing about the psyche – like the body – is that given half a chance it too will detoxify itself so life changing creative energy is released. Spiritual detoxification brings a spiritual new life in its wake – one which echoes throughout the whole of your world. It adds the freshness of a child's vision to the wisdom gained over the years. This combination perennially delights us when we come upon old people whose eyes sparkle.

PSYCHIC DETOX

There are many ways to go about it. Good psychotherapy can help. So can meditation, Feldenkrais, Trager and energy approaches to exercise like tai chi, yoga and marshal arts – provided that they are always taught with a real respect for the spiritual power that underlies them. Autogenic Training is another simple but powerful way of cleansing the psyche of false ideas and emotional rubbish. So are some of the leading-edge binaural technologies such as Holosync – forms of electronic meditation – which alter brain functions and foster a greater sense of wholeness and peace.

All these techniques have something in common: When you practise them regularly they not only bring you greater peace and balance. Periodically they also bring to the surface old feelings of discouragement or depression, frustration or fear. They rise like echoes from the past to be cleared, very much the way physical toxicity rises to the surface when you begin a detox

> We must be willing to get rid of the life we've planned, so as to have the life that is waiting for us.
>
> *Joseph Campbell*

programme. It coats your tongue and spoils your breath *temporarily*. It soon clears and, in its wake, old stress you may have been carrying most of your life has surfaced and been cleared away. Every time it happens, the easier it becomes to hear the whispers of the soul and to *allow* the full expression of your seedpower. Personal growth is nothing more than the passage by which we realise who we have been all along, and welcome it.

Perhaps middle age is, or should be, a period of shedding shells; the shell of ambition, the shell of material accumulations and possessions, the shell of the ego. Perhaps one can shed at this stage in life as one sheds in beach-living; one's pride, one's false ambitions, one's mask, one's armour. Was that armour not put on to protect one from the competitive world? If one ceases to compete, does one need it? Perhaps one can at last in middle age, if not earlier, be completely oneself. And what a liberation that would be!

Anne Morrow Lindbergh

DARKNESS INTO LIGHT

You'll never be able to dance unless you hear your own music ...
the words on your lips must reflect the truth of your
heart. Otherwise your life's breath is muted.

Carl A Hammerschlag MD

The great religions insist the universe is one – an intelligent, loving, aware, perfect loving energy which is the source of all things. Complete in itself, this divine oneness whirls ever outwards to infinity. Each of us *is* that divine energy. Sounds great in theory. But for most of us it remains little more than an idea. How can I be this magnificent loving energy when I struggle so much and feel so lousy?

Why don't I *feel* the peace? And, if this is my true nature, how do I come to live it? The mystics teach that we do not experience our true nature because of the distortions of our mind. False ideas, memories of trauma, repressed or unresolved emotional material – all these things filter reality so we can only see 'through a glass darkly'. How, then, do we polish the lens of perception to see clearly?

HITCHES AND BUMPS

That is where meditation, Autogenic Training and other forms of spiritual practice comes in. These can be as simple as sitting each day to watch your breath or as far out as using binaural sounds fed into the brain to foster its integration. Whatever you choose, a spiritual practice is important if growing older is to mean growing into power, creativity and joy. It is a fascinating process with a lot of hitches and bumps along the way. Even the hitches and bumps are important for human growth. They are a part of Age Power's continual process of dissolving away structures no longer large enough to house your expanding human spirit.

To understand the patterns, it is useful to look at chaos theory models created by Nobel Laureate Ilya Prigogine. They

> As we recognise that the fragmentation to which we are subject is due to a disconnection from the course of our life, the immortal self, it follows that our path to wholeness must involve a 're-membering' of that self.
>
> *Ralph Metzner*

describe how *open systems* transform and reorganise themselves in what can only be described as quantum leaps.

NEGENTROPIC GROWTH

An open system is a system which continually interacts with its environment by taking in energy and giving out energy (see Chapter 12). We are such a system. It is this that makes it possible for us to stay alive. We take in oxygen and water and food as well as information and experience. We give out carbon dioxide, waste, information as well as taking actions which effect the world around us. According to Prigogine, open systems maintain their structure and grow – continually evolving into more complex systems – first because they suck order from their environment as Schrodinger claims, but because things have the ability to *dissipate* entropy – chaos or disorder if you like – into their environment. He looks upon any open system as a flow of energy and his model fits beautifully when applied to a human being who is continually changing, evolving and transforming himself throughout the whole of his life.

Prigogine calls open systems 'dissipative structures'. He points out that, although they are highly adaptable and able to deal with all kinds of fluctuations in input from their environment, each open system – for that matter, each of us – has a limit to how much entropy or disorder it can dissipate into its environment and still maintain its structure. And the more complex a particular open system is, the greater its ability to dissipate entropy into its environment.

Chaos Theory is a new theory invented by scientists panicked by the thought that the public are beginning to understand the old ones.

Mike Barfield

Where there is dismemberment in the beginning there is remembrance at the end.

Alan Watts

BIFURCATION MEANS NEW LIFE

Human beings are highly complex open systems, continually exchanging free energy, with an enormous capacity for dissipating entropy. But, like any open system, when influences from our environment push us beyond our limit, we come to the point at which we can no longer dissipate enough entropy to maintain the current structure of our belief system, our ways of operating, our habit patterns. Then things fall apart. Prigogine calls this the *bifurcation point* (bifurcation means dividing into two branches). When a bifurcation point is reached, he says, the system spontaneously re-orders itself in a brand new way – a way so different that it can seem almost unrelated to the way in which it previously functioned (or for that matter the way we previously experienced ourselves and the world around us). Such a change is a true quantum leap on the road to becoming what we already are, but don't yet know we are.

I RISE IN FLAME

At its essence, Age Power is nothing less than a process of unfolding which enables a human being progressively to become more and more of who he or she truly is – to express more fully the unique divine spark of their soul. Prigogine's bifurcation points happen to all of us as we grow. When we become aware of this and come to welcome them instead of trying to suppress the sense of falling apart, the Age Power process grows more powerful and graceful. The way in which real spiritual growth happens is seldom through a steady process of change. More often it occurs as a series of quantum leaps, each of which resemble the metamorphosis of caterpillars into butterflies or the mythological phoenix whose form is continually consumed by a fire of his own making out of which an entirely new being of greater beauty and glory emerges.

LEAP AFTER LEAP

In physics the word *quantum* has very specific properties. It means a bundle of energy. Quantum leap is the term used to describe the movement of an electron from the orbit of one atom to another in a very special way:

> Are you willing to be sponged out, erased, cancelled, made nothing? Are you willing to be made nothing? Dipped into oblivion? If not, you will never really change.
>
> *D H Lawrence*

It moves from one place to another not by a linear process as we expect change to take place, but by a *discontinuous jump* like that which happens at Prigogine's bifurcation points. In other words, It leaves one place to arrive at the next without passing through the space in between. By doing this, a quantum leap transcends the rules of time and space as well as negating linear laws of Newtonian physics which for so long scientists believed to be inescapable.

Like the quantum leaps recorded in the lives of mystics, artists and scientists, Age Power's quantum leaps are similar in nature. The transformations we experience are discontinuous – progressive 'rebirths' which cannot be described either by the laws of mechanistic science or classic psychological theories. They are changes which happen from within, each in a unique and highly individual way – changes which do not depend on following any external set of values or any religious or philosophical set of beliefs. These are changes from the soul.

TRANSFORMATIONS

The profound changes which take place in life from working with various spiritual practices have certain things in common. First, like quantum leaps, they are discontinuous in nature. Second, the major shifts which occur are not simple changes at all. They are true transformations. They can only be described as passages out of a more *limited* way of being into a more expanded place where you experience your self and life anew. They expand health, creativity and joy and increase our capacity to give and receive love. Simple change implies the ability to change back again to one's previous state. This kind of change is like leaving the womb to be born – a Prigogine leap to a more complex structure which creates a higher order of being.

> Nothing is more dangerous than an idea when it's the only one you have.
>
> *Emily Chartier*

> It is looking at things for a long time that ripens you and gives you a deeper understanding.
>
> *Vincent van Gogh*

MY OWN PATH

For many years I worked with meditation in Tibetan Buddhist practices and was imbued in their traditions. Gradually, my interest turned towards shamanism – the world's oldest collection of tools and techniques for expanding consciousness. Worldwide in origin, they pre-date all the world's great religions by 40,000 years. I became immersed in shamanic training and practices. Eventually I was asked to teach core shamanism in Britain and Ireland as Guest Faculty Member for the Foundation for Shamanic Studies. By then I had spent some thirty years working with meditative practices and methods and experimenting with other techniques for spiritual development. The Journey to Freedom workshops, which I still teach in many countries, grew out of my conviction that shamanism, properly taught and focused towards the expansion of human health and creativity, was the most efficient method of spiritual growth.

I had also long been fascinated with technological methods for expanding consciousness such as the work done by organisations like the Munroe Institute and the Institute of Noetic Sciences in the United States and by independent researchers such as Max Cade and Geoffrey Blundel in London, who together developed the biofeedback-based Mind Mirror.

I never believe anything until I try it myself and experience what it has to offer and I am always on the lookout for other tools and techniques, other methods and practices which I believe can contribute to the full unfolding of a human being's beauty and power. The year before last I discovered something which I believe can make a significant contribution to an individual's growth – and maybe even to the evolution of our relationship to the life of the planet over which we human beings hold the greatest sway.

HOLOSYNC

Called Holosync, this is the most powerful technologically based tool for growth, mind expansion and creativity I have yet to come across. Developed at Centerpointe Research Institute in the United States, it consists of state of the art sound technologies in the form of tapes or CDs designed to enhance the functioning of the brain as well as the development of the nervous system as a whole. Over months and years of use, the Holosync recordings become effective tools for both physical and emotional health and healing as well as personal and spiritual growth.

Everyone may educate and regulate his imagination so as to come thereby in contact with spirits, and be taught by them.

Paracelsus

Belief consists in accepting the affirmations of the soul; unbelief in denying them.

Ralph Waldo Emerson

SHIFTING SOUNDS

Holosync uses an advanced form of neuro-audio technology which, like many of its predecessors, enables the listener to enter a desirable state by shifting brain wave frequencies out of *beta* – our usual state of awareness – into the deeper *alpha*, *theta* and *delta*, each of which brings benefits. But it goes far beyond. It uses these frequencies in specific and progressive ways that can, over time, link up disparate parts of the brain and enhance neurological functions. This can lead to better sleep, to a greater capacity to handle stress positively and to improved health. It can also bring about emotional and spiritual development including the ability to live with expanded awareness, creativity and capacity for joy. In short, using it can foster significant spiritual growth – from within. The programme is designed in a step-by-step way. You use one set of CDs or tapes for, say, three or four months, then move on to the next so that neurological changes take place in an ordered and progressive way.

TOWARDS GREATER ORDER

What I particularly like about the Holosync programme is that, unlike any other form of neuro-audio technology, it encourages what Prigogine calls bifurcation points as well as the quantum leaps which follow them that other similar programmes do not. It does this thanks to the progressive nature of the programme. For the fluctuation of brain waves it induces provide a highly controlled stimulus which challenges the nervous system and is always just beyond its ability to maintain its structures.

The great Hans Selye who identified the nature of stress reactions in the body – he coined the word 'stress' applied to the human experience – used to say, 'Whatever challenges you but does not destroy you, only makes you stronger.' By challenging the nervous system, Holosync triggers quantum leaps in development continually forcing it to reorganise itself at a higher level of functioning and forcing it – both metaphorically and literally – to evolve new structures. Its creator and the director of Centrepointe Research Institute in the United States, Bill Harris, believes that this reorganisation stimulates the

So thou shalt feed on death, that feeds on men And death once dead, there's no more dying then.
Shakespeare

creation of new neurological pathways, creating connections between parts of the brain which had not been communicating optimally before. In this way the Holosync technology attempts to create synchronisation of the brain's two hemispheres. This results, over time, in whole brain thinking with increased learning ability, expanded awareness and creativity and fosters a greater sense of ease and peace. (See Resources, page 480.)

SIMPLY LIFE CHANGING

Far simpler, yet enormously powerful is Autogenics. A comprehensive technique for relaxation and personal transformation, Autogenic Training was developed in the early 1930s by the German psychiatrist Johannes H Schultz. It consists of a series of simple mental exercises designed to turn off the body's 'fight or flight' mechanism and turn on the restorative rhythms and harmonising associated with profound psychophysical relaxation. Practised daily it can bring results comparable to those achieved by serious Eastern meditators. Yet unlike meditation, Autogenics has no cultural, religious or cosmological overtones. It demands no special clothing, unusual postures or practices. When you practise autogenics, emotional and spiritual detoxification can occur in much the same way that physical detoxification does in the body.

Schultz discovered – as have many since – that in a state of passive concentration all activities governed by the autonomic nervous system, once believed to be out of man's control, can be influenced by the person himself. This happens not by exercising any conscious act of *will* but rather by learning to abandon oneself to an ongoing organismic process.

Imagination is not make-believe, it's the journey of an unfettered mind.
Carl A Hammerschlag MD

If only human beings could ... be more reverent toward their own fruitfulness ...
Rainer Maria Rilke

PASSIVE CONCENTRATION

This strange paradox of self-induced passivity is central to the way Autogenic Training works its wonders. It is a skill which Eastern yogis, famous for their ability to resist cold and heat, to change the rate of their heartbeat, to levitate and perform many other extraordinary feats, have long practised. But until the development of biofeedback and Autogenic Training and the arrival of Eastern meditation techniques, this passive concentration largely remained a curiosity in the West, where active, logical, linear, verbal thinking has been encouraged to the detriment of practising our innate ability to simply *be.*
Many experts on the psychological processes of ageing believe that it is this overemphasis on the use of the conscious will in the West that makes us highly prone to premature degeneration and stress-based illnesses in the first place.

No one can live without experiencing some degree of stress all the time. You may think that only serious disease or intensive physical or mental injury can cause stress. This is false. Crossing a busy intersection, exposure to draft, or even sheer joy are enough to activate the body's stress mechanisms to some extent. Stress is not even necessarily bad for you; it is also the spice of life, for any emotion, any activity causes stress. But, of course, your system must be prepared to take it. The same stress which makes one person sick can be an invigorating experience for another.

Hans Selye, MD: The Stress of Life

HEAVY AND WARM

To help his patients induce the Autogenic state, Schultz worked with the sensations of heaviness and warmth. Later he added suggestions about regular heartbeat and gentle quiet breathing – two more natural physiological characteristics of relaxation – and then went on to suggestions of warmth in the belly and coolness of the forehead. These six physiologically-orientated directions – heaviness and warmth in the legs and arms, regulation of the heartbeat and breathing, abdominal warmth and cooling of the forehead – form the core of Autogenic Training.

STEP BY STEP

A person learning Autogenics goes through each of the six steps, one by one: 'My arms and legs are heavy and warm, my heartbeat is calm and regular etc.' each time he or she practises. Because of the body and mind's ability with repetition to slip more and more rapidly into the deeply relaxed yet highly aware Autogenic state, the formula becomes increasingly shortened until after a few weeks or months of practising you can induce a state of profound psychophysical relaxation with ease. Once you have mastered the exercises they can be practised anywhere – even sitting on a bus.

ENERGETIC HOMEOSTASIS

A key principle on which Autogenics is based is that the body will naturally balance its life energies, biochemically and psychologically, when repeatedly allowed to enter a relaxed state. The benefits of being able to do this are virtually endless. Some of them come immediately – such as being able to counteract acute stress and fatigue, refresh yourself and clear your mind. People with high blood pressure who learn Autogenics report drops in systolic blood pressure of between 11 to 25 percent and more, as well as five to 15 percent in diastolic pressure. Brain-wave activity also changes so that you get a better balance of right and left hemisphere leading to improved creativity at work and a sense of being at peace with oneself. Other benefits come more slowly over the weeks and months and years that you practise. Recoveries from bronchial asthma and a whole range of other psychosomatic disorders have been reported, as well as the elimination of self-destructive behaviour patterns and habits such as drug taking, compulsive eating and alcoholism. As a result, Autogenic Training is often given as a standard instruction in schools Germany and Switzerland.

> The two worlds, the divine and the human . . . are actually one. The realm of the gods is a forgotten dimension of the world we know.
>
> *Joseph Campbell*

> Let the beauty we love be what we do.
>
> *Rumi*

HERE'S HOW

The basic Autogenic exercises are simple. Take up one of three optional postures – sitting slumped rather like a rag doll on a stool, lounging in an easy chair or lying on your back with your arms at your side, and make sure you are reasonably protected from noise and disturbances and that your clothes are loose and comfortable. It is easiest to learn Autogenics lying flat on a floor or on a very firm bed. Once you have got the basic exercise under your belt you can do it just about any time, anywhere, sitting up or even very discretely on a bus on the way to work. If you like you can record the Autogenic exercises that follow on tape very slowly and play it to yourself in the beginning. I generally find, however, that it is better to learn it very simply from the words in the box on page 384. If you prefer to learn Autogenics from a teacher, (see Resources, page 478).

ENTER THE DEPTHS

Lie down on your back in bed or on the floor. Make yourself comfortable with whatever pillows or covers you need to do so. Close your eyes gently. Take a deep slow breath and pause for a moment. Now exhale fully and completely. Let yourself breathe slowly and naturally. Feel your body sinking back into the floor. Now repeat the following phrases to yourself slowly and silently letting yourself savour the sensations of heaviness and warmth as you do. The first phrase is: *My left arm is heavy . . . my left arm is heavy . . . my left arm is heavy . . . my right arm is heavy . . . my right arm is heavy . . . my right arm is heavy . . .* Let go of any tension in your arms as you say to yourself: *My left arm is heavy . . . my left arm is heavy . . . my left arm is heavy . . .* repeating each suggestion three times. Continue to breathe slowly and naturally, remembering to exhale fully. Say to yourself: *Both arms are heavy . . . both arms are heavy . . . both arms are heavy.* Let go of any tension in your arms. Then say: *Both legs are heavy . . . both legs are heavy . . . both legs are heavy . . .* As you continue to breathe slowly and naturally, say to yourself: *Arms and legs heavy . . . arms and legs heavy . . . arms and legs heavy . . . arms and legs warm . . . arms and legs warm . . . arms and legs warm . . .*

> Adults are always asking little kids what they want to be when they grow up – cause they're looking for ideas.
>
> *Paula Poundstone*

> Nothing in all creation is so like God as stillness.
>
> *Meister Eckhart*

FLOOD OF WARMTH

Feel the warmth flow through to your arms and legs as you say to yourself: *Arms and legs warm . . . arms and legs warm . . . arms and legs warm . . .* Continue to breathe slowly and freely while you repeat silently to yourself: *My breathing calm and easy . . . my breathing calm and easy . . . my breathing calm and easy . . . my heartbeat calm and regular . . . my heartbeat calm and regular . . . my heartbeat calm and regular . . .* Feel your strong, regular heartbeat as you say the words to yourself. Continue to breathe easily and say to yourself: *My solar plexus is warm . . . my solar plexus is warm . . . my solar plexus is warm . . .* Feel the muscles in your face relax as you say to yourself: *My forehead is cool and clear . . . my forehead is cool and clear . . . my forehead is cool and clear . . .* Enjoy the feeling of softness and calm throughout your body and say to yourself: *I am at peace . . . I am at peace . . . I am at peace . . .*

THE RETURN

When you have finished the exercise you are ready for *the return.* It will bring you back to normal every-day consciousness: Quickly clench both fists, take a deep breath in, flex both arms up in a stretch, then breathe out slowly and completely, returning your arms with unclenched fists to your sides. Now open your eyes. Lie for a moment with your eyes open and just allow yourself to: BE HERE NOW WITH WHATEVER IS, then get up and go about your life.

When first learning Autogenics, you will need to repeat each suggestion three times and the entire exercise itself needs to be repeated at three different periods each day. The best time is just before you get out of bed, just before you go to sleep and at some other moment of the day. If there is no way you can lie down during the day you can always do the exercise sitting in a chair. If you are practising in public such as on a bus or at your desk in an office, draw your fists up to your chest by bending your elbows rather than bringing the whole arm above the head for the *return.*

> Beyond words, in the silencing of thought, we are already there.
>
> *Alan Watts*

> Losing your mind can be a peak experience.
>
> *Jane Wagner*

THE TRIGGERS

Before long you will find that even the simple suggestion *my right arm is heavy* will trigger the psychophysical relaxation process in the whole body. Some people get feelings of heaviness and warmth right away. For others it can take as long as a week or two of practising three times a day for 10 or 15 minutes at a time. To everybody it comes eventually and with it comes a profound sense of relaxation at the end of the series of self-directed instructions. *Cancelling* the training session occurs when you clench your hand into a fist and raise your arm straight above your head or bend your arm and draw your fist to your shoulders, at the same time taking a deep breath and then stretching. This trains your body to return to normal consciousness right away. Meanwhile your temporary excursion into the realm of deep relaxation keeps working its magic.

To become human, one must make room in onself for the wonders of the universe.

South American Indian saying

AUTOGENIC TRAINING MADE SIMPLE

Here is an aid memoir for practice. Repeat each suggestion three times:

MY LEFT ARM IS HEAVY
MY RIGHT ARM IS HEAVY
BOTH ARMS ARE HEAVY
BOTH ARMS ARE WARM
BOTH LEGS ARE HEAVY
ARMS AND LEGS HEAVY
ARMS AND LEGS WARM
BREATHING IS CALM AND EASY
HEARTBEAT CALM AND REGULAR
MY SOLAR PLEXUS IS WARM
MY FOREHEAD IS COOL
I AM AT PEACE

The Return:

CLENCH BOTH FISTS
TAKE A DEEP BREATH
BREATHE OUT SLOWLY
RETURN ARMS
UNCLENCH FISTS
OPEN YOUR EYES
LIE FOR A MOMENT WITH EYES OPEN
BE HERE NOW WITH WHATEVER IS

Repeat each suggestion three times, repeat the exercise three time a day.

DISCHARGE IT

Although Autogenic Training brings about a 'low-arousal' state similar to yoga and meditation, where parasympathetic activity dominates, it stems from exercises meant specifically to induce simple *physical* sensations leading to a state of relaxation of a purely physical nature. The benefits which come with practising it go far beyond the physical: in addition to slowing the heartbeat, reducing blood pressure, regenerating and rejuvenating the body,

> We do not see things as they are but as we are.
>
> *Jewish Proverb*

Autogenics triggers changes in the *reticular activating system* in the brain stem which can result in what are known as 'Autogenic discharges'. These are a spontaneous way of de-stressing and de-ageing the body, eliminating old tensions and wiping away thought patterns that may have been inhibiting the full expression of your being.

Autogenic discharges can manifest themselves as temporary twitching of the arms or legs – much like the twitch experienced occasionally on falling into a deep sleep – during the session itself, or increased peristaltic movement – stomach grumbles – or various transient feelings of dizziness or visual or auditory effects. These phenomena are harmless, quick to come and go, yet an important part of throwing out life-accumulated, stressful material stored in the body or psyche.

INNER CLEANSING

A few people – I among them – when they first begin Autogenic Training, go through two or three weeks where a lot of old stress and emotional rubbish gets released through Autogenic discharge. Old feelings of discouragement or depression, laughter or anxiety can sometimes rise to the surface. It is important to be aware of this possibility and to be aware of what is happening if it does occurs. It is only the psychic side of detox that will help renew, refresh and rejuvenate you as old stress you have been carrying about with you rises to the surface to clear permanently.

Rituals and symbols can provide the structure by which life experiences yield new meaning.

Carl A Hammerschlag MD

As we progress and awaken to the soul in us and things, we shall realise that there is consciousness also in the plant, in the metal, in the atom, in electricity, in every thing that belongs to physical nature.

Sri Aurobindo

Because of this discharge phenomenon some psychologists in the English speaking world who teach Autogenics like to work on a one-to-one basis with their students in order to help them gain perspective on what is coming up from their consciousness. In Germany and Switzerland this is not considered important. There, Autogenic Training is taught as a matter of course both to adults and school children with no such psychological back up. The important thing to remember is whatever surfaces is likely to be very old indeed, stuff you've been carrying around for a long time and which you are far better off without.

THE MAGIC OF THREE

It takes about 10 to 15 minutes to run through Autogenics while you are learning it. Afterwards the exercises can be done much more quickly – eventually in two or three minutes if you are short of time. The magic of Autogenics depends on your continual repetition of the exercise again and again, day after day. Once the initial period of learning is completed you can then choose to practise the exercises once or twice a day whenever you like. In the process you will have gained a life-long skill that is invaluable for de-ageing the body and mind. Within 10 days to two weeks of practising Autogenics, most people feel a steady and increasing release of creative energy and a sense that great burdens are being lifted away so that – often for the first time – they begin to feel more free to live their own life by their own values – spiritual rejuvenation at its very best.

It is only with the heart that one can see rightly; what is essential is invisible to the eye.

Antoine de Saint-Exupery

Fortunately [psycho] analysis is not the only way to resolve inner conflicts. Life itself still remains a very effective therapist.

Karen Horney

The new meaning of soul is creativity and mysticism. These will become the foundation of the new psychological type and with him or her will come the new civilisation.

Otto Rank

SEDONA METHOD

There are hundreds of various techniques, training programmes, CDs and tapes on the market which promise to make us richer, better, more creative and lead more satisfying lives. Sadly, few of the ones I have come across fulfil their promises. The Sedona Method is different. It is a simple technique by which you learn to let go of negative thoughts and feelings – often literally in seconds.

Using the Sedona Emotional Release Techniques over a period of time can literally remove many obstacles that prevent each one of us living out the truth of who we are and achieving the goals we want to reach. On a practical level it helps people to tap their potential for health, for rich and fulfilling relationships, creativity and energy. It can also help you achieve financial security, make better decisions and perform well even under the heaviest stress.

CLEAR IT

The Sedona Method acts much like a 'detoxification instrument' not so much for detoxing your body, but for detoxing your mind. Bit by bit, the technique allow us to clear the burdens we carry of unresolved emotional material, self-limiting belief systems and behaviour patterns, which interfere with simply living out who we are. One of the other things I particularly like about the Sedona Method is that it absolutely respects the individual. It does not ask you to believe anything or buy into any philosophy or psychological system.

LET GO OR NO

The brainchild of American physicist Lester Levinson, the Sedona Method consists of a series of very simple questions that make you aware of what you are feeling right now in this particular moment, how you feel about feeling that you are feeling right now and whether you are willing to let go of what you feel right now. There is no right answer by the way. If you are *not* willing to let go, that's fine. It asks other questions which allow us to become aware of the many limitations in our lives which come from feelings, ideas and limiting beliefs. It also makes us aware that these things do not *belong* to us. Rather, they are ever-shifting experiences, which can change in an instant with no effort.

The psychological rule says that when an inner situation is not made conscious, it happens outside, as fate. That is to say when the individual remains undivided and does not become conscious of his inner contradictions, the world must perforce act out of the conflict and be torn into opposite halves.

Carl Jung

EXPERIENTIAL

It is difficult to describe what it is like to do the Sedona as it is non-linear and highly experiential in nature. It is one of those things you have to experience for yourself to know the rich gifts it can bring.

Sedona is available in the form of tapes and/or in the form of work-shops. The Sedona Method Course consists of 10 tapes and a workbook that can take you through the whole process of learning the technique. Once you have learned it you don't need to rely on the tapes. When you find yourself in a position of fatigue, anxiety, depression, uncertainty, you can then use the technique silently, wherever you happen to be, and the releasing process clears whatever is disturbing your equilibrium. Most people who learn the Sedona Method do it because they want a specific payoff: To get rid of stress and to be more effective in their jobs, for instance. It offers many other benefits not as easily described, when you practise the method over several months – a sense of being free to be who you are, a sense of lightness, a sense of clarity and the feeling that you have been relieved from a burden you have long been carrying.

Another researcher, Dr Elliott Grumner, says, 'The Sedona Method is different from anything I have ever done before. It works on a feeling level and allows people to eliminate negative emotions and thoughts. The Sedona Method is so fast and effective because it goes directly to the heart of the problem . . . it is a short cut for everyone who uses it.' The Sedona Method is widely used by some corporations including Merryl Lynch, ATT and Chase Manhattan Bank.

Levinson lived another 40 years to become enormously healthy and finan-cially successful. Before long he decided to give away the money that he had earned and went to live in the desert of Sedona. That was in the sixties when the town was nothing but dirt tracks. There he remained, living in a trailer, in a state of bliss, as he describes it, for six to 10 years. Later he came to feel that these gifts which has been given to him as a result of his experiments needed to be offered to others. He realised when he met troubled people, it was not enough just to smile at them from his own place of peace. So he began to develop the release technique which later became the Sedona Method. Levinson died in 1994 passing on the techniques to many people in the US, including Hale Dwoskin, whose voice is found on the Sedona Method course tapes.

> There are wildernesses to be tamed within, and hostile beings we may encounter, but even those respond better to a touch of the silk glove than to the slap of the gauntlet.
>
> *Stephen Larsen*

TEST IT

There have been a couple of interesting studies validating the effectiveness of the Sedona Method, such as one carried out by Dr Richard J Davidson, together with Dr David McClelland of Harvard University. They tested three groups of 20 people each – 60 people all told. To one group they taught the Sedona Method, to another group they taught progressive relaxation (a well-tested means of decreasing stress and increasing energy). The third group of people were taught no stress reduction technique at all. Researchers showed all of the subjects a film that involved some pretty horrific visual incidents, before the training, two weeks after the training had begun, and three and a half months after the training had finished. They measured various parameters such as heart rate, blood pressure and muscle tension. The results were pretty remarkable. When it came to a decrease in heart rate the third control group had a reduction of five percent during the third viewing of the film, the progressive relaxation group had a reduction of 10 percent in heart rate, but the Sedona Method group over the same three-and-a-half months period had a reduction of 23 percent. Blood pressure results and muscle tension were similar. Researchers concluded that the Sedona Method 'stands out far above the rest for its simplicity, efficiency, absence of questionable concepts and rapidity of observable results'.

It would be hard to overstate the potential that the Sedona Method has to change people's lives. It is simple, direct and respectful of each human being's individuality and values.

ZEN OF NOW

There are two important aspects to making Holosync, Autogenic Training, the Sedona Method or any other spiritual practice work for you. The first is a real *acceptance* of your current circumstances or position – knowing that anything that you feel just now, whether it happens to be fear, anxiety, joy, frustration, inadequacy or environmental stress, is OK for the moment. It is only through acceptance of what is now that we open the gateways to change. The second is self-discipline. You need to make time to do the practice. It takes a bit of effort at first to make the time. Then doing it becomes easy and pleasurable.

PEACE AND BLISS

Lestor Levinson, who invented the Sedona Method, was a successful physicist and businessman in New York City. Suffering badly from a powerful 'Type A' personality, he developed a serious illness, including two heart attacks, jaundice and stomach ulcers. So ill was Levinson that at one point his physician told him he had but two weeks to live. He began to explore his relationships and, as he described it, 'Square all with love'. By this he meant going back to all of his interactions with people and putting right whatever felt wrong or incomplete. As a result of exploring this process (and knowing he was going to die within a fortnight anyway) he discovered some pretty remarkable things. Needless to say, he did not die. Within three to six months all of the frustration and anger that he had carried was gone. What replaced it was a state of peace and bliss.

But the idea that passionate pursuit of work is harmful has caused many of us to worry that we are too attached to something we love. In one of his more pragmatic moments, Sigmund Freud recognised that the important things in life are love and work. Wouldn't it be ideal to combine the two?

*Robert Ornstein PhD
and DavidSobel MD*

I have the conviction that when the physiology will be far enough advanced, the poet, the philosopher, and the physiologist will all understand each other.

Claude Bernard

PART SIX:
POWER LIFE

MANPOWER

You're a dangerous woman.
Thanks. You look good to me, too.

Paul Cavanagh and Mae West,
Goin' to Town

To be male is to be sexual. To be sexual, is to be hormonal. When hormones go awry, everything in a man's life can seem to fall apart and he can get on a fast track to ageing. For sexuality lies at the core of most men's sense of self.

Sexual problems such as infertility, premature ejaculation, impotence, prostate enlargement and loss of libido can mess up with your life and your sense of self. Eighty-five percent of male reproductive problems stem from physiological causes – poor blood circulation, use or abuse of alcohol, cigarettes, recreational drugs or medications, or metabolic disorders such as diabetes. Syndrome X has a large part to play in male dysfunctions. So does lack of exercise which usually accompanies it.

MOVE UP TO GREAT SEX

A recent study highlighted the way regular exercise not only enhances cardiovascular fitness and builds strength, but heightens libido and improves a man's physiological ability to participate in good sex. Researchers put 78 healthy, but sedentary, men – average age 48 – into a three-to-four-times-a-week programme. These men exercised an hour a day for three months. From beginning to end the men kept a daily journal. The records they kept showed quite clearly that, compared to the control group who did not exercise, they had a much higher frequency of sexual activity than before entering the programme, performed better physically and they experienced a far higher number of satisfying orgasms.

FOOD POWER

Male sexuality relies on many things – from good levels and balance of sex hormones to sensory stimulation and first rate circulation for it all to happen. All of these things are dependent not on just *adequate* but *superb* nutrition, especially as you get older. Most sexual dysfunction and abnormalities associated with ageing have nothing to do with ageing. They are the result of years of poor diet. Vitamins and minerals, which act as co-factors for all of the enzymes that rule your metabolic processes, become depleted. As they do, your body is unable to create the vitality, which is essential for good sexual functions.

Syndrome X, with all its distortions, can put a real dampener on sex. It is little wonder that the diabetic – someone in whom Syndrome X has gone so far that the pancreas itself breaks down – is often unable to perform sexually. Age Power's Insulin Balance way of eating counters Syndrome X, helps lower cholesterol levels, shifts triglycerides, enhances circulation, lowers blood pressure and improves your body's ability to use energy.

COENZYME-A
MALE POWER AT YOUR CORE

Coenzyme-A is your body's most important enzyme for energy, vitality and maintaining production of your sex hormones. Coenzyme-A empowers their biochemical synthesis from cholesterol. It increases your body's ability to handle stress, improves physical performance and counters enzyme deficiencies that develop in men as a result of less-than-adequate nutrition, toxic conditions or the passing of years. Whatever changes you make to increase male power, use Coenzyme-A – three times daily on an empty stomach. It supports sex organ functions, enhances repair, slows ageing and reduces stress damage (see Chapter Four Pillars of Ageing, and Resources, page 479).

THINK ZINC

There are specific foods that are known to enhance virility. They include seeds and nuts, legumes, organic liver and oysters. All of them are good sources of zinc. Zinc is the most important mineral for healthy male sexual function. It exists in great concentration in sperm. The more sexual your life becomes and the more ejaculations that take place, the greater will be your body's demand for zinc. If you have a zinc deficiency, this can lead not only to a lowered libido – since your body will try to conserve its supply of this vital trace mineral – it can also lead to poor quality sperm. All of the anti-oxidants are particularly important for sexual function. Vitamin A, vitamin C, vitamin B_3, vitamin B_6 and vitamin E and of course the phytonutrients

Do I look heavyish to you? I feel heavyish. Put a note on my desk in the morning, 'Think thin'.

Cary Grant to his secretary,
North by Northwest

in low-glycaemic vegetables such as spinach, broccoli, bok choy and cauli-flower. Be sure to get plenty of omega-3 fats by eating the fatty fishes and using flaxseed oil. A good quality multiple vitamin and mineral formula is important, past the age of 25 or 30, if you value your sexuality.

THE FIVE KEY HABITS

A recent Harvard University study indicated that more than 80 percent of heart attacks in men can be prevented by making five simple lifestyle changes. These same changes help prevent sexual dysfunction.

- ❑ Don't smoke.
- ❑ Exercise at least 30 minutes a day.
- ❑ Maintain your ideal weight.
- ❑ Eat more high fibre food, especially low-glycaemic fruits and vegetables rich in B complex vitamins, while cutting back heavily on sugar and all processed foods and favouring fish over fatty meat.
- ❑ Drink half a glass of wine or grape juice each day (not beer). Recent studies indicate that this can be red or white wine.
- ❑ Take a good multiple vitamin and mineral replete with phytonutrients like licopene, the flavonoids, carotenoids and sulpharophane.

HORMONES – GOOD BAD AND UGLY

Testosterone is the big one. This male hormone causes the penis and testicles to develop before birth and to grow large during puberty. Made mostly in the testicles, testosterone triggers the growth of body hair and beards. It deepens a boy's voice, turning him into a man. It can also be the culprit behind male acne and male pattern baldness. Many believe that it is the high levels of testosterone which make men more assertive and aggressive than women. But testosterone is by no means the only sex hormone that men produce. They also secrete small quantities of oestrogen, the female sex hormone, in the same way that women produce small amounts of testosterone. When oestrogen levels become too high in a man, he develops female sex characteristics including the laying down of fat over the pectorals so they begin to resemble female breasts. Beards become scanty. Men lose muscle mass and their testicles can shrink while their fertility diminishes. They can have problems getting an erection.

Ironically, one of the things that increases levels of female hormones in the male body is the habit many body builders have of using steroid hormones to bulk up their muscles. It is a dangerous practice. The cascade of the body's own steroid hormones which include both male and female sexual hormones, is a complex one. When you take too much of an artificial steroid or hormone such as testosterone, it can actually turn into oestrogen in the body, causing what are commonly known among body builders as 'bitch tits'.

POST-MODERN PLAGUE

In the last 50 years there has been a dramatic decrease both in the average quantity and quality of human sperm. In 1940 the average sperm count was 113,000,000 per ml. By 1990, it had fallen to only 66,000,000 per ml. During the same period the amount of seminal fluid also fell by 20 percent. In effect, today's men produce only about 40 percent as many sperm with each ejaculation as men living 50 years ago. Experts believe that some of the drop in sperm count is due to increased use of convenience foods filled with junk fats and sugar and to lack of regular exercise. However, much of it is also attributable to these dangerous oestrogen-mimicking chemicals in our environment.

TOXINS ARE NOT SEXY

More of a worry – this affects just about everyone – is the unwitting intake of chemical oestrogens from environmental pollution, which continues to disrupt our reproductive system. Herbicides, pesticides and plastics as well as industrial pollutants continue to pollute our food chain. These petrochemically derived compounds are in fact oestrogen mimics known as *xenoestrogens*. Oestrogens and testosterone are antagonists. They need to balance each other. And the balance, which is different in men than in women, has to be just right. In most bodies, it no longer is. In many countries livestock continues to be plied with artificial oestrogens to fatten them. You end up with cow's milk containing a substantial amount of oestrogen. Even our drinking waters may be filled with oestrogen. Water purification systems are unable to eliminate from the water supply the oestrogen excreted by women on birth control pills and hormone replacement therapy. Rising levels of oestrogen in the environment have done untold damage to human and animal reproduction. They are a major issue in the development of abnormalities – from infertility in both men and women, to certain forms of cancer.

ORGANIC SOYA CAN HELP

Here's how to help protect yourself from xenoestrogens:

Use organic foods that are not sprayed with these hormone-like chemicals. Eat good quantities of soya products (which have not been genetically modified). Soya milk, soya flour, cooked soya beans and roasted soya nuts, tofu, soy sauce, tempeh etc. are high in natural oestrogens known as *phyto-estrogens*. These plant-based chemicals are very gentle and have protective effects against the environmental oestrogens. Throughout your body, your cells have oestrogen receptors which enable them to take up female hormones from your bloodstream. Xenoestrogens are taken up by these receptor sites and disrupt the system. Oestrogen receptor sites welcome phytoestrogens and let them come into these sites, blocking the uptake of the dangerous chemical varieties in the environment. Soya foods are rich in *isoflavones* such as *genistein* and *daidzeiene* – powerful anti-oxidants, to help protect against cancer and free-radical damage to the body. You could also take supplements of isoflavones. But the best way to get them is through the foods you eat. There are other benefits to soya as well, not related to male reproduction. They help to lower high blood cholesterol levels and may help protect against heart disease as well.

– May I ask what your profession is?
– Certainly, I am a genius.
Clifton Webb to Maureen O'Hara, Sitting Pretty

Now let's look at some of the specific male concerns and natural ways of helping them.

IMPOTENCE

These days they call it erectile dysfunction in order to separate it out from other difficulties like loss of libido, premature ejaculation and infertility or an inability to experience orgasm. Recent studies show that more than 50 percent of men between the ages of 40 and 60 have problems with erection. They are not so much a result of ageing but rather the result of a less than optimal lifestyle for health. In 85 percent of these cases, erectile dysfunction comes from a physiological cause – blood circulation for instance, abuse of alcohol or drugs or some kind of metabolic dysfunction like diabetes. Very occasionally prostate surgery or another abdominal operation has severed the nerves responsible for an erection. For one man in 10, the cause is psychological as a consequence of anxiety, depression or stress. In nearly half of the men who experience erectile dysfunction you will also find evidence of arteriosclerosis – the hardening of the arteries which interferes with blood vessels throughout the body, including those which feed the penis. Age Power's Insulin Balance, combined with a good multiple vitamin and mineral which includes lots of vitamin B$_3$ or niacin, especially in the form of *inositalhexaniacinate*, can improve blood flow throughout the body and help reduce the risk of arteriosclerosis. Be particularly careful of any prescription medications you take. They can interfere with sexual functions of all kinds and often do.

We must be willing to fail and to appreciate the truth that often 'Life is not a problem to be solved, but a mystery to be lived'.

M Scott Peck

It's not the men in my life that count – it's the life in my men.

Mae West

DON'T MIX DRUGS AND SEX

Be particularly wary of using any of these:

- ❑ Anti-hypertensives for lowering blood pressure
- ❑ Diuretics
- ❑ Calcium channel blockers
- ❑ Beta blockers and ACE Inhibitors
- ❑ Alcohol
- ❑ Tobacco
- ❑ Recreational drugs including marijuana, cocaine, amphetamines or heroin
- ❑ Allergy and cold medications containing anti-histamines
- ❑ Sedatives and muscle relaxants such as diazepam (Valium)
- ❑ Some antibiotics
- ❑ Histamine blockers used to treat ulcers
- ❑ Epilepsy drugs
- ❑ Anti-spasmodic drugs for nausea, Parkinson's disease and irritable bowel syndrome

Abuse of alcohol and tobacco are fast tracks to impotence. Drinking a great deal, especially over a long period of time, can actually shrink your testicles and reduce testosterone. Cigarettes interfere with circulation and inhibit a man's ability to achieve erection. Hormones matter too. Testosterone levels tend to drop by about one percent a year. If you have hyperthyroidism, this undermines the functioning of every cell in your body. So do high levels of prolactin – the hormone which, in women, stimulates the production of the breasts. Diabetes increases the risk of impotence dramatically as a result of the nerve damage and the arteriosclerosis it engenders.

I never smoked a cigarette until I was nine.

W.C. Fields

NATURE'S WAY

There are all sorts of natural things that can be enormously effective in banishing erectile dysfunction in men of any age. A diet rich in low-glycaemic fruits and vegetables filled with phytonutrients, some whole grains and legumes is ideal. Eliminate sugar. Sugar kills sexuality and undermines vitality more than anything else. Get plenty of protein from organic meats, game, chicken, turkey and especially from fish rich in omega-3 fats. Use microfiltered whey protein in drinks and snacks. Supplements of zinc can be useful, as can other key nutrients including vitamin A, vitamin B_6 vitamin C and vitamin E.

GINKGO *Ginkgo Biloba*

This ancient tree is enormously useful in treating vascular insufficiency of all kinds, including the brain and the penis. Ginkgo is especially useful for erectile dysfunction that has been caused by poor blood flow. Doctors using it recommend taking between 40 mg and 80 mg of a ginkgo extract standardised to contain 24 percent flavonglycosides. Be patient with ginkgo for it takes time to work its wonders. Expect results within six to 12 weeks.

CAUTION: Ginkgo should not be taken with blood thinning medications.

GINSENG *Panax ginseng*

Panax ginseng has been long used to increase sexual activity and enhance mating behaviour in animals. And while there have never been human studies to support the belief that ginseng is a sexual rejuvenator, there is much anecdotal evidence that this is so. Ginseng boosts testosterone levels in animals. The standard dose is from 100 to 300 mg of ginseng powder or extract containing five to 10 percent of the Panax ginseng root taken one to three times a day. It is best to start with a low dose and then increase gradually. In some people, high doses may cause sleep problems. Ginseng is an adaptogen. Taken over a long period of time it helps strengthen your body's ability to deal with stress as well.

DON'T GO THERE

YOHIMBE *Pausinystalia johimbe*
This bark of the tree from West Africa has long been used as
an aphrodisiac. An alkaloid, it increases peripheral blood flow
and appears to work to promote erections by stimulating
nerves in the genital area as well as in the central nervous
system as a whole. There are no scientific studies that verify
the use of yohimbe but there are many reports of serious
problems in using it, including tremors, palpitations, nausea
vomiting and hallucinations. In very large doses it can even
create paralysis. Although yohimbe is available on prescription
in most countries, it is something best left alone.

POTENCY WOOD or **MURIA PUAMA** *Ptychopetalum olacoides*
This Brazilian plant has a long-standing reputation as an aphrodisiac and
nerve enhancer. A recent French study showed that 1 to 1.5 g of the
extract given daily was helpful to more than 50 percent of men with erectile dysfunction and raised libido in more than 60 percent.

DAMIANA *Turnera diffusa*
For more than 100 years in the United States, Damiana has been used to
enhance sexual performance, despite the lack of clinical studies to support
this belief. You will often find it combined with other herbs to enhance
sexuality for both men and women. It can be taken in the form of a herb
tea. Those who use it claim that even one cup can exert a positive effect.

HORMONES IF YOU REALLY NEED THEM

❑ **Testosterone injections** every two to four weeks can help correct low hormone levels and improve erectile dysfunction. This can also be done with a skin patch attached to the arm or a shaved area of the scrotum.

❑ **DHEA** can be used to boost testosterone. It is usually given daily on an empty stomach in oral doses of 25 to 50 mg. It, too, needs to be used only as an adjunct to improving your diet and lifestyle.

❑ **Androstenedione** This hormone is only one step away from testosterone in the cascade of steroids. Taken on an empty stomach at a dose of 50 mg a day, it is a favourite of physicians who lean towards more natural approaches – particularly in cases where DHEA does not respond.

CAUTION: There is some evidence that androstenedione can raise testosterone levels in older men and women but it should never be used by anyone under 30 years of age. If testosterone levels are high (as they tend to be in young men), the body's metabolic pathways can convert androstenedione into oestrogen. This would only make the condition worse. In a recent study carried out at the University of Iowa, where 300 mg of androstenedione was given to young men, researchers discovered that while the levels of testosterone in their blood remained unaffected by this supplement, their oestrogen levels increased dramatically. Androstenedione is of no benefit whatsoever to young men with normal levels of testosterone. Indeed, it carries significant health risks for them.

Many of us are not getting our minimum requirement of sensual pleasure.

Robert Ornstein, PhD, and David Sobel, MD

MALE INFERTILITY

Most male infertility comes from a low sperm count. With each ejaculation a man produces up to 200,000,000 sperm, even though only one sperm is needed to fertilise the egg. Very occasionally, male infertility is the result of some sort of obstruction in the nerve ducts. Often stress, the abuse of drugs or alcohol and poor diet lowers the sperm count temporarily. So can lack of sleep, exposure to radiation, solvents, pesticides and other toxins. Even having a cold or the flu or not getting enough sleep can affect sperm count. Long-term male sperm count is now seriously affected by xenoestrogens in the environment.

STAY COOL

Testicles are highly sensitive to changes in temperature. This is probably why they are attached to the outside of the body so that they can be kept a degree or two cooler than body temperature. Boxer shorts are much better than briefs in protecting fertility as they do not hold the testicles so close to the body. Tight fitting jeans and trousers, as well as soaks in hot tubs or long bouts of strenuous exercise, should be followed by a period in which the testicles are allowed to hang free to recover their normal temperature. Natural medicine in Germany has long promoted the use of hydrotherapy, especially daily cold showers, as a method for enhancing fertility. Many swear by its effectiveness.

Not only the quantity of sperm matters. So does the quality. A high sperm count of unhealthy or abnormal sperm means poor fertility. There are standard tests available to measure sperm function including motility and the presence of anti-sperm antibodies that sometimes result from infection and can affect male reproduction. Alcohol, tobacco and recreational drugs undermine sperm health. Steer clear of them. So can free radical damage. Forty percent of infertile men have high levels of free radicals. Exposure to heavy metals like mercury, arsenic, cadmium and lead undermines fertility too. This is a major reason why some of the most powerful natural methods for dealing with male infertility are based on giving a high level of free radical protection and detoxifying the body.

NATURAL HELP WHEN YOU NEED IT

TAKE ZINC

Essential for healthy sperm as well as a good sperm count, a deficiency in zinc can lower testosterone levels. One recent study showed that when men with low testosterone levels were given zinc supplements, it not only raised their sperm counts but also increased the pregnancy rate in their partners. Men with normal testosterone levels did not benefit from this. The usual recommended dose of zinc for infertility is between 20 and 50 mg a day, taken at the end of the day. It is often given with 1 mg of copper at the beginning of the day (these two trace element minerals must not be taken together as they are antagonists).

CAUTION: Too much zinc over too long a period of time can be toxic so it is important not to go higher than this.

TRY VITAMIN B$_{12}$

Essential for making new cells, a deficiency in this vitamin can lead to reduced sperm count and lowered motility. In one double-blind study of almost 400 infertile men, supplementation with vitamin B$_{12}$ proved helpful to those with a significantly low sperm count. Other studies show that 1 to 6mg. of vitamin B$_{12}$ a day can significantly improve fertility.

USE L-CARNITINE

This amino acid is used by the body to turn fat into energy, encouraging the breaking down of long chain fatty acids in the mitochondria. Healthy sperm has a very high concentration of carnitine which also appears to promote sperm motility. In addition to the use of carnitine to help the body heal itself in the cases of various muscular diseases as well as heart conditions, supplements in doses of 500 to 1000 mg of L-carnitine three times a day have shown themselves to be useful in infertility.

CAUTION: Make sure that you get L-carnitine, not D-carnitine or DL-carnitine when buying supplements. D-carnitine and DL-carnitine can actually interfere with the metabolism of L-carnitine in the body and cause muscle pain. Carnitine is an expensive supplement. It is probably best to use only as a last resort unless money is no object.

WATCH YOUR FAT
Stay away from hydrogenated plant oils found in margarines as well as processed golden oils on supermarket shelves, especially cottonseed oil which not only can contain toxic residues but also a substance called *glossypoll* – shown to inhibit sperm function. Make sure you get plenty of omega-3 fats by eating fatty fish and using flaxseed oil. Stay away from convenience foods that are riddled with junk fats. Use olive oil for salads and cooking.

USE ANTI-OXIDANT SUPPLEMENTS
Many double-blind placebo-controlled studies of infertile men indicate that anti-oxidants can be of enormous benefit for male infertility. Even 100 international units of vitamin E improve sperm activity and increase the pregnancy rate of partners. Vitamin C, too, can increase sperm count and function, in doses from 500 to 2000 mg a day. Vitamin C helps protect the sperms DNA from damage. So may supplements Co-enzyme Q10, PABA, Selenium, beta carotene and the amino acid L-arginine.

GET INTO HERBS
Most of the herbs used to treat impotence are also helpful for male infertility. There are clinical reports that ashwagandha and pygeum can help.

I am Giacomo, a lover of beauty and a beauty of a lover.

Danny Kaye,
The Court Jester

PROSTATE ENLARGEMENT

If you are male and live long enough you are likely to develop benign prostatic hyperplasia (BPH). Ninety percent of men in the Western world do by the time they are 80. It brings with it annoying symptoms such as a sensation of fullness in the bladder even after you have urinated, difficulty in starting urination and a diminished flow. A man of 20 has a prostate gland which weighs less than an ounce and sits quietly beneath the bladder and in front of the rectum. By the age of 40 or 50, his prostate gland can begin to change and grow bigger, eventually pressing against the urethra, impeding the urine flow and making some prone to bladder infection. No one is quite sure what causes BPH. Some believe it to be hormone changes within the prostate. Others insist that high levels of dihydrotestosterone trigger the development of changed cells which, in a very small number of cases, can lead to malignancy. Should you experience any of the symptoms associated with BPH it is important that you have a checkup with your doctor before beginning any course of treatment, either drug-based or natural.

GET IT CHECKED

Even though most prostatic enlargement is fundamentally harmless, go to see your doctor to rule out any prostatic cancer. Prostate cancer is the most common malignancy among men in the Western world. Its incidence has been rising steadily over the past 30 years. Check up on any prostate enlargement and rule out prostate cancer immediately. Early screening is important too since chances of survival are excellent if cancer does exist, provided it is detected and treated while still confined to the prostate gland. The examination is usually carried out by ultrasound and/or digitally. A sample of urine or prostatic fluid may also be taken and blood tests used to measure levels of prostate specific antigen (PSA). If it is above 4.0 this is generally believed to indicate that a further investigation should be made, often including a biopsy. Once cancer is ruled out there are numerous natural methods available, with good scientific backing, to help clear BPE.

SAY YES TO NATURAL HELP

What anti-oxidants and herbs can do for other reproductive dysfunctions, they can also do for benign prostatic hyperplasia. In fact they usually work far better than drugs and don't carry dangerous side effects.

VITAMIN E – Protector

A study of 30,000 men in Finland showed that those who had taken supplements of vitamin E over several years had a third less prostate cancer than those who did not. Recommended dose of vitamin E is 400 to 1000 international units of alpha-tocopherol.

CAUTION: Vitamin E supplementation should be started at a low dose if you have high blood pressure. Then gradually increased very high doses of the vitamin – above 1500 IUS a day – need to be taken with caution by anyone who is using aspirin or other blood thinners.

ZINC AND SELENIUM – The Magic Minerals

These anti-oxidant minerals work particularly well with vitamin E to give extra protection against free radical damage. They are believed to help slow prostate growth and prevent prostate cancer. The usual supplement dose of selenium is 200 to 400 mcg and of zinc is 15 mg to 50 mg a day.

CAUTION: Doses of selenium above 800 mcg a day can be toxic. Long-term use of doses above 30 mg of zinc taken in the evening should be balanced with 1 mg of copper taken in the morning.

LYCOPENE – Eat Tomatoes

This carotenoid, found in good quantity in tomatoes, as well as other bright coloured fruits and vegetables, tends to concentrate in the prostate. A large scale study of almost 50,000 men carried out over six years showed that the lowest incidence of prostate cancer among men occurred in those who ate at least 10 servings a week of tomatoes, especially in a cooked form such as tomato sauce. Lycopene can also be taken in supplemental form. The usual dose is 60 to 120 mg a day with food.

SOYA FOODS – Plant Hormones Help

Tofu, soya nuts, soya milk and tempeh are all rich in isoflavones.

There is considerable evidence that isoflavones help prevent prostate enlargement because they help protect from xenoestrogens damage. They may also help to detoxify dihydrotestosterone (DHT) which many believe to be responsible for prostate enlargement. Many doctors in natural medicine recommend eating 25 to 50 g of powdered soya protein each day. You can add it to fresh vegetable or fruit juice or soya milk to make a smoothie for breakfast.

CAUTION: Make sure that as many of the soya products you use as possible are organic and free from GMO's (genetically modulated organisms).

HERBS HOLD A KEY
Many plants offer great help, check them out.

SAW PALMETTO *serenoa repens*
At least seven double-blind studies involving more than 500 men comparing the effects of saw palmetto and placebos have shown that in cases of BPH, the herb significantly improved urinary flow rate. So effective is this herb that another double-blind study which followed over 1000 men who received either saw palmetto or the leading drug for the treatment of BPH, had equally good results in stemming urine flow. Recommended dose of saw palmetto is 160 mg twice a day of extract standardised to contain 85 to 95 percent of the plant's fatty acids and sterols. Saw palmetto appears non-toxic and is virtually side-effect free.

PYGEUM *Pygeum africanum*
The bark of this tall evergreen African prune tree has been used for centuries for urinary problems. Good clinical evidence in Europe shows that it is a useful treatment for prostatitis as well as impotence and male infertility. Double-blind studies have shown that pygeum helps reduce symptoms of night-time urination, residual urine volume and urinary frequency. Recommended doses are from 50 to 100 mg twice a day. Pygeum is believed to reduce inflammation of the prostate and to inhibit prostate growth factor. Many practitioners combine pygeum with nettle root as they appear to work best in combination.

> First you forget names, then you forget faces. Next you forget to pull your zipper up. Then finally you forget to pull it down.
>
> *George Burns*

NETTLE ROOT *Urtica dicoica*

A popular European treatment for enlarged prostate, nettle root given over several months can reduce the obstruction of urinary flow and decrease night-time urination. Nettle root extracts contain compounds which inhibit the action of hormones believed to stimulate the growth of prostate tissue. The standard dose – according to Germany's Commission E, the official body that regulates herbal medicines – is from 4 to 6 g of the whole root or a proportional dose of the concentrated extract a day. When using standardised nettle root extract twice a day the usual dose is 120 mg. Nettle root is often taken together with saw palmetto and/or pygeum. This plant is virtually non-toxic, even in large doses.

POWERWOMAN

The age of a woman doesn't mean a thing. The best tunes are
played on the oldest fiddles.

Sigmund Engel

We are riding a wave of revolution in women's anti-ageing
natural health care. This time, it is not pregnancy and
natural childbirth which are its focus but attitudes and
treatments given to women before, during and after
menopause – including the use of drug-based oestrogens
and progestins prescribed as HRT.

Nobody ever prepares you for menopause. Nobody tells you that if you
are going to have hot flushes or emotional instability they are likely to be
far worse *before* you stop menstruating than afterwards. Nor does anybody
explain that waking regularly at two or three in the morning and lying in
bed filled with sadness or fear or anger is likely to be not some aberration
of nature, but a messenger announcing that menopause is near. And because
we are still told so little about menopause – apart from the scaremongering
that equates the menopause with a disease – something that needs fixing
– few women in our culture are prepared for the next phase of their life.
We seldom expect the intensity of emotion – both pain and pleasure – that
can accompany the end of the childbearing years, nor do most of us realise
that such passions can be transmuted into creative power.

LISTEN TO THE WHISPERS

There are many signs that the change is near. Alterations in
menstruation for instance. Periods can become longer, heavier,
shorter, lighter or irregular. You can find your feelings go up
and down very much the way they did in puberty so that one
moment you are completely content with your life and the
next you want to throw everything up and go off to India to
'find yourself'. You may begin to experience a growing dis-
satisfaction with the parts of your life that used to seem fine.
You may find yourself very tired without apparent reason.
You may also begin to get aches and pains in joints or find
your skin suddenly seems to sag or look sallow.

PERIMENOPAUSAL PAUSES

Some or all of these things can happen to a woman in mid-life. They are commonly lumped together with menopause, some can be *temporarily* masked by giving hormone drugs, however most have little to do with the change: Aches and pains in the joints, weight gain and ageing skin for instance as well as the sense many women report that they have climbed to the top of the ladder only to find that it was against the wrong wall. Such symptoms are really signs that a woman's lifestyle – probably her values too – needs revising. It could be time to give up the work you are doing and do something else, to follow your passion, or simply to begin to care for yourself again – to take up weight training, to learn a technique for meditation or deep relaxation, to re-educate the way your body moves through Feldenkais, or to revise your way of cooking and eating.

MY OWN VALUES

My own experience of a natural menopause has made me clear about what I think and what my values are. I believe:

❑ That each woman is born unique and gifted.
❑ That creativity is wild and free and female in nature even when found in a man.
❑ That too often a woman's creativity is kept within. Unless she takes action herself it tends to remain imprisoned.
❑ That every woman has a right to walk her own path and speak with her own voice.
❑ That all life, art, sexuality, wishes and dreams move in cycles as do the flow and ebb of a woman's hormones.
❑ That as women we have tended to allow our own imprisonment and treat it as normal.
❑ That a woman must above all honour her instincts.
❑ That a woman's wild spirit is best fed when she surrounds herself with what she loves and does the things she likes doing best.

FILL THE GAPS

If you have been eating convenience foods or going on and off crash diets over the years in an attempt to keep your weight down you will have inevitably created biochemical imbalances in your body. Deficiencies of minerals such as magnesium and zinc or trace elements such as boron or chromium, along with excesses of heavy metals such as lead or aluminium from your environment, radically interfere with the functions of enzymes in your body which are responsible for the manufacture of hormones, for the digestion of food and assimilation of nutrients and for the production of energy. Our bodies have a remarkable ability to compensate for a deficiency here and there. But, as a result of chemical farming which unbalances minerals, depletes the soils and therefore our foods of trace elements and as well as food processing which further depletes vitamins and minerals and puts chemicals into our bodies that do not belong there, by the time mid-life arrives most women have accumulated many metabolic imbalances. In time these biochemical distortions begin to create symptoms – mood swings or depression that occur because of a resultant deficiency in brain chemicals such as serotonin, low levels of adrenal hormones that we need to cope with stress and to protect against inflammation in the tissues, and fatigue with no apparent cause. Perhaps a woman also begins to get hot flushes or night sweats, both of which are a normal and temporary part of the re-adjustment in hormones that takes place during the profound passage of menopause yet which are often thought of as an illness and so she goes to her doctor for help.

Because few doctors are trained in either nutrition or metabolic biochemistry nor are they aware of how to use effective plant substances and natural hormones to ease a woman's passage through the change they believe there is no alternative but to put the woman on drug-based HRT. He will choose from an enormous variety of combinations of oestrogen and artificial progestin drugs, the latter being added to help protect her from cancer. It has been well established that giving oestrogen on its own is dangerous – predisposing a woman taking it to cancer of the breast and womb.

If you can't beat them
arrange to have them
beaten.

George Clooney

TO DRUG OR NOT TO DRUG

The experience of taking HRT varies widely from one woman to another. Some feel great on it. Others feel lousy and gain weight. More commonly a woman will feel better for a few months and then begin to report unpleasant side-effects from the drugs she is taking. The most common complaints from prolonged HRT are migraine, bleeding, depression, water retention, increased blood pressure, weight gain, thrush, breast problems, varicose veins and chest pains. A Swedish survey in the university town of Linkoping showed that 48 percent of women who go on HRT stop taking the drug within a year. A recent British study examined the reasons most commonly given by women who give up HRT after starting the treatment: About half stop taking it because of side-effects, about one-fifth because they are advised to do so by their doctors and about one-third either because they are afraid of long-term consequences such as cancer or because HRT has shown itself to be ineffective in helping them.

Health educators such as Sandra Coney author of *The Menopause Industry* and Dr Robert Jacobs at the Society for Complementary Medicine in London, scientists such as biologist Renata Klein and doctors such as John Lee MD – the first doctor to carry out a study on 100 women and to have been able to *reverse* osteoporosis naturally – vigorously challenge the wisdom of established medical practices in the treatment of women with drug-based hormones. They also object to the widespread propaganda which accompanies the sale of HRT claiming that the indiscriminate doling out of potent drug-based hormones can undermine a woman's fertility as well as trigger the development of menstrual agonies – from PMS and endometriosis to cancer of the breast and womb. So do I. This practice of making virtually every woman a 'patient' for most of her life by subjecting her to drug treatment not only where it is not necessary but when it can be potentially dangerous is a way of diminishing her personal power and taking away control over her own body. It is biologically, politically and morally reprehensible.

In our modern industrialised world it is easy for a woman's biochemistry to become distorted not only as a result of declining physical activity and from eating a diet of highly processed convenience foods, but as a consequence of the rise of a whole new – as yet largely unrecognised – phenomenon known as *oestrogen dominance*. This is where a woman's oestrogen levels far outweigh progesterone

> Statistics show that there are more women in the world than anything else – except insects.
>
> *Glenn Ford*

CO-A FOR WOMANPOWER

The energy demands on your body made by 20 or 30 years of hormone cycles each month as well as the intense biological expenditure and upheaval of pregnancy and birth can rob your body of life force and create chemical imbalances. Such imbalances can show up as distorted biomarkers – high cholesterol, triglycerides and blood pressure, fat gain and frazzled nerves. For they diminish your body's Coenzyme-A pool. Co-A is central to your ability to cope with stress and remain free of depression and anxiety. It also strengthens immunity and can prevent the energy slump that comes with a period. Co-A also plays a major role in supporting the formation of sex hormones. The changes you will experience in energy, good looks, personal power and emotional balance using Co-A are subtle, yet profound and also cumulative. Three months down the road you look back and can hardly remember what it used to be like having no energy because you feel so good. It takes time to replenish you Co-A after having had it depleted for years but the rewards are wonderful.

Dose: 1 capsule of Coenzyme-A three times a day on an empty stomach (i.e. half an hour before a meal).

in her body making her prone to cancer, menstrual miseries and menopausal difficulties. Oestrogen dominance has developed for many reasons in industrialised countries, including the widespread use of oestrogen-based oral contraceptives and the exponential spread of chemicals in our environment which are oestrogen mimics. These are taken up by the oestrogen receptor sites in a woman's body to throw spanners in her metabolic works.

BEWARE CHEMICAL OESTROGENS

Called *xenoestrogens,* these are found in the petrochemical derivatives we take in as herbicides and pesticides sprayed on our foods, in the plastic cups we drink our tea from, the plastics our foods are wrapped in and even the oestrogens that come through drinking water recycled from our rivers. Oestrogens from the Pill and HRT are excreted in a woman's urine. They end up in water and cannot be removed by standard water purification treatments. Every woman needs to be aware of the potential dangers of the

STOP GAP

Unlike changes in diet and lifestyle, at best HRT is a stop-gap measure which addresses symptoms but offers little in the way of genuinely strengthening and re-balancing a woman's body. And as far as the treatment of hot flushes is concerned – the single major symptom which *is* part of menopause – plant-based treatments from wild yam or angus castus to angelica, will tend to work more slowly but will also tend to eliminate hot flushes completely. The woman who opts for HRT as a way of treating hot flushes finds that the moment she stops taking the oestrogen – whether in a few months or 10 years – her hot flushes return.

'sea of oestrogens' in which we now live. Not long ago, Greenpeace issued a report describing the effect that xenoestrogens are having on men's sperm count. It has dropped by more than 40 percent in 50 years. But far more devastating – and much less publicised – are the effects that the rising sea of oestrogens and oestrogen dominance have on women's lives.

> Women sit or move to and fro, some old some young. The young are beautiful – but the old are more beautiful than the young.
>
> *Walt Whitman*

Oestrogen dominance – too much oestrogen and too little progesterone – makes us more prone to breast and womb cancer, to fibroid tumours, to endometriosis, to osteoporosis and to infertility – not to mention a long list of emotional and mental imbalances. However, because much of the medical profession as well as the general public remains largely ignorant of the effects of xenoestrogens and the growing oestrogen dominance in women's bodies, oestrogens continue to be prescribed heavily as part of HRT. And not only to the handful of women who, around the time of menopause, would choose to use HRT temporarily to counter perimenopausal

> Each reproductive cycle depletes some Coenzyme-A from a resource that is very often deficient from the start. Added to this is pregnancy and nutritional deficiencies. Both of these deplete even more Coenzyme-A, allowing the deficiency to become even more severe. This is why many women gain a significant amount of weight after having children and also when they are peri-menopausal and menopausal. Their Coenzyme-A pool is dwindling.
>
> *Nicholas Skouras PhD*

HORMONES – THE BIG TWO

There are two classes of major reproductive hormones in a woman's body – the oestrogens (which are commonly lumped together and called 'oestrogen') and progesterone. When these two are in good balance, a woman's health thrives. She remains free of PMS and other menstrual troubles. She is fertile and able to hold a foetus to full term and menopause becomes a simple transition instead of a passage riddled with suffering. She is also protected against fibroids, endometriosis and osteoporosis and she is likely to remain emotionally balanced and free of excessive anxiety or depression. When oestrogen and progesterone are not in balance in a woman's body all of these things come a cropper.

symptoms, but for thousands of women whose lives would be far better off without it. Neither do they know that hot flushes, dry vaginas and early ageing can be addressed more safely and successfully – not to mention less expensively – by alterations in diet to eliminate highly processed convenience foods replete with junk fats which can interfere with the production of important hormones and prostaglandins in a woman's body. Changing to a diet such as Age Power's Insulin Balance, for instance. Changes in lifestyle and the use of traditional herbal remedies such as wild yam (from which incidentally many of the drugs sold for HRT are derived), chastetree, motherwort and black cohosh, have a much more lasting effect.

When the sun comes up, I have morals again.
Elizabeth Taylor

PLAGUE OF PLAGUES

A strange and highly dangerous marriage is taking place between the increase of oestrogen-mimicking chemicals in the environment and the rise in various oestrogens prescribed medically to women. It is out of this union that oestrogen dominance has largely developed. The oestrogens and progesterone in a woman's body must balance each other for a woman to remain healthy. In many of us they are becoming more and more out of kilter.

DISEASE ON THE RISE

We are now seeing a widespread rise in many diseases and discomforts for which – with strange irony – doctors are prescribing more oestrogen. Here are a few of the ways in which oestrogen dominance can manifest:

When oestrogen is not balanced by progesterone it can produce weight gain, headache, bad temper, chronic fatigue and loss of interest in sex – all of which are part of the clinically recognised pre-menstrual syndrome or PMS.

Not only has it been well established that oestrogen dominance encourages the development of breast cancer thanks to oestrogen's actions, it also stimulates breast tissue and can in time trigger fibrocystic breast disease – a condition which wanes when natural progesterone is added to a woman's body to balance the oestrogen.

By definition, excess oestrogen implies a progesterone deficiency. This in turn leads to a decrease in the rate of new bone formation in a woman's body. This is the prime cause of osteoporosis.

Oestrogen dominance increases the risk of fibroids. One of the interesting facts about fibroids – often remarked upon by doctors – is that, regardless of their size, fibroids commonly shrink once menopause arrives and a woman's ovaries are no longer making oestrogen.

In oestrogen-dominant menstruating women where progesterone is not peaking and falling in a normal way each month, the ordered shedding of the womb lining doesn't take place. Irregular menstruation cycles result.

Beauty is but the spirit breaking through the flesh.

August Rodin

Endometrial cancer – cancer of the womb – develops only where there is oestrogen dominance. Some of the artificial progesterones may also help prevent it, which is why a growing number of doctors no longer give oestrogen without combining it with a *progestagin* drug during HRT. A natural progesterone cream is better.

Water retention and an increase in sodium levels in the body which predispose a woman to high blood pressure – hypertension – frequently occurs with oestrogen dominance. This can also be a side-effect of taking a progestagin-drug.

The risk of heart disease is increased dramatically when a woman is oestrogen dominant.

I am by no means altogether opposed to HRT. But I want to see it put into perspective. I believe that, while it may be useful for short periods in a small number of women who actually *need* oestrogen, the use of drug-based hormones in most women's cases is costly both in financial and physical terms. Drug-based oestrogens and progestagins in the 'treatment' of menopause is not a good plan because virtually all have been shown to have dangerous side-effects and because, for many who have followed such advice, the use of hormone drugs has ultimately created more problems than it has solved. There are better, more natural, ways.

FOREIGN MOLECULES

Unlike the artificial progestins and progestagins prescribed in conventional HRT, natural progesterone cream has virtually no side-effects since it is an identical molecule to that of the hormone itself. As such the body has the enzymes needed to metabolise it easily. Progesterone is also superior to the progestins because it is a biochemical *precursor* to many other important hormones in the body. This means your body can turn it into other important hormones – hormones which help protect your body from stress damage and hormones which support brain function and balance emotions. Progesterone – the real thing – can even be transformed into the natural oestrogens if your body has need of them. By contrast, progestin drugs are '*end product molecules*'. They cannot be converted into other important body chemicals that are needed for emotional and physical health. As such, their presence in the body may actually interfere with these conversions.

As drugs, the progestins *have* to be unique molecules foreign to the human body to be patented and sold. There are no big profits for anybody in selling a generic substance like a natural progesterone cream. This is another reason why so many doctors remain ignorant of its value in the treatment of women who could benefit from extra hormones. Unlike oestrogen, commonly given in HRT to help slow down bone loss, progesterone actually *increases* bone density. It effectively stimulates the activity of osteoblasts – the cells which make new bone. By contrast no drug has ever been shown to do this to any significant degree.

PROGESTERONE CREAM

One alternative to the currently available HRT appears to offer many new benefits yet is virtually side-effect free. It consists of using plant derived *natural* progesterone – natural in the sense that it is the identical molecule to that found in a woman's body – in the form of a cream applied to the body. Progesterone cannot only help eliminate oestrogen dominance in a woman's body, re-establishing hormonal balance, it can therefore help protect against the many conditions with which oestrogen dominance is associated.

In many countries, the progesterone used for natural HRT is readily available to women for their own use without a prescription. In Britain it is available by prescription from doctors who know about it, but it can also be legally ordered by post by any woman for her own personal use from the United States or the Channel Islands. Not long ago a French study reported that not only is transdermal progesterone in small doses well absorbed, but used monthly reduces the risk of breast cancer.

BAD BLOOD PLAGUE

Mounting xenoestrogenic pollution in our environment and the widespread use of artificial hormones for birth control and HRT have produced an epidemic of female problems which develop out of a state of oestrogen dominance in a woman's body. They have set the stage for the development of a bad blood plague. It is a plague which only women themselves are able to defeat, first by becoming aware of what has been causing it and second by taking actions to counter it personally and politically. Let's look at some of the major challenges and how to help yourself through them.

PREMENSTRUAL SYNDROME

PMS is a big problem. Today somewhere between 40 and 60 percent of menstruating women in the Western world suffer to some degree from premenstrual syndrome. There are no specific laboratory tests for PMS. Neither are there specific clinical signs for the condition, which is why it is called a syndrome – a set of complex symptoms which occur together and don't appear to have one specific cause. Women with PMS can experience symptoms from bloating and depression to mood swings, headaches, weight-gain, irritability, fatigue and lack of interest in sex which begin a week or more before a period starts and last for two or three days into the period before they clear.

INNER WORLD

The causes of PMS are many: Some nutritional, some psychological, many are stress related. Even a woman's attitude towards menstruation has a part to play in the development of PMS. In our culture menstruation has long been associated with the work of the devil. It is often called 'the curse'. The whole cycling in a woman's body involving the build-up and flow of blood has been treated with humiliation. Women grow up fearing that there is something diseased and unclean about their body. Exercise (see Chapters Kiss Sarcopenia Goodbye and Shed Fat) is important for PMS not only because of the physical benefits that regular exercise brings but also because regular exercise can enhance self-esteem and erase the old patterns of feeling like a victim who goes through monthly suffering.

NUTRITIONAL SUPPORT

No nutritional supplement is going to replace a proper diet and lifestyle which supports your energy and is a reflection of the value you place on yourself. However certain supplements – especially magnesium, zinc, vitamin B_6 and the other B vitamins can be instrumental both in clearing PMS and all the other female reproductive complaints listed here and need to be looked at. In an uncontrolled study where women with PMS were given a multivitamin and mineral supplement containing high doses of magnesium and B_6, 70 percent of them showed a reduction in symptoms.

MAGNESIUM

Magnesium is an essential catalyst in many enzyme reactions – particularly those involved in energy production and sugar metabolism. A deficiency in magnesium appears to be a strong factor in the development of PMS.

BONES AT RISK

Here are some of the major factors that put your bones at risk:

❏ Poor calcium absorption as a result of inadequate vitamins and minerals including vitamin C, vitamin D, zinc and magnesium, often from years of living on a diet of processed foods.

❏ Excess phosphorous from colas or processed meats which leaches calcium from bones.

❏ Excess alcohol which renders your blood acidic and causes calcium to be leached from the bones so it can be used to lower the blood's acidity.

❏ Physical inactivity and lack of weight-bearing exercise.

❏ Smoking

❏ Frequent use of diuretics, antibiotics, antacids and drugs such as cortisone, thyroid hormones, heparin and prednisone can also disrupt the formation of good bone.

❏ Progesterone deficiency which reduces the activity of osteoblast cells so that more old bone is broken down and less new bone is being built.

❏ In a few women, inadequate oestrogen after menopause.

Magnesium levels are significantly lower in PMS sufferers than in other women. Low magnesium often produces symptoms of aches and pains as well as nervousness, lowered immunity, breast pain and weight gain. Take 400 to 800 mg chelated magnesium a day in split doses.

Women complain about premenstrual syndrome but I think of it as the only time of the month I can be myself.

Roseanne

HERBS HELP

There are a number of herbs which bring potent help to a woman wrestling with PMS. Some of the best are mother-wort, wild yam (either *Dioscorea villosa* or *Dioscorea mexicana*) black cohosh and Dong Quai.

MOTHERWORT *Leonurus cardiaca*

My favourite plant of all for PMS – particularly for the emotional ups and downs – is motherwort. Ten to 20 drops of tincture of motherwort works wonders when you are feeling unsettled. Alternatively you can take five to 15 drops of the tincture every day for a month or two to stabilise emotions long term. Motherwort is the most comforting herb I have ever come across. It brings a sense of inner security and calm strength that is unequalled by anything except perhaps for a love affair – maybe not even that.

WILD YAM *Dioscorea villosa* or *Dioscorea mexicana*

The most effective single herb for PMS for most women is wild yam from which so many hormones are derived. Taking 3 g of powdered wild yam a day split into two doses works so well on many women that, unless they are seriously oestrogen dominant, this course of action together with changes in diet and lifestyle is often enough to banish the condition permanently. And the nice thing about using wild yam is that often after taking it for three to six months, many women find they can stop using it altogether without a return of symptoms.

DANDELION ROOT *Taraxacum officinale*

Ten to 20 drops of tincture of dandelion root three times a day with meals usually works for eliminating water retention. Or drink three cups of dandelion root tea a day made with 1 teaspoon of dandelion root in a cup of boiling water.

ST JOHN'S WORT *Hypericum perforatum*
Oil of St John's Wort rubbed onto sore breasts relieves pain
thanks to its action on nerve endings.

YELLOW DOCK ROOT *Rumex crispus*
Tincture of yellow dock root – five to 10 drops two or three
times a day – can help counter indigestion, constipation and
intestinal gas.

SAGE *Salvia officinalis*
Drinking sage tea or taking tincture of sage (10 to 20 drops
three times a day) rich in phyto-hormones can help counteract PMS.

VITAMIN B COMPLEX

B complex deficiencies result in depressed liver functions. Much PMS
develops out of an excess of oestrogens in the blood that results from the
liver's inability to clear them from the system. Take a good vitamin B
complex supplement, 50 to 100 mg of the major B vitamins a day.

ZINC

Zinc deficiencies are common in women who have taken synthetic
hormones in the Pill and HRT. Coffee and tea drinking also interfere with
zinc absorption. Take 18 to 22 mg zinc citrate or zinc picolinate a day,
preferably at night.

VITAMIN E

Studies show that women given vitamin E supplements experience significant improvement in other PMS symptoms including headaches, tired-
ness, depression, insomnia and nervous tension. Take 200 to 400 IU of a
drug form of vitamin E a day.

BETA CAROTENE

Precursor to vitamin A, beta carotene is a safe alternative to vitamin A
itself. In studies it has been shown to reduce PMS symptoms. Take 50,000
IU a day.

FLAVONOIDS

Phytonutrients such as *quercetin* and *apigenin* act in the body to inhibit
the actions of excess oestrogen and have been shown to be useful in eliminating many symptoms of PMS. Take mixed flavonoids – 1,000 mg a day.

ESSENTIAL FATTY ACIDS

To manufacture and use hormones properly, essential fatty acids are necessary. The proper metabolism of essential fatty acids demands adequate magnesium, vitamin C, zinc, vitamin B_6 and vitamin B_3. This is a major reason why all of these nutrients are so important in the treatment of PMS. Using borage oil or evening primrose oil supplements which are all high in GLA can be very helpful for PMS in many women. Take 500 mg three to four times a day. You can also use flaxseed oil one to two tablespoons poured over salads or vegetables every day. Finally and most important of all, take a good source of omega-3 fish oils EPA and DHA a day to counter inflammation and cool a fiery brain.

The water retention which occurs near a menstrual period is not simple oedema. Water actually gets blocked within cells. This can mean as much as a six or eight pounds weight gain over the 10 days just before a period. In women who experience such weight gains the use of a progesterone cream for three months from day 12 to day 26 or day 27 of their menstrual cycle will almost invariably clear this up. After several weeks of using the cream, John Lee suggests that women weigh themselves during the time of the month that the oedema was always there. 'When a woman sees that the oedema is now gone,' says Lee, 'It proves to her that the progesterone is working.' After using progesterone cream Lee's patients report that they feel much better, that they feel they have a handle on their life again, they can get on with things without the disturbing effects of their PMS. 'Not all PMS is due to progesterone deficiency or oestrogen dominance,' says Lee, 'but a wide proportion of PMS women have oestrogen dominance and are helped by progesterone.'

PROGESTERONE CONNECTIONS

Underlying all premenstrual syndrome, whether primarily nutritional, emotional or stress-related in origin, is an imbalance in hormones. In most PMS the imbalance in hormones is a simple one – too much oestrogen and too little progesterone. While this is not the case for every woman it is certainly what happens in the vast majority of cases. Many of the common treatments for PMS from the use of extra vitamin B_6 to changes in diet, actually work because through one action or another they are able to influence hormone balance.

PROGESTERONE FOR PMS

Here are some of John Lee's protocols for PMS: Use a 2oz jar of progesterone cream in a 10-day period, ending just before your period. With experience many women discover that the progesterone dose can be applied in a manner to produce a crescendo effect in the four to five days just before menstruation begins. In fact some women prefer to add the use of drops of oil under the tongue during the last four to five days in addition to the progesterone cream. Others find that additional cream can be applied several times a day close to a period depending on their symptoms. 'The important thing to remember about dose,' says Lee, 'Is that the right dose of progesterone for any particular woman is the dose that works.' The way Lee achieves the crescendo dose is for a woman to use a full 2 oz jar in 10 or 12 days from days 14 to 26, or days 12 to 28, aiming to have finished the jar two days before the period. In the last five days Lee adds four drops of progesterone oil under the tongue each day. Taking progesterone under the tongue is a little tricky to get used to as the oil has to be held under the tongue for three to five minutes to allow it to be properly absorbed through the mucous membranes of the mouth. It often takes practice to hold the oil there for long enough without swallowing.

ENDOMETRIOSIS

A mysterious and rapidly increasing condition of modern times in the Western world, endometriosis is where the normal endometrium or uterine lining which develops each month, instead of breaking down and being shed fully during a menstrual period, proliferates inside the uterine cavity. Tiny islets of endometrial tissue can migrate to other areas of the pelvis, the fallopian tubes, the surface of the ovaries, even beyond to the sides of the pelvic wall and occasionally onto the bowel. Because they are of the same endometrial tissue in the womb they swell and diminish with the ebb and flow of monthly hormones, then are shed at menstrual time bringing pain in their wake. Endometriosis can be accompanied by pelvic pain, cramps, infertility and disturbed menstrual cycles. Pain is often worse at ovulation and just before and during a period. The only sure way to diagnose the condition is via *laparoscopy* although sometimes endometrial lesions can be seen during a pelvic examination on the vagina, vulva or cervix. Often endometriosis and fibroids are found together. The incidence of endometriosis has increased dramatically in recent years, partly because women are giving birth later and having fewer children, and because of widespread oestrogen-dominance. For oestrogen is the hormone of proliferation – responsible for the build-up of endometrial tissue. When it gets out of hand endometriosis can be one of the results.

STANDARD PRACTICE

The standard medical treatments for endometriosis include birth control pills, using a progestagen to suppress menstruation, prescribing analgesics and narcotics to kill the pain, or giving drugs which in effect render a woman menopausal so long as she takes them. Other drugs commonly used for the treatment of endometriosis can bring masculinisation such as facial hair growth. None of these treatments have been shown to be very successful. Surgery is another standard treatment for endometriosis – either for the removal of the endometrial lesions themselves or more radically a complete hysterectomy as well as ovary removal. The cause of endometriosis is much debated. Since adequate progesterone inhibits the proliferation of endometrial tissue, it is not surprising that a growing number of doctors, nutritionists and naturopaths prefer to recommend the cyclic use of a natural progesterone cream so that the pain and menstrual flow are adequately reduced and the need for surgery eliminated.

INNER WORLD

Endometriosis is a condition in which there is often a conflict in a woman's life between what she wants to fulfil her needs and what she has chosen to do or feels obliged to do in terms of her day-to-day life. That is perhaps why endometriosis is often called the 'career woman's ailment'. It is a way in which a woman's inner self can be demanding attention through pain or abnormal menstrual cycles – asking her to turn back from total absorption in the externals of her life and look within.

When endometriosis makes life miserable, take a little time for yourself and write down exactly how you are feeling – both physically and emotionally. This works best if it is done without paying much attention to what you are writing or trying to make sense of anything – just letting the words pour out of you. You may be surprised to find some of the impulses that get expressed and some of the desires. See what can be done gradually to create space for yourself. Do you need more time alone? Do you need to allow yourself more freedom of self-expression in your work? Your relation-

> We have women in the military, but they don't put us in the front, don't know if we can fight or if we can kill. I think we can. All the general has to do is walk over to the women and say, 'You see the enemy over there? They say you look fat in those uniforms.'
>
> *Elayne Boosler*

ships? Are you in need of self-care? Time off? Are you resting enough? What changes would you like to see in your life if anything were possible? Are you living somebody else's values – your parents', your boss', your family's – rather than your own? Do you feel helpless – a victim of your condition and your pain or do you conceive of the possibility that you can change your life?

CASTOR OIL PACKS

Castor oil packs are an age-old remedy traditionally used to treat everything from colitis and peptic ulcers to arthritis and female problems from back pains to fibroids, PMS and endometriosis. They work. Preliminary research at the George Washington School of Medicine in the United States has shown that they are likely to improve the functioning of the immune system. They are an excellent helper for endometriosis not only to alleviate discomfort but also to help speed recovery. Use them at least three times a week – preferably every day.

What you need:
- ❏ cotton or wool flannel cloth (a piece of an old sheet is fine but make sure there are no synthetics in the fabric)
- ❏ plastic freezer bag or plastic sheet
- ❏ hot water bottle
- ❏ 2 safety pins
- ❏ 175 ml (6 fl oz) of castor oil
- ❏ bath towel

Your cloth needs to be big enough so when folded you have two to four thicknesses of cloth and it is about 10 inches wide and 12 inches long. Fold you cloth and pour caster oil into it so that it is saturated with the oil but not dripping. Whilst lying down, apply it to the abdomen then lay the plastic bag or sheet over the soaked cloth. Put the hot water bottle on top of that as warm as you can manage then cover with the towel folded lengthways over the whole area. Leave the castor oil pack on for a minimum of an hour – leave it on all night if you can manage it. Afterwards cleanse the skin using water to which a teaspoon of baking soda has been added. Provided it is kept clean the soaked flannel can be used many times.

HERBS HELP

Two herbs are traditionally used with success in the treatment of endometriosis: Raspberry leaves and Chastetree or *Vitex agnus castus*. They work well together.

RASPBERRY LEAVES *Robus idaeus*

Raspberry leaf tea is easy to make. Simply steep a tablespoon of the dried herb in a pint of hot water for five minutes and drink hot or cold throughout the day with a little honey if you like.

CHASTETREE *Vitex agnus castus*

Vitex agnus castus can be taken in the form of fresh powdered berries (three capsules a day with food), made in tea form from the powdered berries or easiest of all taken in tincture form – 20 drops in a little water two to three times a day. Chastetree is slow acting but profound in its effects. It has a reputation for being virtually free of side-effects. It is an enormously useful natural remedy for severe hot flushes, and can help eliminate flooding, spotting, irregular cycles, fibroids and endometriosis while balancing emotions, making skin clearer and improving vaginal dryness. It also counters most of the usual PMS problems from headaches and depression to water retention and breast tenderness. I first learned the virtues of *agnus castus* from Dr Dagmar Liechti von Brasch. Dr Liechti was the niece of the famous natural Swiss physician Max Bircher Benner who founded the Bircher Benner Clinic in Zurich. Dr Liechti was head of the clinic for 40 years during which time she gave birth to and raised five children and ran a big hospital. Chastetree was her preferred remedy for menopausal women because it was so successful on so many levels. A conventionally trained medical doctor, she had at her disposal every possible natural and hormonal treatment yet she most often opted for this one. Results begin to show in two or three months of daily use and can become permanent after a year.

FOOD MATTERS
Throw out the coffee, sugar, colas, dairy products – cut out all milk and milk products – throw out anything containing hydrogenated oils such as margarines, junk fats, cooking oils and convenience foods. Use Age Power's Insulin Balance. Eliminate shellfish. Eat 50 percent of your foods raw especially fruits and vegetables as well as making sure you eat plenty of good quality protein – fish, eggs, microfiltered whey. Use organic tofu often, too. Use a green drink of chlorella, spirulina, green barley or wheatgrass in water or fresh vegetable juice daily.

PROGESTERONE FOR ENDOMETRIOSIS
Used either in the form of a cream rubbed on the skin twice a day, or in oil form taken under the tongue, from day 10 or 12 to day 26 of your menstrual cycle. Says John Lee, 'I recommend that a woman increase the dose of the cream until she is satisfied her pelvic pains are decreasing. Once that dose is reached, a woman can continue for three to five years before gradually lowering it.'

Lee finds that this decreases menstrual flow and gives the body time to heal the endometrial lesions. If the pains come back he advises women to continue the treatment until menopause. Lee has treated patients with mild to moderate endometriosis in this manner for the past 13 years and none of them has ever had to resort to surgery.

ALL CHANGE
Alternate the sites at which you apply progesterone cream – breasts, back, belly, face, neck and thighs. Progesterone oil can also be useful when symptoms are severe since it contains more progesterone. To use the oil put four or five drops under the tongue and keep it in the mouth for at least three minutes without swallowing (this takes a bit of practice). Increase or decrease the dosage of the oil or cream depending upon the severity of the symptoms and on how rapidly the cream is absorbed. Use at least one 2 oz jar each month from day 10 to 26 of your cycle.

FIBROID TUMOURS

Fibroids are benign (non-cancerous) tumours of the uterus. They are made out of lumps of fibrous tissue, very much like the tissue of the womb itself, that grow into unusual shapes which either lace the lining of the womb or are attached by a stump to its outer walls. Probably 50 percent of women in the West have fibroids although most never know they are there. They are more common in black women than in white and if you are going to get them they usually develop in the eight to 10 years before menopause. The size of fibroids can vary from tiny to massive. Sometimes a single fibroid can weigh as much as a new born baby or more. (The biggest reported in medical history weighed 35.5 kg!)

Only if fibroids cause trouble do doctors usually consider that they need to be removed. Many women with fibroids have no symptoms at all. Others experience menstrual cramps, pelvic pains, pressure on the bladder or rectum, a swollen belly or extremely heavy periods which can result in long-term fatigue and anaemia. When a woman's hormones are fluctuating wildly as they can do in the years just before menopause or when she is under a lot of stress, fibroids can grow quickly, sometimes even causing haemorrhaging. Fibroids are responsible for a third of women's gynaecological problems and are the most common reason that hysterectomies are performed for they can often be hard to remove without taking out the womb. Occasionally fibroids are removed without taking out the uterus through an operation called a *myomectomy* but this is generally only done when there is a single large fibroid present or when a woman is wanting to become pregnant, since the operation is difficult. Fibroids are very rarely cancerous.

Fibroids have a tendency to grow and shrink in size as a woman's hormone levels shift during monthly cycles. They are highly oestrogen dependent so are most prevalent in oestrogen-dominant women, particularly women who have not had children early on in life and are in their late 30s or 40s. The good news is that once menopause arrives and oestrogen levels diminish sharply fibroids shrink so small that often they can no longer be detected by pelvic examination. The presence of fibroids in a woman is usually confirmed by a *sonogram* or *ultrasound* since it can be difficult for a doctor to distinguish between an ovarian growth and a fibroid through pelvic examination alone.

> Biologically speaking, if something bites you it's more likely to be female.
>
> *Desmond Morris*

STANDARD PRACTICE

Until recently the best treatment for most fibroids – provided they are not creating too much discomfort in a woman – has been to watch and wait for menopause when they would go away, provided of course that a woman was not given oestrogen replacement. Now, doctors at the forefront of the natural menopause revolution urge women to make dietary changes and recommend the use of progesterone cream or oil. A few prescribe progesterone orally.

INNER WORLD

In some women fibroids almost seem a physical manifestation of plans, projects or dreams that have either outlived their usefulness or have not yet been fulfilled. Fibroids can be like frustrated creative energy stuck in the womb. It can be useful to take a look at your life and ask yourself if a job, a project, a relationship has outlived its value. Have you in some way out-grown the life you are living? If so, would you like to change things? Sometimes fibroids are linked with conflicts over whether or not to have a child, or intimate relationships.

CASTOR OIL PACKS

Use three times a week or more when there is any discomfort, heavy bleeding, abdominal pressure or other symptoms (see page 426).

EPSOM SALTS

Take long epsom salts baths regularly: Take two cups of household grade epsom salts (available from the chemist), pour it into the bath and fill the bath with blood-heat water. Then immerse yourself for 20 to 30 minutes, topping up with warm water when necessary to maintain a comfortable temperature. Afterwards, lie down for 15 minutes or, better still, have an epsom salts bath just before you go to bed.

PROGESTERONE FOR FIBROIDS

Provided dietary changes are also made, when enough progesterone is supplied fibroid growth is arrested and frequently reversed as well. Good herbal support (see above) works well with both. Progesterone cream should be rubbed on different areas of the skin twice a day. It can also be used in oil form taken under the tongue from day 12 to day 26 of your menstrual cycle. Use enough cream so that you get through a 2 oz jar during this two-week period, alternating the sites at which you apply the cream – breasts, back, belly, face, neck and thighs. It is always worthwhile to have your doctor monitor the results of such natural treatment by way of regular sonogram tests three or four times a year to verify

HERB HELP

Lady's mantle *Alchemilla vulgaris* tincture is a long-used natural treatment for fibroids among herbalists. Chastetree or *Vitex agnus castus* is also useful, as is a combination of mistletoe and butterbur.

LADY'S MANTLE *Alchemilla vulgaris*
Lady's mantle is said to carry magical properties offering support to any woman either entering the role of motherhood or leaving it. It is also good for excessive menstrual flow and flooding taken as a tea – 1 oz of the dried herb to 1 pint of boiling water – or in tincture form 10 to 25 drops several times a day. Lady's mantle is excellent for relieving headaches, too.

CHASTETREE *Vitex agnus castus*
Chastetree berries (see page 427) are also good in tincture form 10 to 20 drops two to three times a day. Both of these herbs are anti-oestrogenic in their actions. They can be profitably used together.

MISTLETOE *Viscus album* & BUTTERBUR *Petesites hybrids*
A combination of mistletoe and butterbur is also one of the best herbal remedies to shrink fibroids. It was developed by the Swiss physician Dr A Vogel. It is available in most countries in the form of *Petasan Tincture* made by Bioforce. Normal dosage is 10 to 20 drops three times a day.

CAUTION: *The Chinese herb Dong Quai (Angelica sinensis) which in general is excellent for many female problems should not be used if you have fibroids since it has been shown to increase their size in some women. Avoid oestrogen replacement since this too increases their growth.*

shrinkage. Progesterone plays an important emotional role in women with fibroids by helping to soften the frustration or anger that often comes with them. This is thanks to progesterone's role as a precursor to important brain chemicals and stress hormones.

VAGINAL IRRITATION, DRYNESS AND THINNING

Some women at menopause experience a thinning of the vaginal walls which can lead to irritation and in a few cases even to repeated urinary infection. This thinning of the walls of the vagina and the things which can accompany it – referred to by the patriarchal medical experts as *atrophic vaginitis* or *vulval dystrophy* – is by no means inevitable. Many women, especially those who are physically active and have active sex lives – never experience it at all. Others have had to handle a tendency to dryness since their 20s, whatever their lifestyle.

YOUR INNER WORLD

Forget the feeling that you are some kind of a freak or growing old, or incapable of enjoying intercourse. Many women never give full vent to the power of their sexuality nor experience the full flood of the pleasure an abandoned sexual encounter can bring until menopause when they are free of fear of pregnancy. Vaginal thinning, which is a natural part of lowered oestrogen levels in menopausal women, can be simple to counter without ever having to resort to potentially dangerous hormone drugs. So just in case you have been feeling bad about yourself or timid, lay those feelings aside and do something about it.

I am not the boss of my house. I don't even know how I lost it. I don't know when I lost it. I don't think I ever had it. But I've seen the boss's job and I don't want it.

Bill Cosby

HERBS HELP

Stay away from soaps, bubble baths, shower gels and nylon tights or underwear since all of these things can make this condition worse. There are several herbs which are great to treat it. Motherwort and chastetree taken internally, along with calendula, aloe vera and comfrey used externally. They can also help prevent recurrent vaginal and bladder infections.

MOTHERWORT *Leonurus cardiaca*
Taken as a tincture – 15 to 20 drops in a glass of water several times a day is an excellent way of restoring thickness to vaginal tissues when it has been lost and of remoisturising the vagina.

CHASTETREE *Vitex agnus castus*
While it was used in the middle ages to calm the lascivious thoughts of celibate monks – hence its name – it has a powerful stimulating affect on women's libido taken over a few months. It is also excellent for bringing moisture and circulation to vaginal tissues when they are hungry for them. Take the berries in tincture form, 10 to 20 drops two to three times a day.

CALENDULA *Calendula officinalis*
This herb in a good cream base (see Resources) can help soften yet toughen vaginal tissues and tissues of the vulva. It can also relieve itching when applied three times a day and help protect against infection.

COMFREY *Symphytum officinale*
In a cream base (see Resources) comfrey is the best soother of all for itchy vaginal tissue. It can also be used as a lubricant instead of the usual vaseline or KY Jelly during intercourse. Use it three times a day for three months and you may never need to use it again.

ALOE *Aloe Vera*
Pure Aloe Vera juice is useful when vaginal tissues have become hot, dry and uncomfortable. Simply wipe it on several times a day.

JOURNEYS OF THE SOUL

These are only a few of the exciting alternatives developing as part of the natural medicine revolution for women. But in many ways, what is most exciting of all about the new movement is a growing recognition that menopause is no more a disease than menstruation. Both are a natural and important transition in a woman's life – a passage every bit as important physically and spiritually as puberty was. And like puberty menopause carries with it enormous fluctuations in hormone levels. With them come shifts in mood, attitude and personal values all of which are part of the passage itself.

In other cultures, the transformation which takes place in a woman's life sometime between the ages of 35 and 60 has traditionally been considered a journey towards new freedom and power, a time of celebration. For her creativity, which has been until then bound to her biology, is at last set free for her to use as she wills. It is a time when women cease to give a damn what others think of their eccentricities and can set themselves free to soar into whatever realms they fancy. The passage we make at menopause – like the passage at birth or in giving birth – is a profound one which dissolves the boundaries of a woman's life and can take her deep inside herself on an archetypal heroine's journey to discover the real treasures lying there.

Each woman is biochemically and spiritually unique. So is the inner journey she must make if she is to live her life authentically. Such journeys need to be undertaken with the highest respect for your body, your spirit and the powers of nature which support your unfolding. Such journeys cannot be codified. They are not package holidays where you pay your money, take your anti-diarrhoea pills and know exactly what to expect. These are journeys of your soul.

JOURNEY OF A LIFETIME

I have come to believe that the journey we are called upon to make at menopause is the most important journey a woman ever takes: First because, given her age and maturity, it is taken with the greatest awareness and, secondly, because it marks the end of the childbearing years in a biological way, a woman has become free of the need to channel her energy into propagating the species. Now, at last, she is free to use her energy, creativity and intelligence in any way she wants. We have been far too busy giving birth, raising children and nurturing

> According to a new survey, women say they feel more comfortable undressing in front of men than they do undressing in front of other women. They say that women are too judgmental, where, of course, men are just grateful.
>
> *Robert De Niro*

the creativity of others to be able properly to care for ourselves and explore our own potential. The journey of menopause offers the possibility of changing these patterns in our lives once and for all. This is the secret, and the joy, of a natural menopause.

HERB CUPBOARD

Pathos activates the eyes and ears to see and hear. At times of pathos illness opens doors to a reality which is closed to a healthy point of view.

Jean Houston

Plants hold powerful medicine for the human body. Their ability to enhance health go far beyond their ability to alleviate symptoms. Wise women like to use the whole of a plant, rejecting the ideas of modern medicine which chooses to give isolated active ingredients as drugs.

In medicinal plants there are two kinds of compounds, each of which has an important part to play in treatment. The first are the active ingredients – these are what capture the imagination of chemists and drug producers. The second are the compounds and substances which drug manufacturers ignore altogether and seek to eliminate but which good herbalists insist play a supportive role in the healing a particular herb can bring to the body.

TRUE SYNERGY

These compounds work synergistically with the actives, making them more easily accessible to the body or dampening the effect of what are often very potent plant chemicals – helping to guard against side-effects. Some even help protect from overdose by causing nausea if the body's safe level of tolerance is passed. It is the synergy of these primary active ingredients and their secondary helpers that makes herbs work so well.

RULE OF OPPOSITES

Ginseng, for instance, is useful in treating both high and low blood pressure. Wild yam is useful for low progesterone as well as low oestrogen in a woman's body. Herbs can be taken in many different ways – as infusions, decoctions, syrups, tinctures, suppositories, capsules, and in baths, ointments and creams. You can grow your own herbs or buy then in bulk. Using the dried plant is by far the cheapest way to use herbs since you can buy a large amount at a time very cheaply and make up your own infusions, decoctions, suppositories and ointments as well as tinctures. You can even buy empty gelatine capsules and fill them with dried herb yourself. It is often easiest if you are a complete beginner to rely on good

THE WHOLE PLANT

There are many different substances and compounds in plants and herbs offering health-support. The volatile oils for instance, the tannins, alkaloids, bitters, glycosides and flavonoids. The most important for treating male and female reproductive disorders and enhancing health are the *steroidal saponins*. The steroidal saponins fall into various categories. Some resemble cholesterol, from which your body makes its own steroid hormones – the oestrogens, progesterone, testosterone, pregnenalone and DHEA. Others give the body support to help it regulate hormonal balance, in no small part because they provide the raw materials out of which the body can make whatever hormones and other metabolites it needs to do this. Because of this balancing ability, unlike drugs or isolated ingredients, the same plant can be used to treat two completely opposite conditions.

quality ready-made herbal products from a good supplier (see Resources) – whole herbs, herbs in capsules, herbal extracts and tinctures. Tinctures are made using either water or alcohol to draw out a plant's chemical constituents and preserve them. Take them in a little water. They are best either bought ready made from a reputable supplier or left until you have mastered the use of herbs in other ways as each herb demands a specific ratio of water and alcohol to plant material. This ratio can be found in a pharmacopoeia. It is worth remembering that, just as people have different personalities, so do plants. One plant might work better than another for different people.

THE PLANTS

Here is a small and simple repertoire of herbs. Get to know them. They are like making new friends. Each has its own personality and characteristics. All have been used for centuries for strengthening the body's ability to handle stress, for healing and for reproductive problems. The therapeutic actions of most have been scientifically validated.

MOTHERWORT

Leonurus cardiaca

Also called lion's tail or Yi Mu Cao in the Chinese Pharmacopoeia, motherwort grows in waste places. It has gained its name from its ancient use for reducing anxiety during pregnancy. The plant has good sedative properties which have been well validated by scientific experiments. It is able to calm the nervous system while acting as a tonic to the whole body. Its leaves are full of mind-altering natural chemicals which studies in China have shown to have a regulating effect on the womb and the heart, bringing calm in its wake. This is one of the reasons why, in addition to being used by women to ease hot flushes, banish insomnia and restore elasticity to the walls of the vagina, it is an excellent herb for the treatment of many heart conditions. I find it is the most physically and psychologically comforting plant I know.

HOW TO USE

Motherwort is rich in alkaloids and is bitter when drunk as an infusion. It is easier to take as a tincture or made into a herbal vinegar. Take 10 to 25 drops of the tincture made from the fresh plant every two to six hours or 1 to 2 teaspoons of the herb vinegar as desired.

WHAT IT CAN DO
- Calm the nerves
- Minimise hot flushes
- Promote undisturbed sleep
- Eliminate waterlogging
- Tone up womb and vagina
- Relieve cramps

CAUTION: *Motherwort is not a herb to use when a woman is experiencing menstrual flooding since it can aggravate this tendency.*

GINSENG

Panax ginseng

Oriental ginseng which is widely cultivated in China, Korea, Japan and Russia, is probably the most studied plant in modern times. It is more potent and effective than its American cousin *panax quinquefolium* and best chosen carefully as there is a lot of relatively worthless ginseng on the market. It has been praised for centuries for its rejuvenating properties, its ability to protect against illness, to enhance the body's ability to handle stress – even to prolong life. The herb is a great ally – the most potent of all the plants for handling very severe symptoms in menopausal women. You should be aware that many of ginseng's benefits will be lost if you take more than 2 g of vitamin C a day, while taking vitamin E will enhance ginseng's actions. The most effective ginseng is the dried root which you chew or a good tincture made from it. Extensive research carried out has shown that for ginseng to work it has to be replete with *ginsenosides* – the active compounds from the plant. Ginseng can heighten immunity, improve the functions of the heart and lungs, counter fatigue and balance female hormones thanks to its oestrogenic effects.

HOW TO USE
Always buy the best ginseng you can afford and take it either as a fresh root tincture five to 20 drops one to three times a day, as an infusion or tea in which 1 oz of the dried root is taken in a cup of water a day or by chewing on a piece of the root the size of the tip of your little finger every day. The effects of ginseng are cumulative so you need six to eight weeks of taking the plant to feel its full benefits.

WHAT IT CAN DO
❑   Regulate hormones and banish menstrual flooding
❑   Enhance the ability to handle stress

CAUTION: *None*

ST JOHN'S WORT
Hypericum perforatum

One of the most useful herbs I know, St John's Wort is a natural monoamine oxidase (MAO) inhibitor thanks to a combination of active ingredients the most important of which is probably *hypericin*. As a result of this inhibition, using it increases the levels of feel good neurotransmitters in the brain creating emotional stability and balancing mood. Its effects usually kick in after two or three weeks of use. It is commonly and effectively used as an anti-depressant. But it has other powers too. Hypericin and another of its chemicals *pseudohypericin* have strong anti-viral activity and broad spectrum anti-microbial activity against many forms of bacteria, too.

HOW TO USE

Look for a preparation of St John's Wort extract standardised to contain 0.3 percent hypericin. As an anti-depressant the standard dose is 300 mg three times a day taken with meals. You can also take it in capsules with meals three times a day.

WHAT IT CAN DO

- ❑ Regulate brain chemicals to balance mood and clear depression
- ❑ Strengthen immunity
- ❑ Knock out viral and bacterial infections

CAUTION: *St John's Wort can cause photosensitivity in animals. Reports in humans have been limited to people taking massive quantities of it, such as AIDS sufferers, however. It can interact negatively with MAO inhibiting drugs and should not be taken with them.*

ECHINACEA
Echinacea purpurea

Purple cone flower or Black Sampson is a plant native to the prairies of North America with unequalled properties to stimulate the immune system, heal wounds, enhance skin, counter infection and calm inflammation. The Sioux used it for snake bites, blood poisoning and wound healing. Until the twentieth century its roots and rhizomes were used for the treatment of fever and infections from flu and colds to serious conditions such as typhoid, meningitis, malaria, diphtheria, boils and abscesses. When drugs came into being in a big way the beautiful echinacea plant was almost forgotten – except in Germany. There researchers began to quantify its effects on the body discovering that it has properties equal to and often greater than most antibiotics to prevent and heal infection. Echinacea is a plant product I would never want to be without. I use it to protect from infection through the long dark winters and to treat illness in myself and my family.

HOW TO USE

By capsule of the ground herb – one to four capsules three to four times a day depending on whether it is being used as a prophylactic or treatment for illness. In the form of fresh plant tincture taken in a little water, 15 to 50 drops at a time once or twice a day for prevention or several times a day as treatment – up to 2 teaspoons an hour for a day or two at the onset of illness.

WHAT IT CAN DO
- ❑ Bring health insurance against illness and premature ageing
- ❑ Boost immunity when illness strikes
- ❑ Protect skin and body from degeneration

CAUTION: *Like many plants echinacea should not be used continuously since the body can become accustomed to it and this may negate some of its potent health-enhancing abilities.*

GOLDENSEAL
Hydrastis canadensis

Favourite cure-all of the Cherokee Indians, goldenseal has in recent years won praise from scientists for its widespread benefits which include banishing morning sickness and nausea, calming digestive disturbances and banishing skin diseases and haemorrhoids. It can be used as a douche in the treatment of vaginal infections, as a mouthwash in the treatment of gum problems and to fight off flu and fevers. One of the most generally effective of all remedies, this is another herb I would never want to be without.

HOW TO USE
Use the powdered root preferably in capsules rather than as an infusion since goldenseal does not taste good. Take one to four capsules three times a day, or tincture of fresh herb 10 to 30 drops three to four times a day.

WHAT IT CAN DO
- ❑ Soothe digestion and ease liver problems
- ❑ Counter infection
- ❑ Calm uterine contractions

CAUTION: *None*

DONG QUAI
Angelica sinensis

This is the most prized of all the Oriental plant treatments for women's hormonal problems. Although its oestrogen content is a mere 1/400th of oestrogen-based drugs, studies have shown that this root, which acts like a sister to ginseng in its actions, can not only quickly clear the kind of hot flushes which are the result of too little or the wrong kinds of oestrogen in your body but can perform many other useful tasks as well: lower blood pressure that is too high for instance, fight bacteria and viruses, get rid of water retention, calm menopausal anxiety, stimulate a sluggish metabolism, protect the cardiovascular system and eliminate insomnia, nervousness and depression. This remedy works fast – usually in a week or two. It is often best used together with ginseng since they perfectly balance each other. Western herbal practitioners sometimes suggest taking dong quai for a fortnight then ginseng for the next fortnight alternating use to reap the highest benefits from both.

HOW TO USE
Like ginseng, a thin slice of dried root can be chewed three times a day. As an infusion take 1/2 to one cup a day or fifteen to 30 drops of the fresh root tincture one to three times a day.

WHAT IT CAN DO
❑　Improve sleep
❑　Moisten vagina
❑　Ease hot flushes
❑　De-age skin

CAUTION: *Dong quai is not a remedy to use if bloating, menstrual flooding or diarrhoea regularly occurs nor if you have fibroids. Neither should it ever be used if you are on blood-thinning herbs or take aspirin. Any tenderness or discomfort in the breasts while using it is a sign it should be discontinued.*

WILD YAM
Dioscorea villosa

There are many related species of the *dioscoriaceae* family which have similar properties to *villosa*, including *Discorea mexicana*. Wild yam was traditionally used to prevent miscarriage, as a natural tonic, and for natural birth control without side-effects as it does not interfere with normal periods. The whole plant, which supplies the raw materials for the body to make hormones, has much to offer perimenopausal, menopausal and postmenopausal women. It soothes the nerves, eases menstrual pains and encourages the production of progesterone in a woman's body to counter oestrogen dominance and the many conditions associated with it. It is useful to counter intestinal wind, colic and nausea. It stimulates libido in many women. The root has also been shown to lower blood cholesterol and blood pressure which is too high.

HOW TO USE
An infusion of the dried root, 1/2 to one cup once or twice a day or as a tincture of the dried root 10 to 30 drops three or four times a day. You can also take the ground root in capsules. Also use on the body in the form of wild yam cream which contains converted natural progesterone as an antidote to osteoporosis and to reverse bone loss after it has occurred.

WHAT IT CAN DO
❑ Ease joint and muscle pains and headaches
❑ Reverse osteoporosis
❑ Moisten vagina
❑ Banishing PMS and menstrual pain

CAUTION: *None.*

AGE OF TREASON
Orthodox medicine's almost total disregard for the use of phyto-hormone-rich plants in the treatment of so many ailments is of recent origin. It is as though with the coming of patentable drugs centuries of traditional methods were dismissed with the wave of a hand. 'Uterine tonics' made from hormone-rich herbs and plants were used for centuries to treat all manner of female complaints. They still work. Once you get to know the actions of various herbs – and the best way of doing this is to use them or to watch them work on other people – you begin to develop a feel for the character of each herb and a skill that enables you to call on the plant or plants you need just when you need them. But it is important to remember that plants are slower acting than drugs so you need to be patient. It is often necessary to use a herb for a few weeks or even longer before you will experience its full benefits. Nonetheless, I have frequently found that a herb will bring almost immediate relief. One big advantage of using herbs is that many, when taken over a period of time, will do the job so well for which they were being taken that you no longer need to use them. Another important thing to remember when using herbs is that they often work well in combination.

DIVE DEEP

Insomnia? I know a good cure for it . . . get plenty of sleep.

W.C. Fields

Sleep de-ages. Getting enough is essential. It is not always an easy thing to do as you get older. Many people sleep less and less or their sleep is disturbed. More than half of the population of the Western world has difficulty at some time during the year falling asleep, while 33 percent of us have to wrestle with insomnia in an ongoing way. Many fall into the habit of using prescription drugs with powerful side effects for sleep, just to help them slip into slumber. Don't. There are better ways.

Disrupted or poor quality sleep can be dangerous. I learned this myself first hand after taking a flight that crossed twelve time zones. I found – unusual for me – that my body never readjusted to the new time zone and I was sleeping only an hour or two a night, and at very irregular times. This went on for almost two weeks, at the end of which I was in severe physical pain. I went to see my doctor who is also a skilled acupuncturist, concerned that I may have contracted some fairly serious illness. He treated me with acupuncture and sorted out the pain within two treatments, as well as my inability to sleep. He also told me that he had seen this in patients of his who are pilots.

SUPPRESSED IMMUNITY

Research studies show that when healthy male volunteers were deprived of four hours of sleep for a single night, the activity of the natural killer cells in their immune system fell by as much as 30 percent. That's the bad news. The good news is that a single good night's sleep brought normal functioning back to the cells. It has also long been known that shift workers, whose hours of sleep continually change, have increasing difficulty falling asleep and staying asleep. They also have more accidents, suffer more illness and die younger than people with normal sleep schedules.

> The advice to get a good night's rest to prevent disease may be more than just folklore; a biochemical link has been found between deep sleep and the function of the cells of our immune systems.
>
> *Robert Ornstein, PhD, and David Sobel, MD*

SAY NO TO DRUGS

Sleeping pills, either by prescription or over the counter, are not the way to go. They come in two forms – benzodiazepines, primarily prescription drugs, many of them tranquillisers, such as diazepam (Valium) and chloriazepoxide (Librium) or trizolam (Halcion). These are the major benzodiazepines which doctors prescribe for anxiety, as well as insomnia. Of course there are many more, from lorazepam (Ativan) to alprazolam (Zanax). These drugs put you to sleep because of their ability to increase the calming action of GABA – the neurotransmitter gamma-aminobutyric acid – which blocks the centres for arousal in the brain. The side effects of benzodiazepines – the major group of anti-insomnia drugs – can be daunting. Avoid them.

Sleep-inducing drugs are designed only for very short-term use, as they are highly addictive. In addition to drowsiness, dizziness and impaired co-ordination, benzodiazepines create abnormal sleep problems and often produce a morning hang-over feeling, as well as in many people, indigestion, nausea, constipation, lethargy, blurred vision and diarrhoea. All of them carry a warning that when you take them you should not use heavy equipment or drive. It's a warning to be heeded. But probably the most serious side effects of the benzodiazepines come as a result of the changes in brain function and profound and highly negative behaviour they can bring about. Many people using them find that their memory becomes severely impaired, report that they suffer nervousness and a sense of confusion or irritability and aggressiveness, while a few even report hallucinations and bizarre behaviour. Benzodiazepines have even been shown to trigger depression in some people as well as suicidal thoughts. They are best left alone.

The reward of sleep is often recognised by its absence. Millions of people spend night after night tossing and turning in a sleepless living hell. They stumble about day after day, weary and bleary eyed, the 'walking wounded'. Irritable, listless, robbed of the pleasures of sleep, they also lose a vital mental sharpness and the zest for living. They are victims of a growing 'national sleep debt'. And this deficit may have a profound effect on the health of our society.

Robert Ornstein, PhD, and David Sobel, MD

OVER-THE-COUNTER HELP

The other class of drugs used for insomnia are the anti-histamines, which are also used to control certain allergic reactions such as hayfever. You can buy these over the counter in any pharmacy. They work by blocking the body from producing histamine in the brain. In doing so, they bring about a sense of drowsiness and sleep. Even 50 g of diphenhydramine (Benadryl), a common over-the-counter sedative, can bring about the same impairment in function in drivers as can a 1 percent blood alcohol content, which is the standard for drink driving in most countries. Using the anti-histamines to treat insomnia can also result in nausea, headaches, drying of the nose, mouth and throat, and allergic reactions.

CAUGHT IN A TRAP

One of the worst things about using over-the-counter or prescription drugs for insomnia is that they themselves create abnormal sleep patterns, so that you enter a vicious cycle. You take the drug to induce sleep, and then find there is a further disruption of sleep so that you have to take more of the drug, while each morning you find you need to drink more and more espresso just to wake up and keep going.

DRUG HANGOVERS

The reason that sleeping pills cause a morning hang-over and interfere with natural sleep is that they suppress REM or rapid eye movement sleep. There are two kinds of sleep. *Orthodox* sleep which is dreamless – sometimes called synchronised slow-wave sleep – because of the brain wave patterns that accompany it and *paradoxical* sleep – during which dreaming occurs along with rapid eye movement or REM. REM is sometimes called de-synchronised sleep. Both kinds play an important role in protecting the body from age degeneration and ensuring that you look good and feel great day after day. Orthodox sleep helps restore the body physically. During the periods of orthodox sleep in the night, your body restores DNA on a cellular level that has become damaged by excessive free radicals. It is deeply relaxing on a physical level. Your heart slows down, your blood pressure falls slightly and your breathing gets slower and more regular. At the deepest levels of orthodox sleep, brain waves become more synchronised and everything is at peace.

CAUSES OF INSOMNIA

- ❑ Anxiety
- ❑ Fear of insomnia
- ❑ Stimulants such as coffee or alcohol
- ❑ Eating too many high-glycaemic carbohydrate con-
  venience foods which disturbs blood sugar
- ❑ Low levels of melatonin
- ❑ Low levels of serotonin
- ❑ Use of drugs
- ❑ Depression

MYSTERIES AND PARADOXES

REM sleep is diametrically opposite to orthodox sleep in many ways, but it's just as vital and it more than earns its name 'paradoxical' by a mass of contradiction. For although the body is virtually paralysed during the REM state, the fingers and the face often twitch, and the genitals become erect. Your breathing speeds up to the level of your normal waking state. Heartbeat, blood pressure and temperature rise, and adrenaline shoots through the system. Meanwhile, beneath the lids, your eyes move rapidly from side to side as though you were looking at a film or tennis match. And that's exactly what happens. You are viewing images that come rapidly in succession, travelling deep within. Your brain waves in the REM state show a marked similarity to the rapid, irregular patterns of being awake.

> You cannot travel into yourself without exploring the infinite reaches of eternal consciousness.
>
> *Ken Carey*

MAINTAIN EQUILIBRIUM

Although the exact purpose of REM sleep remains a mystery, scientists know that it is essential for maintaining mental and emotional equilibrium. Just how much REM or paradoxical sleep you need varies tremendously from one person to another. It's related both to your personality and to your general psychological state. Usually longer and more frequent periods of REM sleep take place each night in times of emotional disturbance and psychic pain or when your defence patterns are being challenged by new demands. Women often have increased REM sleep just before a menstrual period. For most women this is a time of increased anxiety, irritability, mood change and unstable defence patterns. In some ways, REM sleep seems to process psychological difficulties so that the body and the mind are protected from damage that they night cause.

Too little REM sleep makes people restless and anxious. It also contributes to a loss of short-term memory and poor concentration. Using benzodiazapines and anti-histamines severely interferes with REM sleep, which is a major reason why people tend to wake up with a 'hang-over' and to feel more exhausted in the morning than they did when they lay down at night. Using these drugs over a long period of time leads to an increase in nightmares and to other sleep disturbances as soon as you stop taking them as your body, desperate for REM sleep, tries to make up for what it has lost. This is one of the reasons why, if you have been taking benzodiazepines for more than a month, it is essential not to stop taking the drug all at once. You need to work with your doctor to gradually diminish the dose gradually to minimise withdrawal symptoms which, in addition to REM rebound, include depression, hypersensitivity to your environment, seizures, memory loss, poor concentration, insomnia, headache, nausea and paranoia. Be patient or have compassion for yourself if you are kicking the sleeping pill habit. Your body and psyche will rebalance themselves soon enough.

> Which would have the greater effect in your life: my compassion for you or your compassion for yourself?
>
> *Running Wolf*

HOW MUCH IS ENOUGH?

How much sleep you need not only varies from person to person, it also varies from one day to the next. There is certainly no truth to the notion that you must have eight hours of sleep to stay well and feel energetic. Some people need ten, while others get on very nicely with four and a half. Usually, the more stress filled your day, the more sleep you will need to balance it. Many high achievers and great minds throughout history – Napoleon, Freud and Thomas Edison for instance – have been poor sleepers. Others, like Einstein, could sleep the day away. For many people the idea that they must get eight hours of sleep a night is so embedded in their belief system that they are convinced they will be exhausted the next day if they don't. Belief is a powerful force in determining how the body functions. If you carry such beliefs you can easily develop all of the signs of sleep deprivation, even if you did have eight hours the night before.

INSOMNIA TRUE OR FALSE

A lot of so called insomnia is nothing more than the result of worrying about getting to sleep. Many people who consider themselves insomniacs are really victims of the general propaganda about sleep, rather than true non-sleepers. Many people seek treatment because they can only sleep four or five hours a night, although that may be all they need. There is nothing more likely to cause sleeplessness than the worry that you won't be able to drop off. Sometimes sleeplessness can be normal. After all, we all experience a sleepless night every now and then, particularly if we are over-tired, worried or excited about coming events.

> You have the power in the present moment to change limiting beliefs and consciously plant the seeds for the future of your choosing. As you change your mind you change your experience.
>
> *Serge Kabili King*

Real chronic insomnia is less frequent. There are many things that can cause it, from taking stimulants such as chocolate, soft drinks, coffee and tea, to not getting enough exercise. Nocturnal hypoglycaemia is another major cause of insomnia in many people.

BEWARE OF BOOZE

Alcohol can severely interfere with sleep for a number of reasons. First, it brings about the release of adrenalin giving you a sense of excitement – a totally inappropriate condition for putting your head down on the pillow. It also interferes with the transport of tryptophan into the brain. And since the brain depends on a good supply of tryptophan in order to produce serotonin – the neurotransmitter that brings about sleep – drinking alcohol late in the evening severely disrupts serotonin levels. Alcohol, of course, also has a relaxing effect which for many people will put them to sleep immediately provided they have drunk enough of it. Then they find two or three hours later they awake dehydrated and unable to sleep for the rest of the night.

BLOOD SUGAR DISTURBS SLEEP

Where Syndrome X is present, you often find low night-time blood glucose levels, or nocturnal hyperglycaemia. A drop in blood sugar that comes from eating too many high carbohydrate foods, and the accompanying high levels of insulin, bring about the release of hormones such as adrenalin, growth hormone and cortisol, all of which stimulate the brain. This can cause you to wake up in the night, with a mind racing and the feeling of undeniable hunger. Following Age Power's Insulin Balance way of eating (see Chapter Age Power's Insulin Balance) eliminates this problem within a week or two. Others find that a slice of rye bread and butter, either before bed or if they awaken in the night, can help put them back to sleep. Deep relaxation techniques such as Autogenic Training also help tremendously to induce regular deep sleep. They train the sympathetic nervous system to move at will from the dynamic, enthusiastic, sympathetic-dominated state associated with stress to the deeply relaxed, restorative, para-sympathetic-dominated state associated with deep calm, reverie and sleep. And this doesn't have to be practised right before bed, by any means. It is simply a question of re-educating your nervous system by practising it a couple of times a day, over a period of two or three weeks. Exercise, too, has an important role to play in deep sleep. But exercise is not something you want to perform just before going to bed. Following Age Power's exercise programme will help a great deal.

> Insomnia can have many causes, but the most common reasons are depression, anxiety and tension. If psychological factors do not seem to be the cause, various foods, drinks and medications may be responsible,
>
> *Michael T. Murray, ND*

> No more words. Hear only the voice within.
>
> *Rumi*

MELATONIN MAGIC

Produced in the pineal gland, deep within your brain, melatonin – which is scientifically known as N-acetyl-five-hydroxy tryptamine – can be a godsend to many people over the age of 35 who have trouble sleeping. Melatonin production in the brain, which occurs primarily at night, decreases with age. Many age researchers believe that lower levels of melatonin are the major reason why people encounter sleep difficulties as they get older. Melatonin production is turned off and on by light entering your eyes. When light is intense during the daylight hours, the pineal gland remains quiet, but during the hours of darkness, the pineal comes to life, releasing bursts of melatonin. This hormone, in addition to its other anti-ageing properties, can help people with insomnia. A night time dose of between 1 and 3 mg of melatonin decreases the time needed to fall asleep and increases the quality of sleep for most people. But each of us is highly individual. Some need more than 10 mg.

Melatonin does not induce sleep itself. It only works in people whose natural levels of serotonin are low, for serotonin is a precursor of melatonin – if you have adequate serotonin your body will be able to make melatonin. It has no sedative effect of its own. A number of studies indicate that melatonin is most effective in treating insomnia in older people, since low levels of melatonin are common amongst people over 60. In one study, 26 such insomniacs were given 1-2 mg of melatonin a couple of hours before

---

MELATONIN FOR SLEEP

Sold in pills, sublingual lozenges or in time-release form, melatonin regulates body clocks. The time-release form works very well for sleep.

DOSAGE: 0.5 mg to 3 mg taken a half hour to two hours before bed. Best on empty stomach – combines well with sedative herbs such as hops, valerian and passiflora.

BONUSES: Works great for jet lag. Its anti-oxidant properties may help protect brain cells from damage.

CAUTION: *In some people more than 0.5mg induces vivid dreams. Higher amounts can cause morning grogginess, decreased libido and low moods.*

bedtime. The researchers used both standard melatonin and slow-release melatonin. Both helped people get to sleep. However, the time-release variety is better at helping people to maintain sleep throughout the night and stop the tendency they had to wake up every two or three hours.

THE SEROTONIN CONNECTION

Serotonin, one of the relaxing neurotransmitters in the brain, plays an important role in initiating sleep. In order for your brain to make serotonin, it needs adequate tryptophan. For many people, supplementing their diet with this amino acid relieves insomnia within a day or two, as well as deceasing the number of times that people wake up in the night. This has been shown in many double-blind clinical studies, where they have used between 1 and 3 g of this natural amino acid. The problem with tryptophan is that back in 1989 in the United States, a few people taking tryptophan reported strange symptoms from high fever and weakness to joint pain, shortness of breath and swellings in the arms and legs. This led to the removal of every product on the American market with more than 100 mg of tryptophan in it. The number of reported cases with this syndrome, dubbed EMS (eosinophilia-myalgia syndrome), was over 1500 including almost 40 deaths. Researchers investigating this strange phenomenon traced every case back to one manufacturer of tryptophan, Showa Denko, which at the time supplied 50–60 percent of the free-form amino acid to the American market. They discovered that what had happened back in 1988 is that Showa Denko changed their manufacturing procedures and as a result, the products they produced became contaminated with the substance now known to have caused EMS. The problem is that tryptophan, despite receiving a clean bill of health on its own, has remained off the market, although contamination of other food products in the past has led to them only being removed from the market and re-introduced once the contamination was corrected.

There is further evidence that sufficient sleep helps protect health. In a study of over 5000 adults over nine years, those subjects who slept seven to eight hours a night had the lowest death rate for heart disease, cancer and stroke – in fact, for all causes of death. The short sleepers (six or fewer hours per night) and the long sleepers (nine or more hours) were 30 percent more likely to die prematurely.

Robert Ornstein, PhD, and David Sobel, MD

NEXT CONVERSION

There is, however, a special form of the amino acid tryptophan, called five-hydroxytryptophan, or 5-HTP, which is the next conversion of the amino acid tryptophan.

Tryptophan is converted by the body into 5-HTP, which is then used in the production of serotonin in the brain. 5-HTP is generally extracted from a natural source as it is found in good quantity in the seeds of an African plant called *Griffonia simplicifolia.* 50-100 mg of 5-HTP on an empty stomach before going to bed often eliminates sleep problems, particularly in people who have insulin resistance and blood sugar disorders. For eating too many high-glycaemic carbohydrates and sugars interferes with the conversion of the amino acid tryptophan from foods into 5-HTP and then on into serotonin. But if you change your diet you may not even need to worry about 5-HTP supplements as a means of getting to sleep.

CALM THOSE LEGS

An interesting reason why many people awaken during the night is a phenomenon called restless leg syndrome or nocturnal myoclonus. This is a neuro-muscular disorder that produces contractions in some of the muscle groups in the legs during sleep, causing the legs to jerk. Usually people are not aware of the jerking, only aware of the fact that they awaken and often feel sleepy during the day. Restless leg syndrome is more wide-

---

HELP FROM 5-HTP

Extracted from griffonia seeds grown in Ghana and the Ivory Coast, 5-HTP is useful in many ways:

❑ **Anxiety and depression** because it converts into serotonin. Used occasionally it brings a sense of peace and letting go.
❑ **Insomnia** because 25 to 50 mg taken half an hour before bed on an empty stomach helps bring on and sustain peaceful sleep.
❑ **Weight loss** because many people find that it acts as an appetite suppressant when used for a few weeks, especially on Age Power Insulin Balance.
❑ Dosage: 10 to 50 mg taken on an empty stomach. Try using four days a week.

CAUTION: *Tolerance to 5-HTP grows after a few weeks. Use for a few weeks then stop using it for a month. Don't take more than 25 mg during the day if you are driving or operating heavy equipment. In some people doses higher than 100 mg create nausea.*

---

spread that you might imagine. It is usually treatable by very high doses of folic acid – from 35 to 60 mg a day or even higher. Such doses are only available by prescription from your doctor. People with restless leg syndrome often have a particularly high need for folic acid.

LOOK OUT FOR IRON DEFICIENCY

Iron deficiency too can interfere with sleep and contribute to restless leg syndrome. Ask your doctor to measure the level of ferritin, the iron storage protein, in your blood. This will indicate the level of stored iron in your system. Finally, if you get cramps in your legs at night, you might try taking 250 mg of magnesium in the form of chelated magnesium or magnesium citrate, together with 400–800 international units of vitamin E a day.

LOOK TO NATURE

Some of the most powerful helpers for insomnia have botanical origins. Many plants, from skullcap (*Scutellaria laterifolia*) to hops (*Humulus lupulus*), can be used to help promote sleep. I use them often. Here are some of the most effective:

VALERIAN *Valeriana officinalis*

A natural sedative and anti-hypertensive, valerian has been used on both sides of the Atlantic for generations, not only to induce sleep but also to help protect people from the negative effects of stress. A double-blind study involving 128 people showed quite clearly that a water extract of valerian root significantly increased the quality of sleep. The study, which was quite thorough, measured night awakening, people's own perceptions of the quality of their sleep, sleeplessness in the morning and sleep latency – that is how quickly a person got to sleep. In another double-blind insomnia study, 20 people were given either a combination of 160 mg of valerian root extract and 80 mg of *Melissa officianalis* extract, or menzodiazapine

> When we are deprived of sleep, it is the brain which suffers most. Thoughts become disorganised; memory lapses, irritability and confusion reign. 'The madman is a waking dreamer,' wrote Immanuel Kant.
>
> *Robert Ornstein, PhD and David Sobel, MD*

(Triazolam 0.125mg) or a placebo. Melissa, by the way, belongs to the mint family and also has a powerful anti-viral activity. Researchers discovered that the valerian-melissa preparation was comparable to the benzodiazepine drug in its ability to increase deep sleep. However, unlike the drug, it did not cause side-effects – diminished concentration, impairment of physical performance or day-time sleepiness.

PASSIONFLOWER *Passiflora incarnata*

This magnificent climbing plant with its white flowers and extraordinary purple centres, is mildly narcotic and a wonderful sedative for the body. It is particularly useful if you are someone who tends to suffer from nervous tension as well as insomnia. Not as strong as valerian in its action, it is more calming than sedating, and therefore is a superb alternative to tranquilliser drugs. Passionflower works particularly well for sleep when taken together with 5-HTP as a herb, a tincture or fluid extract or in dried powered form in capsules. Passionflower was used by the Aztecs as an analgesic and sedative. One of its plant chemicals is called *harmine,* which has an interesting ability to bring about a contemplative state and a feeling of mild euphoria. It was even used during World War II as a 'truth serum'. Harmine and other plant chemicals in passionflower, which work synergistically with it, prevents serotonin levels from falling and therefore works extremely well with 5-HTP against insomnia.

HOPS *Humulus lupulus*

The flowers from this common herb are often used together with other remedies to treat everything from indigestion to edgy nerves. Like valerian, hops has a pronounced sedative effect but it is much milder. You can use hops in the form of a tincture, but it can be particularly useful as a tea for people who awaken in the middle of the night. Prepare it before going to bed by steeping the flowers for 10 minutes in hot water and then straining and allowing to cool. Put the tea, sweetened with a little honey or preferably stevia (if you can get it), by the side of your bed so you can drink it if you awaken during the night. Some people also swear by small pillows stuffed with dried hops blossoms which you put under your neck when you go to bed or if you awaken.

If you want to find the answers to the Big Questions about your soul, you'd best begin with the Little Answers about your body.

George Sheehan

PERCHANCE TO DREAM

❑ **Expose yourself to morning light** 15 minutes a day. This helps shorten the sleep cycle so you can get to sleep more easily when you go to bed.

❑ **Get more exercise** every day. This burns up adrenalin build-up in the brain which can result in a tense nervous feeling where you are up and can't seem to get down. The best time to exercise is late afternoon or early evening.

❑ **Never exercise within two hours of going to bed.**

❑ **Don't go to bed when you're not sleepy.** Instead pursue some pleasant activity, preferably passive. Television is not a good choice. The rays emanating from the set disturb the nervous system when you least need it.

❑ **Don't drink coffee, alcohol or strong stimulants** at dinner. This is not just an old wives' tale. One researcher looking into the effects of caffeine on human beings showed that total sleep times decreased by two hours and the mean total of intervening wakefulness more than doubles when people are given caffeine in the equivalent of a couple of cups of coffee. Alcohol can put you to sleep but it tends not to keep you there, awakening you instead in the early hours of the morning.

❑ **Be careful if you take high doses of energising supplements** such as guarana, L-tyrosine or ginseng. Only use them early in the day.

❑ **Use an ioniser.** This is a small device you put by the side of your bed that pours negative ions into the air. It's a great gift for anyone who has the kind of nervous system that tends to go up and not want to come down and it's an excellent investment. Negative ions stimulate the production of serotonin in the brain and help relax the body.

❑ **Take lukewarm baths.** Particularly, take a lukewarm bath to which you have added 250-500 g of Epsom salts (magnesium sulphate). Submerge yourself as much as possible for 20 minutes, warming up the bath if you start to get chilled or adding cold water if you begin to get hot. Lukewarm water is the most relaxing of all temperatures on the body. A hot bath before bed is a

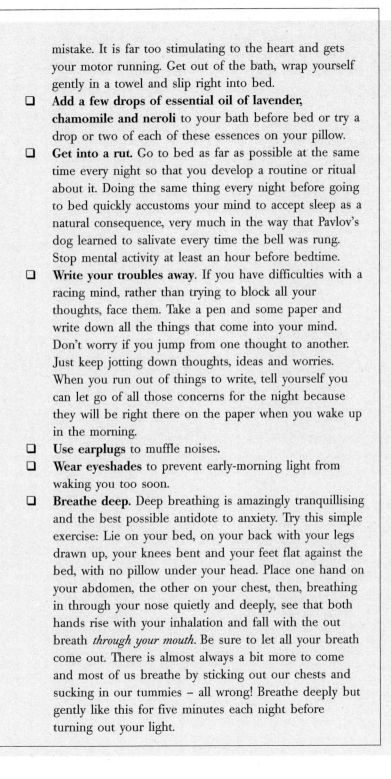

mistake. It is far too stimulating to the heart and gets your motor running. Get out of the bath, wrap yourself gently in a towel and slip right into bed.

❑ **Add a few drops of essential oil of lavender, chamomile and neroli** to your bath before bed or try a drop or two of each of these essences on your pillow.

❑ **Get into a rut.** Go to bed as far as possible at the same time every night so that you develop a routine or ritual about it. Doing the same thing every night before going to bed quickly accustoms your mind to accept sleep as a natural consequence, very much in the way that Pavlov's dog learned to salivate every time the bell was rung. Stop mental activity at least an hour before bedtime.

❑ **Write your troubles away.** If you have difficulties with a racing mind, rather than trying to block all your thoughts, face them. Take a pen and some paper and write down all the things that come into your mind. Don't worry if you jump from one thought to another. Just keep jotting down thoughts, ideas and worries. When you run out of things to write, tell yourself you can let go of all those concerns for the night because they will be right there on the paper when you wake up in the morning.

❑ **Use earplugs** to muffle noises.

❑ **Wear eyeshades** to prevent early-morning light from waking you too soon.

❑ **Breathe deep.** Deep breathing is amazingly tranquillising and the best possible antidote to anxiety. Try this simple exercise: Lie on your bed, on your back with your legs drawn up, your knees bent and your feet flat against the bed, with no pillow under your head. Place one hand on your abdomen, the other on your chest, then, breathing in through your nose quietly and deeply, see that both hands rise with your inhalation and fall with the out breath *through your mouth*. Be sure to let all your breath come out. There is almost always a bit more to come and most of us breathe by sticking out our chests and sucking in our tummies – all wrong! Breathe deeply but gently like this for five minutes each night before turning out your light.

SLEEP THE NIGHT AWAY

Find the right remedy for sleeplessness by identifying the cause. Are you not getting enough exercise? Are you depressed? Do you have low levels of melatonin? Are you eating too much carbohydrate? Do you have an iron or folic acid deficiency? These are all some of the questions you might ask yourself and ask for help from your doctor with.

❏ **SLEEP SUPPLEMENTS**
Try a natural sleep supplement half an hour to an hour before bedtime.

5-HTP	10–50 mg
Melatonin	0.1–3 mg
Vitamin B6	50 mg
Chelated Magnesium	250 mg

❏ **BOTANICAL WONDERS**
Try the plant helpers hops, passionflower or valerian, either singularly or taken together. If you decide to take them together, take one third of the doses recommended below.

❏ **Valerian**

Tincture 1:5	1–1½ tsp (4–6 mls)
Fluid extract	½–1 tsp (2–4 mls)
Dried herb in capsule form	150–300 mg

❏ **Passionflower** (works well with 5-HTP)

Tincture 1:5	½–2 tsp (6–8 mls)
Fluid extract 1:1	½–1 tsp (2–4 mls)
Dried powdered herb	300–450 mg

❏ **Hops**

Tincture 1:5	1–1½ tsp (4–6 mls)
Fluid extract 1:1	½–1 tsp (2–4 mls)
Dried powdered hops	250–350 mgs

NEW DAY – NEW BEGINNING

Don't worry about sleep. Do what you need to do and then just let it happen. If it doesn't happen tonight, so what, it will tomorrow night or the next. Lack of sleep is not likely to kill you, but worrying about it for long enough just might. St. Patrick began each day with a prayer regardless of how much or little sleep he had or how he felt when he awakened. It is my favourite celebration of new beginnings and can wipe away worries following a sleepless night:

> I arise today
>
> Through the strength of heaven
>
> Light of sun,
>
> Radiance of moon,
>
> Splendour of fire
>
> Speed of lightning
>
> Swiftness of wind.
>
> Depth of sea
>
> Stability of earth.
>
> St. Patrick

LIVING WITH AGE POWER

Use the light that dwells within you to regain your natural clarity of sight.

Lao Tzu

In the anti-ageing world of sophisticated biochemistry, complex treatments for body and mind-bending nutrients, how do you gather together what you need in order to begin creating a lifestyle for yourself which will help you live a long, creative and joyous life?

Start by figuring out what you most want to change. You may already be eating well and not too much. It may only be a matter of cutting out the negative things in your diet such as coffee and sugar, increasing the number of fresh foods on your table and using some of the green superfoods to bring you in line with Age Power's Insulin Balance. Maybe you have neglected the state of your muscles and the condition of your body through lack of exercise. Perhaps you too easily stress out by overwork or worry.

You might begin your own Age Power Programme, taking a brisk walk for at least half an hour four or five days a week or begin to learn simple weight training exercises. You might explore what some of the natural anti-anxiety antidotes like 5HTP or St John's Wort can offer you. Someone else, a marathon runner, for example, may be superbly fit and have lots of energy, yet be suffering (as so many athletes do) from haggard-looking skin as a result of living on a low-fat-high-carbohydrate diet which has not been supplying all of the essential nutrients he needs. In this case a substantial programme of nutritional supplements stressing the anti-oxidant nutrients could be a good place to begin, as will tossing out the pasta and sugary sports drinks he has been swallowing.

TWO STEPS FORWARD

For most, change comes in starts and stops. More than 35 years ago I first came upon several physicians who advocated using a high-raw diet. I was fascinated by how such a simple tool could be so transformative. But I am a compulsive experimenter and a great doubter. I have to test something out 20 times before I will believe it. I began to experiment with more fresh foods and found that they changed the way I looked and felt dramatically. But then, because of social convention or basic cynicism, I returned to the usual stodge I had been eating before. It took several

EASY DOES IT

Each of us has unique needs, interests and weaknesses. To make Age Power a part of your life, start with one or two significant changes which are specifically applicable to your needs. Then build your Age Power Programme from there. Leaping into some elaborate regime in which you try to do everything all at once is doomed to failure. Valuable and lasting change almost always comes more slowly and builds gradually on firm foundations. This way, whatever practices you take up for your benefit are not just curious fads to be tried and dropped. They become integrated parts of your life – solid, stable, health-supporting habits which can both bring you closer to the ordered harmony of youthful homeostasis and open up creative possibilities in your life.

years of doubt and experiment – as well as a dawning awareness that at some level I had an unconscious commitment to *worseness* rather than *wellness* – for me gradually to come to a point where a high-raw way of eating became a normal part of my life.

Probably I am slower than most to learn. Several years ago I read in a scientific journal about experiments designed to test animal intelligence. In the 'discussion' part of the paper researchers stated that basic intelligence is directly proportionate to the number of times an animal has to experience a stimulus – say an electric shock every time it touches a switch or a reward of grain whenever it goes through a trap door – before it learns whether the stimulus is of positive or negative value. Only then does the beneficial response become integrated into an animal's behaviour. I remember thinking at the time that I definitely belonged with the lowest level of rats since I often have to beat my head against a brick wall a hundred times before I finally twig to the fact it hurts. The up-side to this is, like a lot of slow-to learn-creatures, once I do know it I actually *know* it, not just theoretically in my head, but at a gut level so it becomes part of me.

Optimism shifts the contents of the mind.
Robert Ornstein PhD and David Sobel MD

GUT KNOWING

It is the gut kind of knowing which is valuable in creating an Age Power life for yourself. And, unless you are one of the very fortunate few who are able to grasp quickly new ideas and techniques and to integrate them into your way of life easily and sensibly, it is going to take time. It also takes experiment to separate out what works best for you from what doesn't work at all. And it may take the help of a doctor or health practitioner who is well versed in nutrition and natural health.

LET YOUR BODY DO IT

Age Power nutritional support is based on an extremely simple nuts-and-bolts hypothesis: We are made of vitamins and minerals, amino acids, fatty acids and other metabolites which all work together according to a living molecular logic. Because we are alive, the life process itself supplies the consciousness to know how to make good use of these nuts and bolts. The nuts and bolts like Coenzyme–A, phytonutrients in fresh foods or alpha lipoic acid are what your body uses to make whatever it needs – energy, oxidation protection, hormones or what have you. Far better to make hormones yourself than supply them as hormone replacement which may undermine the body's ability to make them itself. This simple concept is fundamental to the natural Age Power approach. It is also, I believe, a concept which will eventually change the course of medicine and science in this century.

The results of the Human Genome Project have opened our eyes not to how people will die, but rather to what they need to do to live healthy, full lives based on genetic uniqueness. Nutrition plays a major roll in determining genetic expression, which in turn over the course of our lives determines our health.

Jeffrey Bland MD

It can also be helpful to look at what a good combination of supplemental nutrients designed for Age Power looks like. For although age-researchers can disagree about specifics, the general principles of age-retardation using supplementation are becoming well established. One thing which it is vital to remember is the rule of synergy. It is no good taking large doses of a few vitamins with anti-oxidant properties unless you also provide your body with adequate supplies of *all* the other nutrients you need in smaller quantities, to create an orthomolecular environment which enables it to use them.

PERSONALISE YOUR SUPPLEMENTS

Ideally, if you want to design the best nutritional supplements programme, it is a good idea to consult a good nutritionally orientated doctor or health practitioner who can help you develop one which is personally tailored to your specific needs. Each of us is biochemically unique. Where one person needs only moderate quantities of a specific nutrient such as vitamin B_6 or zinc yet high levels of vitamin C, another may need quite exceptional amounts of zinc and B_6 yet have only a moderate need for vitamin C.

With the information available at this time, it appears that enhancing diet with vitamin and mineral supplements may be of great help to a wide number of individuals. In addition to vitamins and minerals, there are many other nutritional supplements that provide exceptional health benefits, including Co-enzyme-A, Coenzyme-Q_{10}; NADH, alpha-lipoic acid, phosphatidyl serine, pycgenol, DMSO, MSM, aloe vera, n-acetylcysteine (NAC, SAMe, the flavonoids, carnitine); chondroitin sulphate; bee by-products (pollen, royal jelly and propolis); omega-3 fish oils (DHA/EPA) and flaxseed oil; chlorophyll; spirulina, chlorella and other algae products; wheat and barley grass juice; and lecithin.

DAILY OPTIMAL VITAMIN-MINERAL SUPPLEMENTATION

Range for Adults in International Units (IU), micrograms (mcg) or milligrams (mg)

Vitamin	Range
Vitamin A (retinol)	5,000–10,000 IU
Vitamin A (from beta carotene)	25,000–75,000 IU
Vitamin D	100–400 IU
Vitamin E (d-alpha tocopherol in dry form)	400–1200 IU
Vitamin K (phytonadione)	60–1000 mcg
Vitamin C (ascorbic acid)	500–1500 mg
Vitamin B_1 (thiamine)	10–100 mg
Vitamin B_2 (riboflavin)	10–100 mg
Niacin	10–100 mg
Niacinamide	10–100 mg
Vitamin B_6 (pyridoxine)	25–100 mg
Biotin	100–300 mcg
Pantothenic acid	100–500 mg
Folic acid	400–1000 mcg
Vitamin B_{12}	400–1200 mcg
Choline	150–500 mg
Inositol	150–500 mg

Minerals	Range
Boron	1–5 mg
Calcium (calcium citrate or ascorbate)	500–1000 mg
Chromium	200–400 mcg
Copper	1–2 mg
Iodine	50–150 mcg
Iron	15–30 mg
Magnesium	750–1500 mg
Manganese (citrate)	7–10 mg
Molybdenum (sodium molybdate)	10–25 mcg
Potassium	200–500 mg
Selenium (selenomethionine)	100–200 mcg
Silica (sodium metasilicate)	200–1000 mcg
Vanadium (sulfate)	50–100 mcg
Zinc (picolinate)	15–30 mg

LIVING SUPPLEMENTS

Almost all multivitamins and minerals on the market are chemically made. When properly manufactured, packaged to ensure freshness and well formulated in respect to nutrient balance, they offer good nutritional support for age power. But there is another way to go: My own favorite multiple vitamins and mineral supplements, called Vita Synergy For Men™ and Vita Synergy For Women™, are *grown* instead of chemically fromulated. The Vita Synergy ranges are the best of what are known as *food state* nutrients. They are grown in a medium of botanical extracts, food co-factors, enzymes and phytonutrients including wildcrafted and organic flowers and spices. Then they are harvested at low heat to preserve life-enhancing properties and complexities and delivered as a physical mix just as they come in nature. All of this greatly enhances your body's ability to make use of them. Although the levels of nutrients they contain are far lower than those of chemical based vitamins, these multiple ranges are power-fully effective thanks to their high bioavailabilty. Food based nutrients are real foods. You can take them with meals or on an empty stomach to reap the benefits of antioxidant nutritional support of the highest order.

GUIDELINES FOR AGE POWER

Although nutritional supplementation is a highly individual affair, not every aspect of an Age Power lifestyle is so personal. There are lots of 'dos' plus a few simple 'don'ts' which anybody can benefit from adhering to. And while science has not yet provided us with the knowledge which will enable us to live to 200 they should go a long way towards helping us reach 120:

❑ Go for fresh foods – as many as possible eaten raw – and try to get organically grown if you can.

❑ Walk 30 minutes a day, six days a week.

❑ Investigate what nutritional supplements including the anti-oxidant nutrients can do for you, preferably under the guidance of a good nutritionally orientated doctor or health practitioner.

❑ Listen to the messages of your own body. Sleep when you are tired. Eat only when you are hungry. Follow what your inner knowing tells you is best. What works for someone else may not be right for you.

❑ Go easy when incorporating any of the new approaches to Age Power from this book into your own life. Don't try to take on more than you can handle at any one time. It's important to move towards newer methods of health enhancement with caution, wisdom and sensitivity to your own responses.

❑ Never smoke and don't expose yourself to passive smoking.

❑ Drink no more than a glass of *good* wine a day.

❑ Banish any negative expectations you still have about ageing.

❑ Steer clear of drugs, whether prescription, over-the-counter or recreational – unless *absolutely* necessary.

❑ Remove sugar and other high-glycaemic carbohydrates from your diet.

❑ Look at ageing as a positive process which can lead you to even better health, greater stamina and more creativity and happiness than you may have ever known. Such expectations help create your future.

❑ Challenge yourself by learning something new, taking up a new hobby or changing your career.

❑ Let yourself experience joy in your work and play. It is your natural birthright. It can do more to improve your health and longevity than any other single thing.

❑ Seek out new ideas and new people which keep your mind alert and stimulate your interest in life and in other people.

> ❑ Do, as Hans Selye counsels, 'Reach for the highest aim yet never put up resistance in vain.'
>
> ❑ Follow your bliss. Listen to the whispers of your soul and honour them.
>
> Bask in your Age Power freedom. You have earned it.

BRIGHT FUTURE

Thanks to our growing understanding of natural medicine and advanced research into high-tech biochemistry, what was once little more than a pipe dream – the notion that each of us can *die young late in life* – is becoming a reality. Gerontologists challenge the maximum lifespans of many species of animals. Man is next. Already physicians are using anti-oxidant nutrients, electromagnetic techniques and other anti-ageing tools to prevent physical degeneration and to restore health and balance to ailing bodies. Meanwhile psychiatrists and psychologists trained in biochemistry and in the orthomolecular treatment of the brain are not only beginning to cure mental and emotional problems associated with age, they are even using the tools of their trade to expand consciousness. It becomes important to ask the question, 'With what consequences?'

AGEISM DANGERS

The first worry about life extension for most people is, 'What will we do with these old people we are creating?' 'Won't they be yet a further burden to society?' Naturally they want to know about the effect that longevity will have on Housing, medical costs and the rest. Such questions are valid. It is worth examining the assumptions and paradigms which underlie them.

Our society has imprinted its members with negative concepts about being old. In the book for which he won a Pulitzer Prize, *Why Survive? Being Old in America*, Dr Robert Buffer outlined the vast practical problems of dealing with the aged: Housing, pensions, personal security, need for meaningful occupations and the rest, and the horrific conditions in which many old people in modern Western society live. He also pointed out that we hold many unconscious assumptions about the aged which continue to create these conditions. These assumptions are always with us and they greatly distort our view of ageing, old people and their place in society. They include a belief that the aged are inflexible, senile, unproductive people waiting for the inevitable arrival of the grim reaper. Basically not interesting, of little value, they are people worthy of being assigned to a foreclosed existence. Alex Comfort refers to these common views of age and the elderly as 'ageism' which he defines as 'the notion that people cease to be people, to be the same people or become people of a distinct and inferior kind, by virtue of having lived a specified number of years'. 'Ageism' lies behind most of the often asked questions about the social and political consequences of Age Power. They make such questions impossible to answer adequately from our current perspective and with our current views of reality. They also force us to ignore a number of important realities.

We forget the truth of the biomarkers: Chronological age at its best is a very limited indication of biological and functional age. Even our present old people are capable of far more than society allows them to express or contribute – indeed more than they themselves allow. We also forget that every major disease is age-dependent. All of the major causes of death and disability are secondary to the progressive degeneration of ageing. Little wonder, for until now from the age of 30 we have been witnessing a steady and inexorable increase in the probability of morbidity and mortality from one disease or another.

NEW MAPS

People living by the principles of Age Power are different. Highly resistant to the ravages of degeneration which manifest themselves in destructive chronic diseases like cancer, coronary heart disease, arthritis and the rest, they are *less* rather than *more* of a burden to the state in terms of medical, social and psychiatric care. Application of the life-lengthening and life-enhancing principles implicit in Age Power on a wide scale should lead to an increase in the ratio of productive to non-productive men and women with prolonged life spans. This has been the conclusion of Yale's Professor Larry Kotlikoff, one of the few academics to look seriously at the issue. Kotlikoff initiated an inquiry into the economic effects of increased lifespan. He also concluded that this increase in the ratio of productive to non-productive people would result in an increased *per capita* output whether or not the working period increased year for year with life expectancy.

With the increased longevity and the improved resistance to degeneration which

> In one study, a group of elderly subjects considered their future. They listed all the positive things they had to look forward to. Two years later the optimists reported fewer physical symptoms of ill-health and more positive physical and pyschological well-being than did the pessimists. They felt less tension, reported fewer colds, took fewer days off from work and had more energy.
>
> *Robert Ornstein, PhD,*
> *David Sobel, MD:*
> Healthy Pleasures

are the natural outcome of applying the findings of age-researchers to our everyday lives, the population of our old people will also change. So will our attitudes to them. No longer a burden, like the Vilcabamba Indians or the Abkhazians of the Soviet Caucasus they will become not 'old people' but 'long lived people'. Such a simple shift in attitude could revolutionise us as human beings not only in terms of politics and economics, but by shifting us towards a more value orientated society. At that point the question of 'What will we do with all these old people?' begins to take on quite a different meaning. For the challenge now becomes not how we house, feed and care for a growing sector of the non-productive population but rather how we can best use the energy, creativity and wisdom of the older members of our society.

TIME TO REAP

At the moment we have about a quarter of a century allotted to us in which to grow to adulthood. The next 40 years are generally directed towards accomplishment in the outside world, realising the goals of adulthood, procreation and raising a family. Then we tend to slide headlong downhill until we die.

Within the confines of our three-score-years-and-ten and under the pressures of contemporary social values, modern man and modern woman have become quite extraordinarily obsessed with accomplishment. Since for most of us the time for worldly accomplishment is limited to this middle period we push ourselves forward, often at health-breaking and heart-breaking speed. To many of us the concern with fulfilling ourselves in our career, paying the rent, buying the baby a new pair of shoes – during what are supposed to be the best years of our lives – forces us to postpone the pleasures of a time to dream, a time to think and a time to play, in the very highest sense of the word. If we are to find a means of coping with the problems of our society – problems of poor statesmanship, overpopulation, Third World famine, pollution and economic inequities – we desperately need this time to dream. We need this time to recreate our own world and to take our destiny responsibly into our own hands, aside from the demands of adult life.

The diet-heart hypothesis that suggests that high intake of saturated fat and cholesterol causes heart disease has been repeatedly shown to be wrong. The public is being deceived by the greatest health scam of the century.

Dr George M Mann

BEST YET TO COME

Nobel laureate novelist Hermann Hesse wrote about such a time-expanded world in his *Glass Bead Game*. There, time's limits become the rules of the game of life and each human being is freed to order his existential choices. Such a time-expanded world could help us draw together our learning and re-synthesise our knowledge. It might enable the coming together of disciplines such as mathematics, physics, philosophy, biology, medicine, psychology, anthropology, art, literature, politics, theology and law – in fact the whole gamut of human concerns and disciplines – into a kind of connectedness which is urgently needed in the excessively fragmented post-industrial society which has become our home. Healthy longevity – Age Power – would make available to us the steadily maturing wisdom of our old people – people whose experience and awareness have not become distorted by ill-functioning minds and rapidly waning energies. Such wisdom is, I believe, exactly what we need to help guide our species into its further evolution. Moreover, such time expansion takes hold of our personal sense of the present and in a very real way draws it into the future. For when we are able to project ourselves into the future, that future becomes not an abstract consideration but something of active concern to all of us. The future of the earth is our future. We become responsible for it and we will live to see it as caretakers instead of as irresponsible tenants of a rented property. Age Power will help us become its owners and like all owners we are far more likely to look after our property.

Man is not simply a machine. He is not just a physical mechanism. It is clear that there is an ethereal part to man, just as most religions have taught for centuries and medicine has acknowledged with the advancement of psychology. This non-corporeal aspect houses the mind, the emotions, the will, memories and desire. None of these functions can be assigned to any specific organ, yet they are what make us truly human.

James F Balch MD

POWER OF AGE

In George Bernard Shaw's preface to *Back to Methuselah* – the play in which his character Dr Conrad Barnabas promotes an extended lifespan of 300 years – he writes: 'Men do not live long enough; they are, for the purposes of high civilization, mere children when they die'. He then goes on to consider some of the creative possibilities of our being able to lengthen life: 'This possibility came to me when history and experience had convinced me that the social problems raised by millionfold national populations are far beyond the political capacity attainable in three score and ten years of life by slow growing mankind. On all hands as I write the cry is that our statesmen are too old, and that Leagues of Youth must be formed everywhere to save civilisation from them. But despairing ancient pioneers tell me that the statesmen are not old enough for their jobs . . . We have no sages old enough and wise enough to make a synthesis of these reactions, and to develop the magnetic awe-inspiring force which must replace the policeman's baton as the instrument of authority.'

FULL HUMAN LIFE

For me this magnetic awe-inspiring force of which he speaks is nothing less than man's potential to become the creator of his destiny on earth. The situation in which we live with all the global dangers to which we are exposed, from the possibility of mass nuclear extinction to world economic collapse – are not accidents of nature. They have been created by us. And no act of God can suddenly remove their potential destructiveness from our future. Only we ourselves have the potential to do that. If we are to succeed, we will need to call forth every resource which we have – intelligence, wisdom, strength, courage, patience, wit, compassion – and work with them. Age Power can help us do that.

Age Power, and the freedom from mental and physical degeneration which it brings, is no curious artefact of late twentieth-century science. Who cares if, at the age of 85, we are all capable of running a marathon or if we look 30 years younger? Such things matter little on their own. But the high-level health, mental clarity and well-being which are the rewards of Age Power are of urgent concern to our future as residents of the earth. They form the foundation on which we as human beings can build if we are to make use of our full potential for creativity. In the full use of such creativity lies the future of ourselves, our children and our planet. In the words of Capek's Vitek: 'Let's give everyone a three-hundred-year life. It will be the biggest event since the creation of man; it will be the liberating and creating anew of man! God, what man will be able to do in three hundred years! To be a child and pupil for fifty years; fifty years to understand the world and its ways and to see everything there is; and a hundred years to work in; and then a hundred years, when we have understood everything, to live in wisdom, to teach and to give example. How valuable human life would be if it lasted for three hundred years! There would be no fear, no selfishness. Everything would be wise and dignified. Give people life! Give them full human life!'

> Our attitude to life and our relationship with other people often counts far more than fitness or medical regiments.
>
> *Robert Ornstein, PhD, and David Sobel, MD:*
> Healthy Pleasures

An idealistic plea in the midst of the

profound disillusionment with man that is so much a part of early twenty-first century life? A dream? Perhaps. Yet our dreams become the myths by which we live. And right now we urgently need new myths to give our life direction – dreams which, having been tempered by the wisdom of age and experience, are large enough and rich enough to take us forward. Such dreams have power. They also have a remarkable way of becoming reality:

> All men dream; but not equally. Those who
> dream by night in the dusty recesses of their
> minds wake in the day to find it was vanity: but
> dreamers of the day are dangerous men, for
> they may act their dream with open eyes, to
> make it possible.
>
> *T.E. Lawrence*

Leslie Kenton's Website: www.lesliekenton.com. Here you will find a mass of helpful tools, techniques, inspiration and resources for practitioners and products as well as links to other websites which Leslie has found valuable to people. The website is highly active. Information changes weekly including messages from Leslie, herbs of the week, recipes of the week, news about forthcoming events and workshops Leslie is doing throughout the world. There too you have the opportunity to *become a friend* and submit your questions. Those chosen each month are answered personally by Leslie.

RESOURCES

For all the vitamins, minerals and nutraceutical supplements mentioned in *Age Power* the following companies supply a selection of good quality natural products.

The NutriCentre
7 Park Crescent
London W1N 3HE
Tel: +(44) 0207 436 5122
Email: enq@nutricentre.com
Website: www.nutricentre.com

The best suppliers of nutritional supplements and information unique in the world. The NutriCentre is not only the UK's leading supplier of supplements, it also has one of the finest collections of books on holistic health and nutrition including spiritual and psychological books related to health. This small shop in the basement of The Hale Clinic is always at the cutting edge of what is happening in holistic health. Their products can be ordered easily on line or by telephone. The NutriCentre carries more than 20,000 health and natural beauty care products including both those which are available in health-food stores as well as those sold only through practitioners. What you order is dispatched within 24 hours throughout the world. They have become Britain's largest supplier of complementary medicine textbooks to British colleges and universities. They print an interesting newsletter on holistic health with extracts printed on line. The centre is dedicated to service. No order is too small or too large. Almost all of what you need for natural health and beauty you will find here. I can't recommend them highly enough.

Xynergy Health Products
Elsted
Midhurst
West Sussex GU29 0JT
Tel: +(44) 01730 813642
Fax: +(44) 01730 815109
Email: naturally@xynergy.co.uk
Website: www.xynergy.co.uk

This company specialises in selling the finest aloe vera products and green nutritional products – such as spirulina and cereal grasses – you can buy. They also do the only fully natural multiple vitamin and mineral formula derived from plants in the world. They are available in sophisticated health-food stores or can be ordered by post direct from them. Pure Synergy and other good green products, such as Vita Synergy for Women™ and Vita Synergy for Men™, are available mail order from Xynergy Health Products.

BioCare
The Lakeside Centre
180 Lifford Lane
Kings Norton
Birmingham
West Midlands B30 3NT
Tel: +(44) 0121 433 3727
Fax: +(44) 0121 433 3879
E-mail: biocare@biocare.co.uk
Website: www.biocare.co.uk

Solgar Vitamin & Herb
Aldbury
Tring
Hertfordshire HP23 5PT
Tel: +(44) 01442 890 355
Fax: +(44) 01442 890 366
Website: www.solgar.com

An American company founded in 1947 which produces good quality nutritional supplements and standardised single herbs and formulas under strict pharmaceutical standards of manufacture – in many cases stricter than USA government requirements. These include standardised full potency Herbal Female Complex (containing soy isoflavones), Feverfew Willow Complex, Milk Thistle Dandelion Complex, Ginger Fennel Complex, Olive Leaf Echinacea Complex and Herbal Male Complex. Solgar products are available from top health-food stores, some chemists and the Nutri Centre.

Higher Nature Ltd
The Nutrition Centre
Burwash Common
East Sussex N19 7LX
Tel: +(44) 01435 882880
Fax: +(44) 01435 883720
Email: sales@higher-nature.co.uk
Website: www.higher-nature.co.uk

Thorne Research
Interlink House
Asfordby Business Park
Melton Mowbray
Leicestershire LE14 3JL
Tel: +(44) 01664 810 011
Fax: +(44) 01664 810 012
Email: info@health-interlink.co.uk
Website: www.health-interlink.co.uk

Nature's Best
Century Place
Tumbridge Wells
Kent TN2 3BE
Tel: +(44) 01892 552 117
Fax: +(44) 01892) 515 863
Website: www.naturesbestonline.com

Natures Plus
2500 Grand Avenue
Long Beach
CA 90815-1764
USA
Tel: +(1) 562 494 2500
Website: www.natureplus.com

Twinlab Laboratories Inc.
150 Motor parkway
Suit 210
Hauppauge
NY 11788
USA
Tel: +(1) 631 467 3140
Fax: +(1) 631 630 3489
Email: product@twinlab.com
Website: www.twinlab.com

For all the herbs mentioned in *Age Power* the following companies below supply a selection of good quality products.

Phyto Products Ltd
Park Works
Park House
Mansfield Woodhouse
Nottinghamshire NG19 8EF
Tel: +(44) 01623 644 334
Fax: +(44) 01623 657 232

An excellent company originally set up to supply herbalists with high-quality herbs and plant products. Every plant and herb they sell states the source of origin. All Phyto Products' plants are purchased only from recognisable sources. They do a full range of tinctures, herbal skin creams (including Calendula Cream, Comfrey Cream, Arnica Ointment and St John's Wort Oil), fluid extracts, herbs and the Schoenenberger plant juices. Virtually all the herbs mentioned in this book are supplied by this company in both tincture form and the loose dried herb. They do not supply herbs in capsules but they now do some herbs in tablet form. Write to them for their price list. They have a minimum order of £20 (before VAT) plus carriage.

Weleda (UK) Ltd
Heanor Road
Ilkeston
Derbyshire DE7 8DR
Tel: +(44) 0115 944 8200
Fax: +(44) 0115 944 8210
Website: www.weleda.co.uk

Weleda grew out of the work of Rudolf Steiner and have been making medicines and body care products for 75 years. Weleda UK grow over 400 species of plants organically and biodynamically for use in their medicines and body care range. They do an excellent arnica cream and a delightful skin-care range. Available from good health stores and pharmacies. Or order direct on 0115 944 8222.

Simmonds Herbal Supplies
Freepost (BR1396)
Hove
West Sussex BN3 6BR
Tel: +(44) 01273 202 401
Fax: +(44) 01273 705 120
E-mail: sales@herbalsupplies.com

This company has been supplying high-quality additive-free herbal aids to health practitioners in the UK and abroad since 1982. They now do a range of good-quality products for the general public as well, offering single herbs and mixtures as capsules, tinctures or extracts. Write to them for their catalogue.

Bioforce (UK) Ltd
2 Brewster Place
Irvine
Ayrshire
Tel: +(44) 01563 851 177
Fax: +(44) 01563 851 173

Suppliers of herbal extracts, tinctures, homeopathic remedies and natural self-care products and foods, Bioforce is a Swiss company started by the Swiss expert in natural health, Alfred Vogel. The company always use fresh herbs in preparing their products at the Bioforce factory in Roggwil. They do over 100 different herbal and homeopathic preparations, all of which are very high quality. They can be ordered by post but are often also available in good health-food stores and pharmacies carrying herbal products.

Bio-Health Ltd
Culpepper Close
Medway City Estate
Rochester
Kent ME2 4HU
Tel: +(44) 01483 570813

Bio-Health do an excellent range of single herbs, ointments and multi-herb compounds in tablet and capsule form which you can purchase from good health-food stores or order by post. Write to them for a catalogue.

Solgar Vitamin & Herb
Aldbury
Tring
Herts HP23 5PT
Tel: +(44) 01442 890 355
Fax: +(44) 01442 890 366
Website: www.solgar.com

An American company founded in 1947 which produces good quality nutritional supplements and standardised single herbs and formulas under strict pharma-ceutical standards of manufacture – in many cases stricter than USA government requirements. These include standardised full potency Herbal Female Complex (containing soya isoflavones), Feverfew Willow Complex, Milk Thistle Dandelion Complex, Ginger Fennel Complex, Olive Leaf Echinacea Complex and Herbal Male Complex. Solgar products are available from top health-food stores, some chemists, and the NutriCentre.

AGE POWER SPECIFICS

Aloe Vera: The best is from Xynergy Health Products. See suppliers on page 488.

Autogenic Training: To work with a trained practitioner or to find a trained prac-titioner local to you, contact the British Autogenic Society, Royal London Homoeopathic Hospital, Great Ormond Street, London WC1N 3HR. Tel: 020 7713 6336. Website: www.autogenic-therapy.org.uk

Base Cream: A good quality base cream can be purchased from Phyto Products Ltd. See suppliers on page 476.

Candida: Candida Research and Information Foundation, PO Box 2719, Castro Valley, CA 94546, USA.

Cell Therapy Contact Dr Claus Martin, The Four Seasons Clinic, Parkresidenz Bachmair-Weissach, D-83700 Rottach-Egern, Wiesser Strasse, 1 PO Box 244, Germany. Tel: + 49 8022 24041. Fax + 49 8022 24042. Reservation & Information Tel: + 49 8022 26780. Fax: +49 8022 24740.

Coenzyme-A You will find a handful of products on the market which provide pantethine or other precursors to Coenzyme-A. Coenzyme A™ is the only one formulated with the complex advanced delivery system (Modulator Matrix I™) which makes it possible for the natural ingredients to be transported direct to the cells and across the mitochondrial barrier where they can efficiently initiate ATP energy production. This formula over-rides inhibitory enzymes and enables the body to make more CoA within its own cells. Coenzyme A™ is produced by Coenzyme-A Technologies. Contact Coenzyme-A Technologies, 12512 Beverly Pk. Road., B1, Lynnwood, WA 98037, USA. Tel: +1 425 438 8586. Fax: +1 425 438 8766. Website: www.coenzyme-a.com

Coenzyme-A Technologies also produce the following products:

Body Image™ Incorporating the same cutting-edge technology used in the manufacture of Coenzyme A™, Body Image™ with its Modulator Matrix II™ initiates metabolic functions needed to spur fat burning for energy. It is good for weight loss and is a favourite of athletes as it enhances aerobic performance and helps stabilise blood sugar levels.

Healthy Cholesterol Image™ Incorporating the same cutting-edge technology used in the manufacture of Coenzyme A™, Healthy Cholesterol™ with its Modulator Matrix III™ supports healthy cholesterol and fatty acid metabolism. It helps regulate cholesterol and triglycerides, stabilises blood sugar, detoxifies drugs and synthesises hormones.

Clear Skin Image™ Incorporating the same cutting-edge technology used in the manufacture of Coenzyme A™, Clear Skin Image™ is the most potent anti-acne product I have ever come across. Addressing acne at its causes, it supports acetylation reactions for detoxifying the body, shifts distorted fatty acid metabolism and helps rebalance hormones.

Healthy Joint Image™ Incorporating the same cutting edge technology used in the manufacture of Coenzyme A™, Healthy Joint Image with its Modulator Matrix IV™, brings support for bones, joints, ligaments, cartilage and connective tissue. It supports immune functions and facilitates repair of DNA and RNA and physical injuries. It contains N-acetyl D-glucosamine – a superior form of glucosamine which is a precursor to hyaluronic acid found in skin and synovial fluids in joints. As such Healthy Joint Image™ offers superb nutraceutical support for arthritic and rheumatic problems as well as leaky gut troubles.

Flaxseeds (Linseeds): Vacuum-packed whole flaxseeds (linseeds) are available in most health-food stores. I use Linusit Gold as they are well packed and fresh. They are available from The NutriCentre. Organic flaxseeds are also available from Higher Nature Limited. Keep them refrigerated. See suppliers on pages 474 and 475.

Flaxseed Oil (Linseed Oil): Organic Flaxseed Oil is available from Savant Distribution Ltd, FREEPOST NEA 701, Leeds LS16 6YY. Order line: 08450 60 60 70. Fax: 0113 230 1915. E-mail: info@savant-health.com Website: www.savant-health.com In capsule form this is available mail order from BioCare Ltd. See suppliers on page 475.

Feldenkrais: To find a practitioner local to you in the UK contact: The Feldenkrais Guild, PO Box 370, London N103XA. Tel: 07000 785506. Email: enquiries@feldenkrais.co.uk Website: www.feldenkrais.co.uk

Hair Analysis: For hair analysis contact Biolab, 9 Weymouth Street, London W1N 3FF. Tel: 020 7636 5959. Fax: 020 7580 3910. E-mail info@biolab.co.uk Website: www.biolab.co.uk

Holosync™ Audio Technology: Available in the UK and Europe from LifeTools, Tel: 01189 483444 (from outside the UK: +44 1189 483444). Fax: 01189 462505 (from outside the UK: +44 1189 462505). website: www.lifetools.com 230 Peppard Road, Emmer Green, Reading, Berkshire RG4 8UA. Office hours are 9am to 5pm Monday to Friday.
From other countries contact Centerpointe Research Institute, 4720 SW Washington Street, Suite #104, Beaverton, OR 97005, USA. Tel: +1 (800) 945 2741. Fax: +1 (503) 643 3114. Outside the US and Canada: 001 503 672 7117. Email: support@centerpointe.com Website: www.centerpointe.com

Green Supplements: Pure Synergy™ and other good green products are available mail order from Xynergy Health Products, Elsted, Midhurst, West Sussex GU29 0JT. Tel: +(44) 01730 813642. Fax: +(44) 01730 815109 Website: www.xynergy.co.uk Email: naturally@xynergy.co.uk Pure Synergy is simply the best green nutritional supplement I have ever seen, a mix of 62 organically grown superfoods working together synergistically to support life-energy in its purest form. Vita Synergy for Women™ and Vita Synergy for Men™ is the first truly 100 percent all natural vitamin, mineral and herbal supplement made entirely from food source nutrients. They also supply top quality wheatgrass. bluegreen algae, spirulina, seaweed supplements and condiments.

Hormone Creams: You can purchase progesterone cream from Wellsprings Trading Ltd, PO Box 322, St Peter Port, Guernsey, Channel Islands GY1 3TP. Tel: 01481 233370. Fax: 01481 235206. Website: www.progesterone.co.uk
You can purchase Progest by post from: Woman's International Pharmacy, 5708 Monova Drive, Madison WI, USA. Tel: 001 608 221 7800. Fax: 001 608 221 7819.

For information on the multiple uses of natural progesterone for women's health contact the Natural Progesterone Information Service (NPIS), PO Box 24, Buxton SK17 9FB. Tel: 07000 784849. Fax: 01298 70979.

For information about natural health developments including information on progesterone products, contact Well Woman's International Network, La Brecque, Alderney, Channel Islands GY9 3TJ. Tel: 07000 8359946. Fax: 07000 3299946.

Microfiltered Whey Protein: Solgar produce Whey to Go Protein Powder in vanilla, chocolate, honey nut and mixed berry flavours. I prefer the vanilla and chocolate. BioPure Pure Protein by Metagenics or Twinlab Super Whey Powder are also good sources of microfiltered whey protein. Whey to Go and BioPure can be purchased from the NutriCentre. See suppliers on page 474.

Microhydrin™: To order microhydrin in the UK contact Steve Calliaghan. Tel: 0141 423 7578 Website: www.synergy-health.co.uk or Karuna Flame Holistic Health, RBC Ind. Distributors, Knocknahur, Sligo, Ireland. Tel: +353 (0) 71 68699. E-mail: karunaflame@eircom.net

Crystal Energy is a water treatment formula used with microhydrin which lowers surface tension (from 75 dynes to 45 dynes) of any liquid to which it is added. It makes water 'wetter' making it more like biological fluid ready for full absorption and super hydration. If you want more information on Crystal Energy and Microhydrin, and how to use it for optimum benefit then visit www.royal-fitness.com/karuna.

Multi-vitamin & Mineral Supplement: Vita Synergy for Women™ and Vita Synergy for Men™ is the first truly 100 percent all natural vitamin, mineral and herbal supplement made entirely from food source nutrients and is available from Xynergy Health Products. It is highly bioavailable and is my favourite. Solgar also do excellent multiple vitamins and minerals such as Omnium, so do Nature's Plus and Higher Nature. See suppliers on pages 474, 475 and 476.

Organic Foods: The Soil Association publishes a regularly updated national directory of farm shops and box schemes called *Where to Buy Organic Foods* that costs £5 including postage from: The Soil Association, Bristol House, 40–56 Victoria Street, Bristol BS1 6BY. Tel: 0117 929 0661. Fax: 0117 925 2504. E-mail: info@soilassociation.org Website: www.soilassociation.org.

Organics Direct: Offers a nationwide home delivery service of fresh vegetables and fruits, delicious breads, juices, sprouts, fresh soups, ready-made meals, snacks and baby foods. They also sell the state-of-the-art 2001 Champion Juicers and the 2002 Health Smart Juice Extractor for beginners. They even sell organic wines – all shipped to you within 24 hours. Organics Direct, 1-7 Willow Street, London EC2A 4BH. Tel: 020 7729 2828. Fax: 020 7613 5800. Website: www.organicsdirect.com You can order online.

Clearspring: Supply organic foods and natural remedies as well as macrobiotic foods by mail order. They have a good range of herbal teas, organic grains, whole seeds for sprouting, dried fruits, pulses, nut butters, soya and vegetable products, sea vegetables, drinks and Bioforce herb tinctures. Write to them for a catalogue: Clearspring, Unit 19a, Acton Park Estate, London W3 7QE. Tel: 020 8746 0152. Fax: 020 8811 8893. You can order by telephone, fax, post or shop online at www.clearspring.co.uk

Organic Meat: A UK Guide to where to buy organic meat is available from Organic Butchers, Crescent Consulting, 1 The Crescent, Northampton NN1 4SB. Tel: +(44) 01604 459962. Fax: +(44) 01604 459963. Website: www.organicbutchers.co.uk

Eastbrook Farms Organic Meat: Eastbrook Farms Organic Meats, Bishopstone, Swindon, Wiltshire SN6 8PW. This is my favourite supplier of all sorts of organic meat because they take such care over every order. Order online: 01793 790460. Helpline: 01793 790340. Fax: 01793 791239. Email: info@helenbrowningorganics.co.uk Website: www.helenbrowningorganics.co.uk

Longwood Farm Organic Meats: Good-quality organic beef, pork, bacon, lamb, chicken, turkey, duck and geese, a variety of types of sausage, all dairy products, vegetables and organic groceries (2000 lines), are available mail order from: Longwood Farm Organic Meats, Tudenham St Mary, Bury St Edmunds, Suffolk IP28 6TB. Tel: 01638 717120. Fax: 01638 717120.

Fibre in powder form: Powdered psyllium husks available from good health-food stores or by mail order from The Nutri Centre. See suppliers on page 474.

Probiotic Supplement: Available form the Nutri Centre. Good quality probiotic supplements are made by BioCare and Thorne Research. See suppliers on page 475.

Pure Synergy™: and other good green products are available mail order from Xynergy Health Products, Elsted, Midhurst, West Sussex GU29 0JT. Tel: +(44) 01730 813642. Fax: +(44) 01730 815109 Website: www.xynergy.co.uk Email: naturally@xynergy.co.uk
Pure Synergy is simply the best green nutritional supplement I have ever seen, a mix of 62 organically grown superfoods working together synergistically to support life-energy in its purest form.

Resistance Training: Michael Colgan, one of the most knowledgeable men in the world in the field of nutrition and weight training created a series of four videos for USANA called *The Get Lean Series*. Each video lasts about 30 minutes and trains a different body part using nothing more than dumbbells. They are excellent. The best I have found. Sadly USANA are no longer producing this set of videos. If you cannot get the Michael Colgan videos in your country try USANA's new series of videos called Lean Band Workout. Nancy Popp, a national aerobic champion who has trained thousands of people and who worked with Michael Colgan on the first video has created them. They use resistance bands and provide a system that allows safe improvement of muscular strength and endurance.

Find an independent USANA sales person in your area to order them or visit their website: www.usana.com Email: dist.servuk@us.usana.com for information on distributors in your area. USANA UK distributor www.healthscienceuk.com

Sedona Method™: Audio tapes are available from LifeTools, 230 Peppard Road, Emmer Green, READING, Berkshire RG4 8UA. Tel: 01189 483444 (from outside the UK: +44 1189 483444). Fax 01189 462505 (from outside the UK: +44 1189 462505). Website: www.lifetools.com Office hours are 9am to 5pm Monday to Friday, they have live operators taking orders and messages outside of these hours.

Soya Milk: The best soya milk I have come across is called Bonsoy. It is a particularly good soya milk, unusual in that it is not packed in aluminium. It is organic and available from good health-food stores. Contact: Freshlands, 196 Old Street, London EC1V 9FR. Tel: 0207 250 1708 or Wild Oats, 210 Westbourne Grove, London, W11 2RH. Tel: 0207 229 1063.

Stevia: In most countries, not in the UK alas, stevia is readily available in health-food stores in many forms. It comes as clear liquid extract in distilled water, powered stevia leaf or as full strength (very sweet) stevioside extract. In shaker form you can use stevia as you would sugar to sprinkle on foods and drinks. It even comes in tiny single serving packets which you can carry around with you in your pocket or handbag. From the UK, where stevia is unfortunately no longer available, you may be able to order it direct from abroad by looking on the web or asking a friend who lives in the US to send you some. Stevia is unquestionably the best form of sweetener in the world. Far from doing harm it actually has many beneficial properties.

Water: Getting pure water can be difficult. One in ten of us drink water which is contaminated with poisons above international standards. I have finally found a water purifier which I think is good – the Fresh Water 1000 Water Filter System. It removes more than 90 percent of heavy metals, pesticides and hydrocarbons such as benzene, trihalmethanes, chlorine, oestrogen and bacteria without removing essential minerals like calcium. Available from The Fresh Water Filter Company Ltd, Gem House, 895 High Road, Chadwell Heath, Essex RM6 4HL. Tel: +(44) 020 8597 3223. Fax: +(44) 0870 056 7264. E-mail: mail@freshwaterfilter.com Website: www.freshwaterfilter.com

GLOSSARY

Acetylcholine A chemical formed by the choline and acetyl group. It is a neurotransmitter in the nervous system used to transmit nerve impulses. Acetylcholine slows down heart rate, dilates blood vessels and increases activity of the gastrointestinal systems. In the brain, acetylcholine is involved with learning and memory.

Adrenaline The major hormone of the adrenal gland, epinephrine increases heart rate and contractions, constricts or dilates blood vessels, relaxes the muscles in the lungs and smooth muscles in the intestines, and helps process sugar and fat.

Aerobic Capacity How well the body processes oxygen is determined by lung capacity, the size of capillaries, the pumping action of the heart and the transfer of oxygen to target tissues.

Aerobic Exercise Repetitive exercise that gets the heart and lungs moving while bringing about only a modest increase in breathing, so that the exercise may be maintained over a long period. This form of exercise facilitates adequate oxygen transfer to muscle cells so that no build-up of lactic acid occurs. Aerobic exercise is useful for reducing insulin levels and lowering blood glucose.

Age-Related Cognitive Decline (ARCD) The gradual loss of mental abilities with age.

Alzheimer's Disease A progressive brain disease leading to memory loss, interference with thinking abilities and other losses of mental powers. Brain cells show degenerative damage. Neurons that use the neurotransmitter acetylcholine are most affected.

Amino Acids Building blocks of proteins. There are twenty common amino acids: alanine, arginine, asparagine, aspartic acid, cysteine, glutamic acid, glutamine, glycine, histidine, isoleucine, leucine, lysine, methionine, phenylalanine, proline, serine, threonine, tryptophan, tyrosine and valine.

Amyloid Any of a group of proteins that deposit in the brain and cause amyloidosis. Amyloidosis is often associated with Alzheimer's disease.

Anti-oxidant Any substance that helps protect against free radical damage. Some, such as vitamin A, C, E and D, minerals selenium and zinc, as well as phyto-nutrients such as lipuric acid and the flavonoids from vegetable foods are nutritional anti-oxidants, while others are produced in the body as enzymatic anti-oxidants.

Arachidonic Acid An omega-6 long-chain polyunsaturated fatty acid found primarily in animal fats that is often too high in modern diets. Arachidonic acid can be converted into powerfully inflammatory prostaglandins, such as PGE_2. The omega-3 fatty acids EPA and DHA counter the effects of arachidonic acid. High carbohydrate diets can activate an enzyme called delta-5-desaturase, causing the body to make too much arachidonic acid and feed the inflammatory pathways.

Arteriosclerosis Also called hardening of the arteries, this includes a number of conditions that cause artery walls to thicken and lose elasticity.

ATP (Adenosine Triphosphate) The primary fuel used by cells to generate the bio-chemical reactions necessary for life.

Axon The tubelike part of a neuron that transmits outgoing signals to other cells.

Benzodiazepine A class of medicines such as Valium, Dalmane and Xanax, that act on GABA receptors to induce the relaxation and sleep. Too much, used too often, can lead to memory loss. There are also receptors in the brain for benzodiazepines.

Blood Glucose Primary source of energy for the body. Raised blood glucose levels can result in accelerated ageing and in some people may cause diabetes.

Blood-Brain Barrier The filtering system that prevents some of the substances in the regular circulatory system easily getting into the brain.

Blood-Sugar Tolerance (or glucose tolerance) The body's ability to control the amount of blood sugar (or glucose) in our blood after eating or drinking a defined amount of sugar. Blood-sugar levels tend to rise with age, although impaired glucose tolerance, like high blood pressure, has no symptoms. Age-related blood-sugar impairment is probably the result of the sedentary lifestyle of the average ageing person and a diet too high in junk fats and high-glycaemic carbohydrates. Poor glucose tolerance can lead to Syndrome X and Type II diabetes.

BMR (basal metabolic rate) The rate of the body's chemical processes when it's at rest. The BMR tends to decline with age, largely because the amount of muscle tissue in people's bodies tends to decline with advancing age, a situation that can be reversed through regular exercise.

Body Composition How much fat, muscle, bone and so forth, there is in our bodies. Using the most traditional techniques for measuring body composition, physiologists can assess the amount of fat and non-fat (also called 'lean-body mass') tissue. Ageing is associated with increasing amounts of fat and decreases in lean-body mass, specifically muscle.

Candidiasis A complex medical syndrome produced by a chronic overgrowth of the yeast *Candida albicans.*

Capillaries Very small, hairline-thin vessels supplying blood to tissues.

Carbohydrates A macronutrient made out of carbon, hydrogen and oxygen. These are often simple sugars and bigger molecules made up of joining simple sugars together. Examples are lactose, glucose, sucrose, maltose, starch and glycogen. Fibre is also considered a carbohydrate although it is not digestible by humans and does not constitute usable carbohydrate and therefore it is not important in calculating usable carbohydrate levels of a food.

Carcinogen A substance that causes cancer.

Cell Membrane A thin layer consisting mostly of fatty acids that surrounds each cell.

Central Nervous System The brain and the nerves in the spinal cord. The peripheral nervous system refers to the nerves in the body outside of the central nervous system.

Cerebrum The upper, main part of the brain, consisting of left and right sides. It controls voluntary thought and movements.

Cholesterol A waxy substance or sterol, manufactured by all animal cells. Cholesterol is an essential component of the body's biochemistry. It is used to make steroid hormones such as cortisone, testosterone and oestrogen.

Coenzyme-A The most active metabolic enzyme in the human body. Coenzyme-A operates in the body's cells and blood where it is needed to initiate more than 100 important processes. One of the most crucial functions performed by Coenzyme-A is its initiation of the body's energy cycle (known variously as the ATP, TCA, Krebs or citric acid cycle) which produces over 90 percent of the body's energy. Coenzyme-A is expended and constantly needs replenishing.

Coenzyme-Q$_{10}$ Also known as ubiquinone Co-Q$_{10}$ is a nutrient which has two important properties. It is a key player in the mitochondrial generation of ATP – in other words, the body's ability to burn fuel as energy.

It is also a powerful anti-oxidant. Supplements of Coenzyme-Q_{10} can be helpful for some people in the fat burning process.

Collagen The protein that is the main component of connective tissue.

Dehydration A lower amount of body water than normal. Ageing tends to be associated with chronic dehydration due to age-related decreases in kidney function and thirst. The result is a reduction in the body's vital thermoregulatory ability.

Dendrites Spiderlike projections from the cell body that receive and send messages between nerve cells.

DHA Docosahexanoic Acid. A long chain polyunsaturated fatty acid of the omega-3 group. DHA is found in foods such as salmon, mackerel, herring, tuna and sardines.

DHEA Dehydroepiandrosterone. Produced in the adrenal glands, it is a weak male hormone and a precursor to some other hormones, including testosterone and oestrogen.

DNA Deoxyribonucleic Acid. The genetic material in the nucleus of every cell, which provides the blue print for cell reproduction and all body functions, which is very sensitive to oxidation damage from excess free radicals.

Dopamine A neurotransmitter critical to fine motor co-ordination, immune function, motivation, insulin regulation, physical energy, thinking, short-term memory, emotions such as sexual desire and autonomic nervous system balance.

Double-blind study A way of controlling against experimental bias by ensuring that neither the researcher nor the subject know when an active agent or a placebo is being used.

Endorphins Self-made tranquillisers and painkillers. Each endorphin is composed of a chain of amino acids and acts on the nervous system to reduce pain.

Enzymes Proteins that bring about metabolic changes in biological systems. They help change one substance into another. Enzymes usually require minerals and vitamins to act as co-factors and catalysts for them to do their work.

EPA Eicosapentanoic Acid. A long-chain polyunsaturated fat which like DHA is found in foods such as salmon, mackerel, herring, sardines and tuna. It can be made into prostaglandin E_3, a substance that helps counter inflammation in the body.

Essential Fatty Acids The fats that the body cannot make for itself and therefore must be taken in the foods that you eat. Essential fatty acids are the building blocks of prostaglandins. There are two groups – omega-3 and omega-6 fatty acids, each of which produces different prostaglandins.

Excitotoxin Toxins that bind to certain receptors such as glutamate receptors in neurons, and cause injury or death to these neurons.

Flavonoid A generic term for a group of flavone-containing compounds that are found widely in nature. They include many of the compounds that account for plant pigments (anthocyanins, anthoxanthins, apigenins, flavones, flavonols, bioflavonols, etc). The plant pigments exert a wide variety of physiological effects in the human body.

Free Radical A highly reactive molecule, atom or molecular fragment that has free or unpaired electrons. Free radicals interact with proteins, fats and carbohydrates in the body as well as cells and tissues and can cause free radical damage or oxidation associated with degenerative disease and early ageing. Problems happen when free radical production exceeds the body's ability to protect against them, which occurs in many disease processes. Anti-oxidants help protect against free radical damage.

GABA Gamma-aminobutyric acid, a brain chemical that causes sedation. Medicines such as Valium act on receptors for GABA to induce relaxation. GABA also refers to the receptors themselves.

Gene The smallest genetic unit of a chromosome. It is a piece of DNA that contains the hereditary information for the production of a specific protein.

GLA Gamma-linolenic acid. An omega-6 family long chain polyunsaturated fatty acid sometimes used to increase the production of the body's PGE_1 anti-inflammatory system. It should however be used with care, as in some people, supplements of GLA can produce more arachidonic acid and therefore more inflammation in the body.

Glucagon A pancreatic hormone that causes the release of stored carbohydrate in the liver to help regulate blood glucose levels.

Glucose The simple carbohydrate, sometimes known as blood sugar, that circulates in the bloodstream. It can also be stored in the muscles and the liver as glycogen.

Glucose Tolerance The ability to metabolise sugar properly.

Glutamate An amino acid found in proteins that also acts as a neuro-transmitter in the brain.

Glycaemic Index The potential of a sugar or carbohydrate to raise blood sugar levels. High-glycaemic foods tend to raise insulin and can also stimulate the conversion of omega-6 fatty acids into the inflammatory arachidonic acid. This can interfere with fat burning as well as causing many inflammatory problems in the body. Ironically some simple sugars, such as table sugar, have a lower glycaemic index and enter the bloodstream more slowly than many complex carbohydrates such as potatoes and bread. The faster a carbohydrate enters the bloodstream the higher will be its Glycaemic Index. The higher the Glycaemic Index, the greater will be the increase in insulin levels it brings about. Some fruits and most vegetables tend to have low Glycaemic Index, whereas pasta, grains, breads and starches tend to have a high Glycaemic Index.

Growth Hormones The hormone released from the pituitary, which interacts with fat cells to release fatty acids, and also with the liver to produce insulin growth factors. Exercise enhances growth hormone release which is one of the reasons it also helps clear insulin resistance, lower insulin levels and spur fat burning in the body.

HDL High-density lipoprotein, a protein and lipid particle in the blood which functions to remove cholesterol from the cells. Higher blood levels are more desirable. If insulin levels go up, then HDL levels go down. The lower the HDL level the more likely you are to age rapidly and the more at risk you are of heart disease.

Homocysteine An intermediary compound in the metabolism of the amino acid methionine. High levels in the blood can cause arteriosclerosis. Recently it has been suspected that high amounts of homocysteine can also be toxic to neurons. B vitamins, particulary folic acid, B_{12} and B_6, can lower homocysteine levels.

Hormone Replacement Therapy (HRT) The use of oestrogen combined with progestin for the treatment of menopausal symptoms and the prevention of some long-term effects of menopause.

Hormones A substance formed in an organ which excites some vital process by communicating information at a distance. Each hormone demands specific receptors to be able carry out its biological functions. Hormones also use secondary messengers to initiate the cellular changes that use the information they carry.

Hydrogenation The process of adding hydrogen to unsaturated fatty acids in order to make them harder. Many processed foods are hydrogenated, making them potentially unhealthy.

Hyperinsulinaemia A state in which the body continually maintains abnormally elevated levels of insulin. The word literally means 'high insulin'. This is usually the result of insulin resistance where the cells are not responding to insulin to reduce blood glucose levels.

Hypothalamus A small area of the brain above and behind the roof of the mouth. The hypothalamus is prominently involved with the functions of the autonomic nervous system (the independent nervous system outside of voluntary control) and the hormonal system. It also plays a role in mood and motivation.

Hypoxia An inadequate supply of oxygen.

Immune System The cells, biological substances (such as antibodies) and cellular activities that work together to provide resistance to disease.

Inositol An essential nutrient made from glucose that forms part of phosphatidylinositol, one of the phospholipids in the cell membrane. Inositol is widely available in foods and can be made in the human body when needed.

Insulin The 'storage hormone'. A hormone secreted by the pancreas, which helps shuttle glucose from the blood into the cells for storage. Excess insulin is the primary reason for obesity and early ageing. Insulin is also one of the body's most important chemical messengers which directs the activities of the cells.

Insulin Resistance A condition where the cells no longer respond to insulin. This results in the body secreting more insulin into the bloodstream in a brave attempt to lower blood glucose levels.

Insulin Sensitivity The normal healthy state where the body's cells remain receptive and responsive to insulin's action.

Ketogenic Diet A diet that causes ketone bodies to be produced by the liver, shifting the body's metabolism away from burning glucose as fuel, towards burning stored body fat. A ketogenic diet restricts carbohydrates below a certain level – generally below 75 g per day – bringing about a series of adaptations. The ultimate determinant of whether a diet is ketogenic or not is the level of carbohydrate that it contains.

Krebs Cycle The cycle by which nutrients for our foods are converted into energy. It takes place in the mitochondria and is also called the TCA cycle or citric acid cycle.

LDL Low-density lipoprotein. A protein and lipid particle in the blood which carries most of the blood's cholesterol. When damaged it can be deposited in the artery wall. Lower values of LDL are more desirable.

Lean Body Mass The total body weight minus the fat mass. Lean body mass is made up of water, bones, collagen, muscle and organs.

Life Expectancy This is a statistical estimate of how long a person can expect to live based on such variables as his or her year of birth, infant mortality, societal disease rates, sex and environment. Unlike the human 'life span' which is fixed, life expectancy changes. For example, in 1900 we had a projected life expectancy of over 77 years. A 90-year-old nursing-home patient has a remaining life expectancy of about one year.

Life Span Every living species has a distinct life span. For dogs, it's 13 to 17 years depending on size; for elephants, around 70 years.

Linoleic Acid One of the essential fatty acids, which means that the body cannot make it. Linoleic acid belongs to the omega-6 family and must be obtained in small quantities from the daily diet. The Western diet is far too high in linoleic acid and the other omega-6 fatty acids in relation to the omega-3 group.

Lipid Fatty acid molecules derived from the diet, including triglycerides, phospho-lipids, fatty acids and waxes. Cholesterol is often considered a lipid as well, although it is technically not a fat, but a sterol.

Lipofuscin 'Wear-and-tear' brown pigment granules consisting of lipid-containing residues of metabolism. These granules can be found in liver, brain and heart muscles, and are a sign of ageing.

Lipoproteins Compounds that contain lipids and proteins. Almost all of the lipids in blood, including cholesterol, are transported as lipoprotein complexes. There are a number of these lipoproteins in blood. The two best known by the public are HDL (high density lipoproteins, the 'good' cholesterol) and LDL (low density lipoproteins, the 'bad' cholesterol).

Melatonin This hormone from the pineal gland responds to light and seems to regulate various seasonal changes in the body. As it declines during ageing, it may trigger changes throughout the endocrine system.

Metabolism The continuous chemical and physical processes in the body involving the creation and breakdown of molecules; for instance, glucose can be metabolised to release its energy as ATP.

Mitochondria Minute *organelles* within a cell that act as energy factories. It is here that the body takes in the fuel provided by the diet or by the body's fat reserves and converts it into energy that drives every process in the body.

Molecule The smallest possible combination of atoms that retains the chemical properties of the substance. For instance, a molecule of water consist of three atoms – two are hydrogen and one is oxygen.

Monoamine Oxidase The enzyme that breaks down dopamine, norepinephrine and epinephrine in synapses. Two types are present, types A and B. Certain drugs can inhibit the action of MAOs; these drugs are called MAO inhibitors.

Muscle The largest component of lean body mass. Ideally, it should be the largest component of our entire body composition. It is responsible for vitality and health to a much greater extent than most people realise. It can be increased and strengthened through exercise.

Nerve A cell which carries information to and from the central nervous system.

Neuron A cell in the brain. There are billions of neurons in the brain that communicate with each other, using neurotransmitters, through connections called synapses.

Neurotransmitter A biochemical substance, such as norepinephrine, serotonin, dopamine, acetylcholine and endorphin, that relays messages from one neuron to another.

Noradrenalin Known also as norepinephrine. A neuro-transmitter involved in concentration, alertness and self-assertion. Athletes and people who get a lot of exercise tend to have high levels of norepinephrine, sometimes called the feel good neuro-transmitter. Chronically depressed people tend to have low levels. Exercise alone increases the levels of noradrenalin in the body.

Oestrogen A hormone made by the ovaries, adrenal glands and also in various cells of the body. Oestrogen promotes female characteristics. The most common oestrogens are estrone, estradiol and estriol. Premarin, the product name of conjugated oestrogens, is actually derived from the urine of pregnant horses.

Omega-3 Fatty Acids Polyunsaturated essential fatty acids which are found especially in purified fish oils and cold water fish, such as wild salmon, rainbow trout, eel, tuna, mackerel and herring. These fatty acids are in great demand to balance the high levels of omega-6 fatty acids in the modern convenience food diet. Omega-3s are especially beneficial against heart disease, inflammatory conditions and premature ageing, in no small part because they promote the formation of protective anti-inflammatory prostaglandins.

Omega-6 Fatty Acids Polyunsaturated essential fatty acids found in nuts and seeds. Omega-6 fatty acids can produce both inflammatory prostaglandins, such as prostaglandin E_2 and also anti-inflammatory prostaglandins such as prostaglandin E_1. The omega-6 and the omega-3 fatty acids are both necessary to life but need to be properly balanced.

Omega-6 to Omega-3 Ratio An important comparison of the amount of omega-6 fatty acids to omega-3 fatty acids in the diet. Ancient diets were estimated to contain between 1:1 and 4:1. Modern diets sometimes contain as high as 30:1 ratio. This is a balance that needs to be rectified for lasting health.

Omegas Fatty acid families of which there are three – omega-3, omega-6 and omega-9. The number given to each family describes the length of the fatty acid, the number of double bonds it contains and the position of the first double bond. For instance, the fatty acid DHA is written in numeric terms as 22:6n-3. This means it has 22 carbons, 6 double bonds and is in the omega-3 family.

One Repetition Maximum (1RM) The most weight a person can lift with one try.

Osteoporosis An age-related condition, resulting from the gradual loss of bone mineral content that increases risk of bone fracture. Osteoporosis is characterised by weaker, less dense, more brittle bones. Loss in bone mineral may be affected by diet and exercise.

Oxidation The process by which a compound reacts with oxygen and loses a hydrogen or electron.

Parkinson's Disease A chronic disease of the central nervous system caused by lowered levels of the inhibitory neurotransmitter dopamine. Symptoms include muscular tremors and weakness.

Percentage Body Fat That percentage of your total body weight which is body fat. The higher your percentage of body fat, the greater the likelihood of chronic disease, such as cancer, diabetes and heart disease. The level of body fat to lean body mass, has little to do with how 'fat' or 'thin' you appear. Many thin people have a high percentage of body fat. Ketogenics decreases body fat and increases muscle mass.

Phytoestrogens Plant compounds that exert oestrogenic effects.

Pineal Gland A cone-shaped structure about the size of a pea that lies very nearly in the centre of the brain. Once thought to be a left-over from some earlier age of mankind, it is now believed to be a biological clock. It produces melatonin.

Precursor A chemical which can be converted by the body into another is a precursor of the latter chemical.

Prostaglandins Hormone-like substances derived from fatty acids. Some are inflammatory, some such as prostaglandin E_2, made from arachidonic acid are powerfully inflammatory, while others – prostaglandin E_1 and prostaglandin E_3 – are anti-inflammatory.

Receptors Sites on the surface of cells where neuro-transmitters, hormones and other substances, can attach to bring about change, rather like keys which fit into receptor locks. Each receptor is of a specific shape and size needed to react specifically to another molecule. As soon as the molecule attaches to the receptor, a nerve signal can be sent. Receptors are strongly influenced by the fatty acid structure of the cell membrane.

Sarcopenia An overall weakening of the body caused by a gradual, decades-long change in body composition, with loss of muscle mass.

Saturated Fats Fat molecules that contain no double bonds. An excess of saturated fats can interfere with the production of fatty acids essential for brain function, as well as harden cell membranes.

Serotonin A brain chemical (neurotransmitter) that relays messages between brain cells (neurons). It is one of the primary mood-regulating neurotransmitters. It is derived from the amino acid tryptophan. Serotonin can also be converted to melatonin.

Stem Cells Cells from which all blood cells derive.

Sterol A steroid of 27 or more carbon atoms with one OH (alcohol) group.

Strength The maximum amount of force your muscles can generate. The ability to increase muscle strength through muscle-conditioning exercises does not appear to be diminished with age.

Synapse The minute space between two neurons or between a neuron and organ across which nerve impulses are chemically transmitted.

Syndrome X A cluster of symptoms and health problems which include insulin resistance, obesity, blood fat abnormalities, glucose intolerance and hypertension. Syndrome X does not necessarily mean that all these conditions are present, however, they often occur together.

Synergy When compounds are combined and their effects are more than the sum of their individual effects, the compounds are said to have positive synergy.

Testosterone A hormone made by the testicles and adrenal glands and also found in various cells of the body, that promotes masculine traits.

Tinctures Alcoholic or hydro-alcoholic solutions usually containing the active principles of botanicals in low concentrations. They are usually prepared by maceration, percolation or dilution of their corresponding fluid or native extracts. The strengths of tinctures are typically 1:10 or 1:5. Alcohol content will vary.

Toxic Poisonous. Everything, including water and oxygen, is toxic in sufficiently high doses.

Trans-fatty Acid An unsaturated fatty acid that has been altered in a way to bring about a molecular reversal at the position of the double bond on the molecular producing a 'junk fat'. This is what occurs when polyunsaturated fats are processed via heat or solvents to produce the fats used in almost all convenience foods. It changes the essential fatty acid from its normal curved shape to an arrow shape. Trans-fatty acids are very harmful to the body. They alter cell membrane fluidity and have been found to enter the brain in animal studies and are to be avoided at all costs.

Triglycerides Fat molecules composed of three fatty acids attached to a glycerol molecule – the kinds of fat found in different lipoproteins in blood. High levels of triglycerides usually accompany high levels of insulin. The ratio of triglycerides to high-density lipoproteins is an important indicator of insulin levels and can be used to predict the likelihood of heart disease in the future.

Unsaturated Fats Fats that contain double bonds between their carbon atoms in one or more locations. Common unsaturated fats include linoleic and linolanic acid, with two or three points of unsaturation or double bonds – DHA and omega-3 fatty acid from the omega-3 group is a highly unsaturated fatty acid containing 6 double bonds.

VLDL Very low-density lipoprotein. A protein and lipid particle in the blood whose purpose is to transport non-dietary triglycerides around the body. Lower blood values are more desirable.

VO$_2$max The maximum amount of oxygen a person can take in during heavy exertion. VO$_2$max, is measured in laboratories by asking subjects to breathe into a special apparatus while they exercise to the point of exhaustion on a treadmill or a stationary bike. Older people have to exercise regularly over a longer period of time to achieve VO$_2$max levels equivalent to those of younger adults.

Western diet A diet characteristic of Western societies (i.e. a diet high in fat, refined carbohydrates and processed foods, and low in dietary fibre).

Xenoestrogen Found in petrochemically derived pesticides, herbicides and plastics which behave like the female hormone oestrogen when taken into the body. They are responsible for a lowering of the male sperm count, and for wreaking havoc with women's reproductive systems.

FURTHER READING

*I particularly recommend these books.

Allan, Christian, B, Lutz, Wolfgang, *Life Without Bread. How a Low-Carbohydrate Diet Can Save Your Life*, Keats Publishing, Los Angeles, 2000.

*Andes, Karen. *A Woman's Book of Strength.* Perigee Books, 1995.

Appleton, Nancy. *Lick The Sugar Habit.* Garden City Park, NY: Avery Publishing Group, 1989.

Atkins, Robert C. *Dr. Atkins' Age-Defying Diet Revolution.* Bantam Books, 2000.

Atkins, Robert C. *Dr Atkin's Vita-Nutrient Solution.*, Simon & Schuster. New York, 1998.

Audette, R. *Neanderthal.*, Paleolithic Press, Dallas,1996.

Audette, Ray. *NeanderThin.* St Martins Press. 1999.

Barnes, Broda MD and Gayton, Lawrence. *Hyperthyroidism: The Unsuspected Illness.* Littlebrown, Boston, 1997.

*Batmanghelidj, Dr. *Your Body's Many Cries for Water.*, Global Health Solutions, 1992; 800/759-3999.

Beachel, Thomas and Westcott, Wayne. *Strength Training Past 50*, Human Kenetics, Leeds, 1998.

Becker, R.O. *Electromagnetism and Life.* State University of New York Press, Albany, NY, n.d.

Becker, Robert O. and Selden, Gary. *Body Electric: Electromagnetism and the Foundation of Life.* New York: William Morrow & Co., 1987.

*Benson, Herbert. *Beyond the Relaxation Response.* Times Books, New York, 1984.

*Berkson, Burton, M.D., Challem, Jack, Smith, Melissa Diane. *Syndrome X. The Complete Nutritional Program to Prevent and Reverse Insulin Resistance.*, John Wiley & Sons, Canada, 2000.

Bertalanffy, L. von. *Robots, Men and Minds.* George Braziller, New York, 1967.

Bertalanffy, L. von. *Problems of Life: An Evaluation of Modern Biological Thought.* Harper Torchbook, New York, 1980.

Beutler, Jade, and Murray, Michael, T. *Understanding Fats and Oils: Your Guide To Healing With Essential Oils.*, Apple Publishing Company, Vancover, 1996.

Bircher, Ralph. *'A Turning Point in Nutritional Science.'* Lee Foundation for Nutritional Research, Milwaukee, Wisconsin reprint, n.d.

Bircher-Benner, M.O. *Food Science for All.* C.W. Daniel, London, 1928.

Bircher-Benner, Max. *'The Prevention of Incurable Disease.'* Unpublished translation by Hilda Marlin.

Bircher-Benner, Max. *The Meaning of Therapeutic Order*. Unpublished translation by Hilda Marlin.

Bland, Jeffrey. *Medical Applications of Clinical Nutrition*. New Canaan, CT: Keats Publishing, 1983.

Bland, Jeffrey S. *The 20-Day Rejuvenation Diet Program*. Keats Publishing, LA, 1999.

Brand-Miller, Jennie, et.al. *The Glucose Revolution*. Marlowe, New York, 1999.

Bratman, Steven. *Natural Health Bible*. Prima Publishing. 2000.

Brekhman, I.I. *Man and Biologically Active Substances*. Pergamon Press, Oxford, 1980.

Browner, W.S., J. Westenhouse, and J.A. Tice. "What if Americans ate less fat." JAMA 265: 3285–3291, 1991.

Budwig, Johanna. *The Oil-Protein Diet*. Apple Publishing, Vancouver, 1994.

Buist, Robert. *Food Chemical Sensitivity*. Garden City Park, NY: Avery Publishing Froup, 1988.

Buist, Robert. *Food Intolerance*. Garden City Park, NY: Avery Publishing Group, 1989.

Burkitt, Denis. *Refined Carbohydrate Foods and Disease*. Academic Press, New York, 1975.

*Carson, Rachel. *Silent Spring*. Penguin, London, 1962.

*Challem, Jack, Burt Berkson, M.D., Ph.D & Melissa Diane Smith. *Syndrome X: The Complete Nutritional Programme to Prevent and Reverse Insulin Resistance*. John Wiley & Sons, Inc, 2000.

Check, William A. and Anne G. Fettner. *The Truth About AIDS: Evolution of an Epidemic*. New York: Holt, Rinehart & Winston, 1985.

Childre, Don and Howard Martin. *HeartMath Solutions*. Harper, San Francisco, 1999.

Cichoke, Anthony J. *Enzymes & Enzyme Therapy*. Keats Publishing Inc., New Canaan, Connecticut. 1994.

Cohen, Gene D. *The Creative Age*. HarperCollins Publishers, 2000.

Colgan, Michael. *Hormonal Health: Nutritional & Hormonal Strategies for Emotional Well-Being & Intellectual Longevity*. Apple Publishing, Vancouver, Canada, 1996.

Colgan, Michael. *Prevent Cancer Now*. CI Publications, San Diego, 1992.

Colgan, Michael. *The New Nutrition: Medicine for the Millennium*. Apple Publishing, Vancouver, Canada, 1994.

*Cousins, Norman. 'How Doctors Cause Disease', *Medical Self Care*, 1983.

Crayhon, Robert. *Nutrition Made Simple*. M. Evans and Co, Inc, 1994.

Crayhon, Robert, *The Carnitine Miracle*, M.Evans & Co. Inc, New York, 1998.

Crile, George. *The Bipolar Theory of Living Processes*. Macmillan, New York, 1926.

Crile, George. *The Phenomenon of Life.* W.W. Norton, New York, 1936.

*Crook, William G. *The Yeast Connection: A Medical Breakthrough,* rev. ed. New York: Vintage Books, 1986.

*Davidson, Paul. *Are You Sure It's Arthritis?* New York: Macmillian Publishing Co., 1985.

Davis, Adelle. *Let's Eat Right to Keep Fit.* Penguin Books, 1954.

Dean, Ward M.D. & Morgenthaler, John. *Smart Drugs & Nutrients.* Health Freedom Publications, US, 1990.

Dean, W., Morgenthaler, J., and S. Fowkes. *Smart Drugs II: The Next Generation.* Health Freedom Publications. Menlo Park, California, 1993.

*Dennis, Sandra Lee. *Embrace of the Daimon.* Nicolas-Hays, NY, 2001.

Dull, Harold. *Watsu – Freeing the Body in Water.* 2nd ed., Harbin Springs Publishing, 1998.

Eades, Michael, M.D., and Eades, Mary Dan, M.D. *The Protein Power Lifeplan.* Warner Books, New York, 2000.

Eades, Michael, M.D. and Eades, Mary Dan, M.D. *Protein Power* Bantam, New York, 1996.

Eaton, B., M. Shostak, and M. Konner. *The Paleolithic Prescription,* Harper & Row, New York, NY, 1988)

*Erasmus, Udo. *Fats and Oils.* Vancouver: Alive Press, 1987.

Evans, W., and I.H. Rosenberg. *Biomarkers.* Simon & Shuster, New York, NY, 1991.

Fallon, Sally, Mary Enig, PhD and Pat Connolly. *Nourishing Traditions.* New Trends Publishing, 1999.

Feingold, Ben F. *Why Your Child Is Hyperactive.* New York: Random House, 1985.

Finch, C.E. *Longevity, Senescence, and the Genome.* University of Chicago Press, Chicago, IL, 1990.

Frankel, P., and F. Madsen. *Stop Homocysteine Through the Methylation Process.* TRC Publications, Thousand Oaks, California, 1998.

Frawley, David. *Ayurveda and the Mind: The Healing of Consciousness.* Lotus, 1997.

*Galland, Leo. *Power Healing.* Random House, 1998.

Gittleman, Louise Ann, with Nunziato, Dina, R, *Eat Fat, Lose Weight: How the Right Fats Can Make You Thin for Life.* Keats Publishing, 1999.

*Grof, Stanislav. *Psychology of the Future.* Sate University of New York Press, 2000.

Hanh, Thich Nhat. *Anger: Buddhist Wisdom for Cooling the Flames.* Rider Books, 2001.

Hanh, Thich Nhat. *Being Peace.* Rider Books, 1987.

Hanh, Thich Nhat. *Going Home: Jesus and Buddha as Brothers.* Rider Books, 1999.

*Hanh, Thich Nhat. *The Sun My Heart.* Rider Books, 1988.

Hayflick, L. *How and Why We Age.* Ballantine Books, New York, NY, 1994.

Hillman, Anne. *The Dancing Animal Woman.* Bramble Books, Connecticut, 1994.

*Hoffer, Abram and Morton Walker. *Orthomolecular Nutrition.* Keats Publishing, New Canaan, Conn., 1978.

Howell, Edward. *Enzyme Nutrition.* Avery Publishing Group Inc., Wayne, New Jersey. 1985.

Ibid. *DHEA: A Practical Guide.* Avery Publishing Group, Garden City Park, New York, 1996.

Ibid. *5-HTTP: Nature's Serotonin Solution.* Avery Publishing Group, Garden City Park, New York, 1998.

Ibid. Kava: The Miracle Antianxiety Herb. St. Martin's Press, New York, 1998.

Keleman, Stanley. *Love: A Somatic View.* Centre Press, Berkeley, 1994.

Kent, Saul. *The Life Extension Revolution.* Quill, New York, 1983.

*Kenton, Leslie. *Passage to Power.* Vermilion, London, 1996.

Kenton, Leslie. *The New Ageless Ageing.* Vermilion, London. 1995.

Kenton, Leslie. *The X Factor Diet.* Vermilion, London, 2002.

*Kenton, L and S. *The New Raw Energy.* Vermilion, London, 1995.

Kirschmann, Gayla J. and John D. Kirschmann. *Nutrition Almanac.* Fourth edition. McGraw-Hill, 1984.

Knaster, Mirka. *Discovering the Body's Wisdom.* Bantam Books, 1996.

Kuhnau, W. *My Three Decades with Live Cell Therapy.* Kuhnau, Tijuana, Mexico, 1983.

Lakhovsky, G. *L'Origine de la Vie.* University Press, Texas, 1947.

Lamb, M.J. *Biology of Aging.* John Wiley & Sons, New York, NY, 1977.

Lance, James W. *Migraine and Other Headaches.* New York: Scribner, 1986.

Leaf, A. *Youth in Old Age.* McGraw-Hill, New York, 1975.

Levine, Stephen A. and Parris M. Kidd. *Anti-Oxidant Adaptation:* Its Role in Free Radical Pathology. Biocurrents Division, Allergy Research Group, San Leandro, Calif., 1985.

Linus, Pauling. *How to Live Longer and Feel Better.* Avon Books, 1986.

Lombard, J., and C. Germano. *The Brain Wellness Plan.* Kensington Press, New York, 1997.

Lopez, D.A., R.M. Williams, M. Miehlke. *Enzymes The Foundation of Life.* The Neville Press Inc., Charlestone, S.C. 1994.

Mackarness, R, *Eat Fat and Grow Slim.* Doubleday & Co, Garden City, New York, 1959.

Macy, Joanna & Molly Young Brown. *Coming Back to Life: Practies to Reconnect Our Lives, Our World.* New Society Publishers, 1998.

*Margulis, Lynn & Sagan, Dorian. *What is Life.* University of California Press, 2001.

Marti, James E. *The Alternative Health Medicine Encyclopedia.* Gale Group, 1994.

McCarrison, Sir Robert. *Nutrition and Health.* The McCarrison Society, London, 1953.

McCullough, Fran, *Living Low-Carb: The Complete Guide to Long-Term Low-Carb Dieting.* Little, Brown and Company, New York, 2000.

McCullough, Fran. *The Low-Carb Cookbook.* Hyperion, New York, 1997.

McDonald, Lyle. *The Ketogenic Diet.* Morris Publishing, Kearney, Nebraska,1998.

McKeown, T. *The Role of Medicine.* Princeton University Press, Princeton, NJ, 1979.

McKully, Kilmer. *The Homocysteine Revolution.* Keats Publishing, New Canaan, Connecticut, 1997.

McNeill, W. H. *Plagues and People*s. Doubleday, New York, NY, 1977.

*Mendelsohn, Robert. *Confessions of a Medical Heretic.* Contemporary Books, 1979.

Mindell, Earl, L. & Virginia Hopkins. *Prescription Alternatives.* Keat, NTC, Lincolnwood, Illinois, 1998.

Montagu, J.D. "Length of life in the ancient world: Controlled study." *J Royal Soc Med* 87:25–26, 1994.

Montignac, Michel. *Dine Out and Lose Weight.*, Montignac USA, Inc., 1991;

800/932–3229.

Montignac, Michel. *Eat Yourself Slim.* Translated by Daphné Jones, 5th ed. , Montignac Publishing, London, 1996.

Moore, T.J. *Lifespan.* Simon & Schuster, New York, NY, 1993.

Morgenthaler, John and Simms, Mia. *The Low-Carb Anti-Aging Diet.*, Smart Publications, Petaluma, California, 2000.

Murray, Michael T. *Dr. Murray's Total Body Tune-Up.* Bantam Books, 2000.

*Murray, Michael T., and Joseph E. Pizzorno. *Encyclopedia of Natural Medicine,* revised 2nd Edition. Prima Publishing, 1998.

Murray, Michael, T, *Encyclopedia of Nutritional Supplements: The Essential Guide for Improving Your Health Naturally.* Prima Publishing, USA, 1996.

Murray, Michael T. *Natural Alternatives to over the counter and prescription drugs.* William Morrow & Co., 1994.

Murray, Michael T. *Stress, Anxiety and Insomnia.* Prima Publishing, CA, 1995.

Nelson, Miriam. *Strong Women Stay Young.* Bantam, New York, 2000.

*Odent, Michael. *Water and Sexuality.* Arkana, 1990.

Olshansky, S.J., B.A. Caranes, and C.K. Cassel. "In search of Methusalah: Estimating the upper limits to human longevity." *Science* 250: 634–640, 1990.

Packer, Lester & Carol Colman. *The Antioxidant Miracle.* John Wiley & Sons, Inc., 1999.

Parcells, Hazel. *The Electromagnetic Energy in Foods.* Par-X-Cell School of Scientific Nutrition, Albuquerque, New Mexico, 1974.

Pauling, Linus, *How to live Longer and Feel Better.* Avon Books, 1986.

Peirce, Andrea. *The American Pharmaceutical Association Practical Guide to Natural Medicines.* William Morrow & Co., 1999.

Pelletier, Kenneth. *Longevity: Fulfilling Our Biological Potential.* Delacorte Press/Lawrence, New York, 1981.

Pelletier, Kenneth. *Mind as Healer – Mind as Slayer.* Delta, New York, 1977.

Pfeiffer, Carl. *Mental and Elemental Nutrients.* Keats Publishing, New Canaan, Conn., 1975.

Pfeiffer, Carl. *Nutrition and Mental Illness: An Orthomolecular Approach to Balancing Body Chemistry.* Rochester, VT: Inner Traditions, 1988.

Philpott, William H. and Dwight K. Kalita. *Victory over Diabetes.* Keats Publishing, New Canaan, Conn., n.d.

*Price, W, *Nutrition and Physical Degeneration.* 6th ed., Keats Publishing Inc., New Canaan, Connecticut, 1997.

Quas, Dr Vince. *The Lean Body Promise.* Synesis Press, Oregon, 1989.

Randolph, Theron G. *Human Ecology and Susceptibility to the Chemical Environment.* Charles C. Thomas, Publisher, 1981.

Rapp, Doris J. *Allergies and the Hyperactive Child.* New York: Sovereign Books, 1979.

Roose-Evans, James. *Passages of the Soul: Rediscovering the Importance of Rituals in Everyday Life.* Element Books Ltd, 1994.

Roy, A.K., and Chatterjee, eds. *Molecular Basis of Ageing.* Academic Press, Orlando, FL, 1984.

Sahelian, Ray. Creatine: *Nature's Muscle Builder.* Avery Publishing Group, Garden City Park, New York, 1997: updated 1998.

Sahelian, Ray, M.D. *Mind Boosters: A Guide to Natural Supplements That Enhance Your Mind, Memory and Mood.* St Martin's Griffin, NY, 2000.

*Sahelian, Ray, M.D., Gates, Donna, *The Steva Cookbook: Cooking with Natures Calorie-Free Sweetner.* Avery, 1999.

Sapolsky, Robert. *Why Zebras Don't Get Ulcers.* W.H. Freeman and Company, 1998.

Schachter F., L. Faure-Delanef, F. Gueno, H. Rouger, P. Froguel, L. Lesueue-Ginot, and D. Cohen. "Genetic associations with human longevity at the apo E and ACE loci." *Nature Genetics* 6: 29-32, 1994.

Schmidt, Michael A, *Smart Fats. How Dietary Fats and Oils Affect Mental, Physical and Emotional Intelligence.* Frog Ltd, Berkeley, California, 1997.

*Schrödinger, Erwin. *What Is Life?* And *Mind and Matter.* University Press, Cambridge, 1980.

Sears, Barry, *Enter the Zone*. Harper Collins, 1995.

Sears, Barry. *The Age-Free Zone*. Regan Books, 1999.

Sears, Barry with Bill Lawren, *The Zone, A Dietary Road Map*. Regan Books, 1995.

*Seigel, Bernie S., M.D. *Peace, Love & Healing*. Harper & Row, New York, 1989.

*Selye, Hans. *Stress without Distress*. Hodder & Stoughton, London, 1974.

Selye, Hans. *The Stress of Life*. McGraw-Hill, New York, 1975.

Shealy, C. Norman. *The Illustrated Encyclopedia of Healing Remedies*. Element Books, 1996.

Sheehan, George. *Personal Best*. Rodale Press, 1989.

Shils, M., Olson, J., and M. Shike, eds. *Modern Nutrition in Health and Disease*, 8th edition. Lea and Gebiger, Philadelphia, 1994.

Shute, Wilfred. *Dr Wilfrid E. Shute's Complete Updated Vitamin E Book*. New Canaan, CT: Keats Publishing, 1975.

Simms, Mia. *The Smart Guide to Low-Carb Cooking*. Smart Publications, Petaluma, California, 2000.

Simontacchi, Carol. *Your Fat Is Not Your Fault*. Tarcher, New York, 1997.

Spencer, Kate. *The Magic of Green Buckwheat*. Romany Herb Products Limited, 1987.

Spino, Mike. *Beyond Jogging*. Celestial Arts, Milbrae, Calif., 1976.

Stefansson, V. *The Fat of the Land*. Hill and Wang, New York, 1957.

Steffanson, V. *Cancer, Disease of Civilization.*, Hill and Wang, New York, 1960.

Szent-Györgyi, A. *Bioenergetics*. Academic Press, New York, 1957.

Szent-Györgyi, A. *Introduction to a Submolecular Biology*. Academic Press, New York, 1960.

Szent-Györgyi, A. *Bioelectronics*. Academic Press, New York, 1968.

Szent-Györgyi, A. *The Living State*. Academic Press, New York, 1972.

*Trungpa, Chögyam. *Journey Without Goal*. Shambhala, Boston & London, 1981.

Turner, Lisa. *Meals That Heal: A Nutraceutical Approach to Diet and Health*. Healing Arts Press, Rochester, Vermont, 1996.

Tyler, V.E. *The Honest Herbal*. Pharmaceutical Product Press, Binghamton, New York, 1993.

Walford, Roy. *Maximum Life Span*. W.W. Norton & Co., New York, 1983.

Weber, Marcea. *Whole Meals*. Dorset: Prism Press, 1983.

Werbach, Melvin. *Nutritional Influences of Illness*. 2nd Edition, Keats Publishing, 1990.

Wescott, Wayne & Thomas Baechel. *Strength Training Past Fifty*. Human Kenetics, Leeds, 1998.

Wharton, Jim & Phil Wharton. *The Wharton's Strength Book*. Random House, New York, 1999.

Williams, Roger J. and D. Kalita. *A Physician's Handbook on Orthomolecular Medicine.* Keats Publishing, New Cannan, Conn., 1977.

Williams, R. *Nutrition Against Disease.* Pitman Publishing Co., New York, 1971.

Wright, Jonathan V. M.D. & Lane Lenard. *Maximize Your Vitality & Potency: For Men Over 40.* Smart Publications, CA, 1999.

Ziff, Sam. *Silver Dental Fillings: The Toxic Timebomb.* Aurora Press, 1984.

*Zukav, Gary. *The Seat of the Soul.* Rider Books, 1990.

INDEX